D1358728

Return Due Return

CRC Handbook of Ultrasound in Obstetrics and Gynecology

Volume II

Editor

Asim Kurjak, M.D., Ph.D.
Professor and Head
Department of Obstetrics and Gynecology
University of Zagreb
J. Kajfes Hospital
Zagreb, Yugoslavia

CRC Press
Boca Raton   Ann Arbor   Boston

Library of Congress Cataloging-in-Publication Data

Handbook of ultrasound in obstetrics and gynecology/editor, Asim
   Kurjak.
         p.   cm.
      Includes bibliographical references.
      ISBN 0-8493-3253-2 (v. 1). — ISBN 0-8493-3254-0 (v. 2)
      1. Ultrasonics in obstetrics. 2. Diagnosis, Ultrasonic.
   3. Generative organs, Female—Diseases—Diagnosis. I. Kurjak,
   Asim.
      [DNLM: 1. Fetal Diseases—diagnosis.   2.Genital Diseases. Female—
   diagnosis.   3. Pregnancy Complications—diagnosis.   4. Prenatal
   Diagnosis—methods.   5.Ultrasonic Diagnosis. WQ 209 H236]
   RG527.5.U48H36   1990
   618′.047543—dc20
   DNLM/DLC
                                                                         89-23921
                                                                             CIP

   This book represents information obtained from authentic and highly regarded sources. Reprinted material is
quoted with permission, and sources are indicated. A wide variety of references are listed. Every reasonable effort
has been made to give reliable data and information, but the authors and the publisher cannot assume responsibility
for the validity of all materials or for the consequences of their use.

   All rights reserved. This book, or any parts thereof, may not be reproduced in any form without written consent
from the publisher.

   Direct all inquiries to CRC Press, Inc., 2000 Corporate Blvd., N.W., Boca Raton, Florida 33431.

© 1990 by CRC Press, Inc.

International Standard Book Number 0-8493-3253-2 (v. 1)
International Standard Book Number 0-8493-3254-0 (v. 2)

Library of Congress Card Number 89-23921
Printed in the United States

1322904

TO IAN DONALD — FRIEND AND TEACHER

PREFACE

It is now 40 years since Ian Donald first started to use ultrasound in obstetrics and gynecology. In a relatively short period of time ultrasound has improved in what seems to be a logarithmic progression, and it can with good reason be said to have changed the way of thinking of our age. The magnitude of this step alone is incalculable. Moreover, more than any other modern technique ultrasound has made it obvious that the fetus is an individual virtually from conception.

The original excitment is, of course, still felt by many of us. One cannot stop wondering how many applications of this relatively simple invention the future is hiding. Even now fetal medicine, prenatal diagnosis, infertility, and assisted conception are totally dependent in expertise on ultrasound screening and the diagnostic horizon is constantly expanding into new areas such as cancer screening and urodynamics. To quote Ian Donald: ''We live in an age when today's improbability becomes tomorrow's reality.''

The most exciting recent developments are color Doppler and transvaginal sonography. The combination of these two modalities in the same vaginal probe provides for superb simultaneous visualization of structural and flow information and offers new insight in dynamic studies of blood flow within the female pelvis. Our group has been the first to introduce this new technique into the clinical practice and to the best of my knowledge this is the first book containing a chapter on transvaginal color Doppler.

The waves of interest created by present possibilities are spreading rapidly through a large numnber of specialities. We see their solid evidence in the form of hundreds of scientific contributions to almost all major journals. Any interested individual will find it difficult to read or even scan these articles, although he will feel this to be his duty. It is the purpose of this book to offer some relief from this responsibility.

This handbook is the result of my personal efforts to weigh and consider, stemming from my clinical and ultrasonic experience and reading over the years. As such it must be accepted as a personal view with inevitable biases and idiosyncrasies.

A. Kurjak

THE EDITOR

Asim Kurjak, M.D., Ph.D., is Chairman of the Department and Professor of Obstetrics and Gynecology at the University of Zagreb, Zagreb Yugoslavia. He is also Head of the Ultrasonic Institute of Zagreb which is the World Health Organization Collaborating Centre for diagnostic ultrasound.

Dr. Kurjak obtained his training at the University of Zagreb, receiving his M.D. degree in 1966 and his Ph.D. degree in 1977. He served as an assistant professor at the Department of Obstetrics and Gynecology, University of Zagreb from 1968 to 1980. In 1971, as a British scholar he was Research Assistant for one year at the Institute of Obstetrics and Gynecology, University of London under Prof. Stuart Campbell. From 1983 to 1985 he was External Examiner at the University of Liverpool. It was in 1983 that he assumed his present position.

Dr. Kurjak is a member and past president of the Yugoslav Society of University Professors. He is a member of the advisory board of five international scientific journals. He served as Vice President of the European Federation for Ultrasound in Medicine and Biology. He is also the President of the International Society "Fetus as a Patient". He has been the recipient of many research grants from the Scientific Council from Yugoslavia and is currently the WHO coordinator for the use of ultrasound in developing countries. Recently he has been elected as a member of the Executive Bureau of World Federation for Ultrasound in Medicine and Biology. Among other awards, he is an honorary member of the Ultrasonic Society of Australia, Italy, Egypt, and Spain, and of the Society of Obstetrics and Gynecology of Italy, Poland, Hungary, Egypt, Spain, and Chile. He is also an honorary fellow of the American Institute of Ultrasound in Medicine. Recently, he has been elected the Secretary of the International Society for Ultrasound in Obstetrics and Gynecology.

Dr. Kurjak has presented over 90 invited lectures at major international meetings and approximately 100 guest lectures at universities and institutes. He has published more than 200 research papers and 14 books in the English language. Lately, in conjunction with Prof. Kazuo Maeda, he published *Textbook of Ultrasound in Obstetrics and Gynecology* in Japanese. *Ultrasound and Infertility* and *Fetal Growth Retardation—Diagnosis and Therapy,* were published by CRC Press.

His current major research interests include conventional and color Doppler studies of fetoplacental and maternal circulation.

ADVISORY BOARD

Dr. A. D. Christie
Department of Obstetrics Ultrasound
Ninewells Hospital & Medical School
Dundee, Scotland

Dr. Vincenzo D'Addario
Clinica Obstetrics & Gynecology
Universita di Bari
Bari, Italy

Prof. Pentti Jouppila
Department of Obstetrics & Gynecology
University of Oulu
Oulu, Finland

Dr. H. E. Thompson
Louisiana State University
Shreveport, Louisiana

CONTRIBUTORS

Volume II

A. Akaiwa, M.D., Ph.D.
Department of Obstetrics & Gynecology
Tottori University
Nishimachi
Yonago, Japan

Žarko Alfirević, M.D.
Ultrasonic Institute
University of Zagreb
Zagreb, Yugoslavia

Gerhard Bernaschek, M.D.
2nd Department of Obstetrics &
  Gynecology
University of Vienna
Vienna, Austria

Josef Deutinger, M.D.
2nd Department of Obstetrics &
  Gynecology
University of Vienna
Vienna, Austria

Wolfgang Holzgreve, M.D.
Zentrum für Frauenheilkunde
Westf. Wilhelms-Universitat
Munster, F.R.G.

Joseph Itskovitz, M.D., D.Sc.
Department of Obstetrics & Gynecology
Rambam Medical Center
Haifa, Israel

Sanja Kupesic-Urek, M.D.
Department of Gynecology
University of Zagreb
Zagreb, Yugoslavia

Asim Kurjak, M.D., Ph.D.
Professor and Head
Department of Obstetrics & Gynecology
J. Kajfes Hospital
Zagreb, Yugoslavia

Aby Lewin, M.D.
Department of Obstetrics & Gynecology
Hadassah University Medical Center
Jerusalem, Israel

Kazuo Maeda, M.D., Ph.D.
Professor
Department of Obstetrics & Gynecology
Tottori University
Nishimachi
Yonago, Japan

Mladen Miljan, M.D.
Department of Obstetrics & Gynecology
Dr. J. Kjafes Hospital
Zagreb, Yugoslavia

Shraga Rottem, M.D., Ph.D.
Department of Obstetrics & Gynecology
Rambam Medical Center
Haifa, Israel

Joseph G. Schenker, M.D.
Professor
Department of Obstetrics & Gynecology
Hadassah University Hospital
Jeruselem, Israel

Ilan E. Timor-Tritsch, M.D.
Department of Obstetrics & Gynecology
Columbia Presbyterian Medical Center
New York, New York

James van Eyck, M.D., Ph.D.
Department of Obstetrics & Gynecology
Academic Hospital Rotterdam
Rotterdam, The Netherlands

Juriy W. Wladimiroff, M.D., Ph.D.
Professor
Academic Hospital Rotterdam
Rotterdam, The Netherlands

Efram Zohav, M.D.
Department of Obstetrics & Gynecology
Hadassah University Medical Center
Jerusalem, Israel

TABLE OF CONTENTS

Volume I

Volume II

Chapter 1

FETAL ECHOCARDIOGRAPHY

Asim Kurjak and Mladen Miljan

INTRODUCTION

Echocardiography has had a major impact on the health care of the infants and children born with congenital heart disease (CHD) by providing accurate, noninvasive anatomic and functional information for diagnosis and follow-up. Recent improvements in resolution have resulted in the prenatal diagnoses of various birth defects. Although diagnostic ultrasound has been utilized antenatally in the detection of the anomalies of other organ systems, the cardiovascular system has not been adequately evaluated. Fetal cardiac imaging has been attempted in the past using M mode[1,2] and two-dimensional techniques.[3,4] Use of static B scanners for cardiac imaging is limited because the heart is a moving structure. M mode echocardiography has limited value for fetal echocardiography because it lacks spatial orientation and is very difficult to interpret when the examiner has no information about changing fetal position within the uterus. With the recent development of high-resolution, real-time, cross-sectional scanners, previously unrecognized capabilities in fetal cardiac imaging appear to warrant investigation. During the last decade, a number of papers has been published about ultrasonic assessment of fetal cardiovascular anatomy and function.[5-11] Quantitative assessment of growth of particular cardiac structures became possible,[10,12-17] as well as antenatal diagnosis of fetal heart rhythm disturbances.[18-26] In recent times, new technology has influenced fetal echocardiography, too. The introduction of color Doppler technique enables visualization of intracardiac flow.[27-29] This method offers new possibilities for easier and more accurate antenatal detection of congenital heart defects. With this approach, the clinician has the potential of improving overall perinatal survival because, once diagnosed as having CHD or altered cardiac function, the fetus can be optimally managed at a perinatal center equipped to provide maximal antenatal and postnatal care.

HIGH RISK PREGNANCIES FOR CONGENITAL HEART DEFECTS

CONGENITAL HEART DEFECTS AND CHROMOSOMAL ABNORMALITIES

It has been estimated that 0.5% of all live-born infants have a chromosome abnormality. Although the overall incidence of heart defects among patients with chromosome abnormalities is 30%, involvement of the heart may range from a few to nearly 100% in specific syndromes, with 90% and above in trisomies 13 and 18 and 40 to 50% in trisomy 21.[30] Since heart anomalies occur in about 1% of the population in general, the contribution of chromosome abnormalities to the total number of cases with structural heart defects can be considered appreciable.[31] A number of chromosomal defects are characteristically associated with CHD.[32]

The above results show the necessity to perform amniocentesis for chromosome studies in all pregnancies in which a fetal cardiac abnormality has been demonstrated, especially when the cardiac defect per se is considered amenable to surgical treatment and other major structural abnormalities have been ruled out. This will influence both the counseling of the parents and management of pregnancy and delivery.[33]

ULLRICH-NOONAN SYNDROME

The Ullrich-Noonan syndrome encompasses features of Turner's syndrome (such as short stature, characteristic facies, hypertelorism, webbed neck, and shield chest), but in the presence of a normal karyotype. These phenotypic features may not be diagnosable *in utero*; however, CHD is found in 50 to 55%, with right heart involvement in 80% of these, usually pulmonary valvular or infundibular stenosis.[30,34] Asymmetric left ventricular free wall hypertrophy may be seen and should be amenable to diagnosis *in utero* if present at the time of examination.[35] Tetralogy of Fallot, Ebstein's anomaly, ventricular septal defects, and total anomalous pulmonary venous return have also been described.[35,36] As the syndrome is transmitted as autosomal dominant, couples at risk may request prenatal diagnostic testing, and fetal echocardiography may be useful.

ENVIRONMENTAL FACTORS

Both embryonic consideration and epidemiologic evidence support the concept that teratogenic exposure prior to implantation of the fertilized human ovum does lead to malformation. If the teratogenic insult is major, viability is not maintained. Implantation and differentiation must progress to about 14 d of conceptual age before maldevelopment may be produced by teratogens.

It is thought that the most sensitive, vulnerable period for almost all cardiac structures occurs from the 18th to 60th d of embryonic development. Limits are variable in relation to the involved cardiac structure and the teratogenic agent to which fetus has been exposed.

Drugs

A number of drugs have been implicated as the primary cause of various syndromes of congenital malformations often including the heart. Now only of historic interest, thalidomide was primarily known for its association with phocomelia when ingested in the first trimester. If the exposure was between days 20 and 36 after conception, a 5 to 10% incidence of CHD was identified, especially tetralogy of Fallot, truncus arteriosus, and septal defects.[37]

Alcohol

A number of papers were published concerning the increased frequency of stillbirths, infant mortality and prematurity, decreased birthweight, and retardation of growth and psychomotor development. A fetal alcohol syndrome, consisting of mental retardation, microcephaly, intrauterine growth retardation (IUGR), hypertelorism with other facial abnormalities, and joint anomalies, has usually been seen in women consuming more than 60 ml of absolute alcohol per day, but more moderate alcohol consumption may carry some risk as well.[38] CHD has been identified in 25 to 30% of infants with the full syndrome, especially ventricular and atrial septal defects.[37,39,40]

Anticonvulsants

Approximately 0.5% of pregnant women have epilepsy; thus, the obstetrician if often faced with women who require anticonvulsants during the period of organogenesis.

In 1968, Meadow reported the increased risk of malformations (particularly cleft lip and palate and CHD) to offspring of epileptic mothers on anticonvulsants. A large number of reports followed, and eventually the data from the collaborative perinatal study were analyzed for the association of diphenylhydantoin, and selected malformations were reported.[41]

The questions arises as to whether teratogenicity is caused by the maternal illness itself or by the effect of the drugs given to the mother. Several studies have compared untreated epileptic patients with the general population and found no difference in overall malformation rates.[42-44] CHD has been described in 2 to 3% of offspring whose mothers were under the hydantoin treatment, particularly ventricular septal defect, pulmonary stenosis, aortic stenosis, and coarctation of the aorta.[37] Trimethadione has been reported to be associated with a high incidence of CHD, with as many as 15 to 30% of exposed fetuses found to have transposition of the great arteries, tetralogy of Fallot, or hypoplastic left heart.[37,45,46]

Lithium

Lithium has won increasing acceptance in the treatment of manic-depressive psychoses. In a study of 118 infants whose mothers were under lithium therapy during the pregnancy, 6 of them were found to have congenital heart defects (a 5-fold increase over expectation).[47] In another study of 143 cases, 11 newborns had a cardiovascular anomaly.[48] It is interesting that the incidence of Ebstein's anomaly showed a 400-fold increase in the group of lithium-exposed infants. That leads us to believe that this drug is a potent teratogen in susceptible individuals.[49]

Sex Hormones

Exposure of the fetus to sex steroid hormones as a cause of CHD has been a source of controversy in the literature. An association between maternal unspecified sex hormone use and multiple anomalies, including cardiovascular, skeletal, gastrointestinal, and genitourinary, was first suggested by Nora et al.[50,51] Similar effects were found by other investigators.[52,53]

The data are somewhat contradictory, but a twofold increase in congenital heart disease appears to be present in fetuses exposed to combination oral contraceptives or sex steroid analogues.[54,55] No pattern of specific malformations was found,[54,55] although some others have suggested a relative increase in truncoconal defects.[40] A recent update of the perinatal collaborative study revealed a risk of congenital heart disease 2.3 times as high in the maternal sex hormone-exposed groups, as compared with those not exposed to these agents.[54]

Nora's conclusion, based on personal experience and on the detailed evaluation of the literature on this subject, is that sex hormones appear to be agents that cause a small increase in risk of cardiovascular maldevelopment to individuals, but because of their widespread use, may be responsible for large numbers of malformations in the population.[56]

Vitamin A Analogue

The most recent addition to the list of possible cardiac teratogens is the vitamin A analogue isotretionoin. A survey conducted by the American Academy of Dermatology and the U.S. Food and Drug Administration found 35 instances of pregnancy exposure, and 5 of the 10 anomalous infants had CHD especially septal defects and great artery abnormalities. Exact risks are hard to assign as the true number of exposed fetuses is unknown. Some bias is inevitable because of selective reporting, but the defects were remarkably similar between infants and similar as well to those abnormalities seen in experimental animals.[57]

Immunodepressants and Chemotherapy

The findings here are somewhat surprising. One would anticipate that these agents would be highly teratogenic to the heart as well as to other structures. This should be clinically relevant because more infants are being born to mothers who have been taking immunosuppressants after kidney transplantation. Abnormalities include prematurity, small size for gestational age, immunologic deficiency, increased neonatal mortality, and CHD. The numbers of patients are still small, and the presence of 1 congenital heart lesion (pulmonary valve stenosis) in 20 cases is insufficient to indict these drugs as important cardiovascular teratogens.[58]

Infectious Agents
Rubella

Rubella as a cause of CHD was discovered in Australia in 1941.[59] Maternal rubella infection during the first trimester of pregnancy can lead to a variety of congenital malformations, cardiovascular being among them. From a prospective study by the British Ministry of Health, it appears that CHD occurred in 7% of the children whose mother had rubella in early pregnancy; this was 14 times as common as among controls.[60]

Data about the incidence of CHDs due to maternal rubella infection varied from 2% to 10%.[61,62] They differ according to the places in which the patients were examined (referral, etc.) and to the time the observations were made (relation to rubella epidemics).

Campbell concluded that rubella is not one of the major causes of congenital heart defects and that it is responsible for only 2 to 4% of all cases of congenital heart defects.[63] Although maternal rubella accounts for only a small percentage of the cases of congenital heart defects, the discovery of this infection as an etiologic factor was of great theoretical importance. It pointed to the possibility that other viral infections may play a similar role in the etiology of CHDs. In 1941, Gregg was the first who recognized a triad of abnormalities — cataracts, deafness, and patient ductus arteriosus — that afflicted infants of mothers who had rubella in the first trimester of pregnancy. Recent studies have demonstrated that not only patent ductus arteriosus is found in those children, but also other cardiovascular defects.[30,38,63-68] With the improvement in diagnostic methods and with necropsy experience, the knowledge of cardiovascular lesions following prenatal rubella was augmented. It was found that sometimes patent ductus arteriosus may dominate the disease picture and conceal associated cardiac anomalies.[69] Stenosis of the main pulmonary artery or its branches has become increasingly recognized.[70-74]

According to the experience of Nora and Nora, a sizable series revealed that 71% of patients with the rubella syndrome acquired during the pandemic of 1964 to 1965 had some form of cardiovascular disease.[75] The risk of some abnormality, in review of Sever, was 50% for an exposure in the 1st month, 22% in the 2nd month, and 6 to 10% in the 3rd, 4th, and 5th months.[76] Peripheral pulmonary artery stenosis, with or without pulmonary valve stenosis, was the most common problem, being present in 55% of their patients. Patent ductus arteriosus was present in 43%, and a variety of other lesions in 8% (including ventricular septal defect, atrial septal defect, aortic stenosis, and tetralogy of Fallot). It is important to know that subclinical rubella can also cause congenital heart defects.[77,78] Sometimes women who are exposed to rubella without clinical signs have children with the fully developed rubella syndrome.[77] In rare cases, the syndrome is seen in children of mothers who are not aware of either exposure or illness during pregnancy.[79,80]

Although women inadvertently vaccinated during early gestation have been shown to have virus cultured from the products of conception at abortion, no teratogenic effect of vaccination have been found.[81,82]

Other Viruses

Placental transmission of a number of viruses is well established.[83] An association between certain enteroviruses and CHD was suggested in one study based on early and late serologic testing, particularly Coxsackie virus B3 and B4,[84] but others have disputed these findings.[30] Some authors reported that infection with Coxsackie group B virus may produce myocarditis in the late fetal or neonatal period.[85,86]

The role of intrauterine mumps virus infection in the etiology of endocardial fibroelastosis has been discussed in recent years. Some of the patients with the primary form of this disorder have cutaneous delayed hypersensitivity to the mumps virus antigen, and in a number of cases, the patients' mother had parotitis or exposure to mumps during pregnancy, yet virus-neutralizing antibodies are uncommon in the patients and the virus has not been recovered from them after birth.[87,88] The association of maternal infections with cytomegalovirus, herpes, and Asian influenza viruses have also been implicated in large studies, but there have been some conflicting results. Much remains to be learned regarding the influence of maternal viral infections on intrauterine development of many systems, including cardiovascular.[49]

MATERNAL CONDITIONS

Several maternal conditions demonstrate a higher risk for maldevelopment of the cardiovascular system of the unborn. These are diabetes mellitus, phenylketonuria, and maternal connective tissue disorders. Rh hemolytic disease will also be presented because of its effect on fetal cardiovascular system.

Diabetes Mellitus

A considerable amount of debate has surrounded the teratogenic potential of maternal diabetes because the incidence of CHD is increased fivefold among infants of diabetic mothers (4 to 5% risk).[89] Since these mothers are being treated with hypoglycemic agents in almost every case, it is difficult to separate the effects of the maternal illness from the effects of, or interaction with, the mother's medication.

Cardiovascular defects include structural abnormalities such as transposition of the great arteries and ventricular septal defect.[89] Another common pattern in diabetic pregnancies is cardiomyopathy and asymmetric septal hypertrophy which may be seen in the newborn infants of diabetic mothers. The overall frequency of congenital anomalies has been related to first-trimester hemoglobin A1c levels, an indicator of long-term glucose levels.[90] Recent evidence strongly supports the concept that meticulous control of diabetes, beginning before conception and being maintained throughout pregnancy, reduces the risk of malformation in infants of diabetic mothers.[91]

Phenylketonuria

During the past decade, there has been an increasing awareness of the significant teratogenicity of high maternal blood levels of phenylalanine. It has recently become evident that hyperphenylalaninemia during organogenesis results in a number of malformations (microcephaly, CHD, etc.) and IUGR.[92] When maternal levels exceed 15 mg/dl, the frequency of CHD has been reported to be 12 to 16%.[93] Some authors refer to even higher rates of congenital heart defects.[94,95] Tetralogy of Fallot and other truncoconal malformations are the most common, perhaps reflecting the early timing of the teratogenic insult. Ventricular and atrial septal defects and coarctation of the aorta may also be found in this group of patients.

Connective Tissue Disorders

McCue et al. noted retrospectively that 63.6% of mothers of infants with congenital heart block had a clinical or laboratory diagnosis of connective tissue disease.[96] Recently, fetal echocardiography allows diagnosis of congenital heart block *in utero*. Multiple siblings have been affected by presumed antigen/antibody complex directed against the fetal conducting system. In general, these infants have done well, although a pacemaker has often been needed.

Rh Hemolytic Disease

The importance of Rh immunization is not concerned with a higher risk of congenital heart defects, but because in severe cases of the disease congestive heart failure may be commonly seen. Thus, the severely sensitized fetus requires close ultrasound surveillance to detect congestive heart failure and other signs of fetal compromise (ascites, hepatomegaly, pericardial effusion, etc.). In such cases, intrauterine transfusion and other therapeutic methods may be performed to prolong the stay *in utero* until pulmonary maturity may be achieved. This approach has minimized hydrops and has resulted in the survival of all severely sensitized infants.[97]

FAMILY HISTORY OF CHDs

The incidence of CHD in first-degree relatives can be predicted by testing the polygenic model mathematically.[98] Initial family studies were undertaken by Nora et al. and corresponded well with the theoretic prediction that the recurrence risk for first-degree relatives was between 1 and 5%.[99] Thus, the polygenic model for inheritance has become widely accepted. Whittemore et al.[100] reported a 16% recurrence risk for offspring of patients with congenital heart defects, and Rose et al.[101] reported a 9% recurrence in patients with specific defects. This represents a higher recurrence risk than would be expected in a polygenic model.

Not only do CHDs as a general category of anomalies run in families, but specific heart defects cluster in families.[102-104] Recurring lesions in a family are by no means always identical. Sometimes recurrence of the developmentally related anomalies may be found.[105] A familiar recurrence of a heart lesion that apparently bears no developmental relationship to a previously encountered defect may indeed be unrelated or may be a manifestation of a common mechanism of maldevelopment that is obscure to the observer.[49]

PREVIOUS INFANTS WITH CONGENITAL HEART DEFECTS

It is well known that mothers who had one or more offsprings with CHD have a higher risk of giving birth to another child with congenital heart defect than those mothers who had healthy children from the previous pregnancies. Repeated occurrence of congenital heart defects in siblings probably is more frequent than transmission through several generations.[106] However, such familial cases in the same generations are not convincing proof of genetic etiology, since repetitive or persistent environmental or maternal factors could be responsible for cardiac defects in several children born to the same mother. In such cases, the risk of CHD is between 2 and 10%.[30] It is important to bear in mind that the risk for disease in the following children depends on the type of congenital heart defect in the sibs and on the number of previously affected sibs.

FETAL ARRHYTHMIAS

Recently, diagnosis of fetal cardiac arrhythmias became feasible during intrauterine life using M mode echocardiography (see later). Although many fetal cardiac arrhythmias are benign, disappear in the neonatal period, and are unassociated with CHD, others are potentially life threatening and have led to fetal demise or resulted in the birth of an infant requiring immediate and intensive neonatal care. When the fetal cardiac arrhythmia is noted during routine ultrasound examination, II level echocardiographic examination has to be performed. This is to exclude possible associated congenital heart defects and to plain, if possible, intrauterine therapy in cases when the fetus cannot be delivered.

TWINS

An excess of monozygotic twins has been noted in a retrospective review of CHD among offspring of multiple births. Anderson[107] looked at 107 children identified because of the presence of CHD in patients who were also twins. He found that of the 107 sets of twins, 67 were monozygotic (63%) and that there was a higher concordance rate for CHD among those judged to be monozygotic (6.8%) than among judged to be dizygotic (2.2%; similar to the expected concordance rate for nontwin siblings). Similar findings were reported by other authors.[107-109] It is estimated that twins had a 17.5 per 1000 risk of CHD as compared with 7.57 per 1000 among singletons. Although specific figures are not included, most of the increase occurred among monozygitic twins.

NONIMMUNE HYDROPS FETALIS

A number of papers reported the high rate of CHDs among the fetuses with nonimmune hydrops. Data obtained on autopsied series vary from 5 to 18%.[110-112] Recently, Allan et al.,[113] in review of 52 fetuses with nonimmune hydrops, found cardiovascular etiology in

21 cases (40%); 13 of them had structural heart defects, and in 8 cases, fetal tachyarrhythmia was diagnosed. The higher incidence of cardiac causes for fetal hydrops in this series is probably due to the fact that this report was based on the prenatal examinations, which enable elucidation of some causes unobtainable postnatally (like disturbances of the fetal heart rhythm). Therefore, in each fetus with a nonimmune hydrops, fetal anatomy has to be examined carefully, including echocardiographic examination of the fetal heart.

GROWTH-RETARDED FETUSES

Isolated congenital heart defect is not generally considered to be strongly associated with IUGR,[114] but the association of chromosomal abnormalities with IUGR, as well as the high percentage of congenital heart defects among fetuses having chromosomal defects, is well known. Few reports were published in which congenital heart defects were found in growth-retarded fetuses.[115,116] According to Stewart et al.,[117] ultrasonic evaluation of the fetal cardiovascular system in cases of severe IUGR is mandatory, as the diagnosis of serious cardiac malformation may substantially alter plans for further management of these fetuses, particularly as Cesarean section may be avoided when the prognosis for the fetus is considered hopeless.[117]

ASSOCIATED EXTRACARDIAC ANOMALIES

Fetal echocardiography is also recommended for the evaluation of any fetus with extracardiac malformations.[118,119] Some extracardiac malformations carry a high risk of associated CHD, while for others the risk is low.[32] The overall incidence of extracardiac malformations in children identified as having CHD varies from 25 to 45%.[120-122] This variation appears to depend on the means of identification, with a lower incidence in clinical studies than in autopsy studies. The incidence also appears to be related to the type of cardiac defect.[32]

We feel that ideally, echocardiography should be performed in all fetuses identified as having extracardiac malformations. At present, there are a limited number of laboratories with extensive experience in fetal echocardiography. Consultation with such centers may be advisable when anomalies known to have a high association with CHD are found.

Based on their review, Copel et al.[32] suggest that the anomalies found in Table 1 represent those with a particularly high frequency of association with CHD. If such anomalies are identified *in utero*, fetal echocardiography should be sought, as the information obtained may have a significant impact on subsequent care. Future epidemiologic or clinical studies may result in modification of this list.

TWO-DIMENSIONAL FETAL ECHOCARDIOGRAPHY

Although the fetal heart can be visualized as early as 6 weeks of gestation, optimal visualization of the cardiac structures cannot be achieved until 18 weeks of gestation. At that age, the heart is large enough, and the amniotic fluid compartment is relatively large, providing an excellent medium for transmission of the ultrasound beam. The best period of pregnancy to perform fetal echocardiography is between 18 and 25 weeks. Later on, the fetal spine tends to lie anteriorly, and the bone ossification is more pronounced, so that the spine and ribs are producing shadows which make imaging of the fetal heart difficult. Excessive fetal movements, maternal obesity, or oligohydramnios are other factors that make visualization of the fetal heart difficult.[7]

Before the heart is examined, the fetal head, abdomen, and extremities should be imaged, and biometric measurement of those fetal structures performed. Once gross anomalies of the above organ systems have been excluded, identification of the fetal stomach on the left side of the abdominal cavity should be made, and liver situated on the opposite side (Figure 1).

TABLE 1
Antenatal Sonographic Diagnoses that Should Prompt Cardiac Evaluation[32]

Abnormalities of cardiac position
Central nervous system
   Hydrocephalus
   Microcephaly
   Agenesis of the corpeus calosum
   Encephalocele (Meckel-Gruber syndrome)
Mediastinal
   Esophageal atresia
Gastrointestinal
   Duodenal atresia
   Situs abnormality
Ventral wall
   Omphalocele
   Ectopia cordis
Diaphragmatic hernia
Renal
   Bilateral agenesis[a]
   Dysplastic kidneys
Twins
   Conjoined
   Monoamniotic[b]

[a] Uniformly fatal; presence of congenital heart disease unrelated to prognosis.
[b] Possible relationship to congenital heart disease; firm association not established.

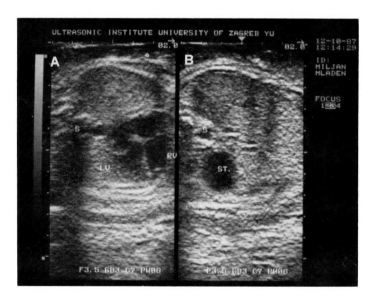

FIGURE 1.   In the left part of this figure (A), cross-section through the fetal chest is present, and on the right side (B), cross-section through the fetal abdomen at the level of fetal stomach. Note that heart apex is oriented to the left, e.g., on the same side where the fetal stomach is situated. LV = left ventricle; RV = right ventricle; S = spine; ST = stomach.

TABLE 2
Standard Echocardiographic Planes for
Evaluation of Fetal Heart

Four-chamber view
Long axis through the left ventricle
Short axis through the basis of the heart
Aortic arch (sagittal section)

Unlike the adult heart, in which the longitudinal axis of both ventricles lies in a plain passing between the right shoulder and the left iliac crest, the fetal heart lies almost perpendicular to the fetal trunk. This is due to the relatively large size of the fetal liver, causing the apex of the heart to be more horizontal and the right ventricle to be more anterior to the left ventricle. The methods for estimation of the fetal heart position and axis will be discussed later in this chapter.

Echocardiographic examination starts with a two-dimensional visualization of the fetal heart. The fetal heart can be viewed in planes unobtainable postnatally, because the fetal lungs are fluid filled and present no obstruction to the ultrasound beam. Besides that, ossification of the surrounding bones (spine and ribs) is not as pronounced as in late pregnancy and during postnatal life. Finally, the fetus is surrounded with amniotic fluid which is an excellent conductor of the ultrasound beam. To visualize fetal heart structures, four main two-dimensional echocardiographic planes are used (Table 2).

FOUR-CHAMBER VIEW

The four-chamber view is the most easily obtained echocardiographic plane. First, the longitudinal section through the fetal trunk has to be obtained, then the fetal spine has to be seen along its full length. Thereafter, the probe is rotated 90°, and the sagittal section through the fetal chest is visualized. The four-chamber view of the fetal heart will be seen.

Before the fetal heart structures are evaluated, the fetal heart position inside the thorax and its axis has to be estimated.

Estimation of Fetal Heart Position and Axis

Unlike the adult heart, in which the longitudinal axis of both ventricles lies in a plane passing between the right shoulder and the left iliac crest, the fetal heart lies almost perpendicular to the fetal trunc. This is due to the relatively large size of the fetal liver, causing the apex of the heart to be more horizontal and the right ventricle to be more anterior to the left ventricle. The fetal heart axis may be expressed as the evaluation of the cardiac long axis from the midline of the fetal trunk. According to Comstock,[123] the angle between the interventricular septum and the line dividing the fetal thorax on two equal sides amounts to 45° (1 SD = 10.4°; range 22 to 75°) and is constant from the 13th week of gestational age onward.[123]

The fetal heart normally occupies the middle and the left part of the chest. If a line is drawn through the interventricular septum and it is extended to the most posterior border of the fetal heart, the point at which it intersects the posterior border is found to be located in the right thorax, just anterior or posterior to a line dividing the thorax into equal-sized anterior and posterior portions.[123]

After the position and cardiac axis is estimated, it is important to determine which side of the heart is left, and which is right.

Identification of the Right and Left Side of the Fetal Heart

To recognize the left from the right side of the fetal heart, some guidelines should be used. They are listed in Table 3 (see also Figures 1, 2, and 3A and B). By observing some

TABLE 3
Identification of the Right and Left Side of the Fetal Heart

	Right	Left
Ventricles		
Position	Beneath anterior chest wall	Nearer to the fetal spine, on the same side of trunk as stomach
Shape	Conical or oval	Ellipsoidal
Wall thickness	Thicker than left	Thinner than right
Atria	—	Ovale foramen flap present within left atrium
Atrioventricular leaflets insertion	Lower	Higher

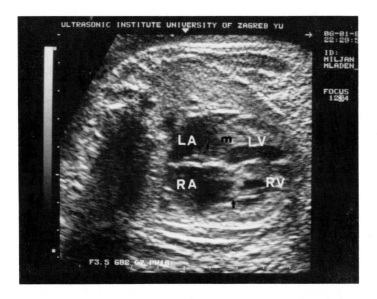

FIGURE 2.   Typical four-chamber view of the fetal heart. Fetal heart structures are clearly visualized: interventricular septum divides left (LV) from the right ventricle (RV), and interatrial septum is situated between the left (LA) and right atrium (RA). Ventricular wall is much thicker than atrial. Note different insertion of mitral (m) and tricuspidal (t) valve and different appearance of ventricular cavities.

characteristics of the ventricles, e.g., their position in relation to the anterior chest wall, spine and stomach, ventricular shape, and wall thickness, it is possible to distinguish the right from the left ventricle. Once the ventricles are identified, movement of the foramen ovale flap within the left atrium should be confirmed (as in normal) intracardiac circulation blood is flowing from the right to the left atrium). Finally, the different insertion of atrioventricular valve leaflets on interventricular septum can be useful in identification of the right and left side of fetal heart. The tricuspid valve is inserted more apically than mitral. After the identification of the heart sides is performed, each cardiac structure seen in this plane has to be investigated.

Four-Chamber View of Heart Anatomy

Heart structures visible in this echocardiographic plane are listed in Table 4 and may be seen in Figure 2.

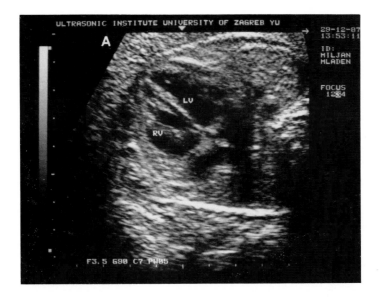

A

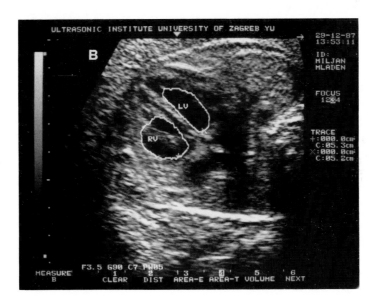

B

FIGURE 3.   Echocardiographic pictures of the same heart, presenting ventricular chambers. Left ventricle (LV) is more elongated than right ventricle (RV); it allows easier recognition of the sides of fetal heart. In B, the lines follow the inner borders of ventricular chambers; thus, the different shapes of the ventricles may be observed.

Ventricles and Atrioventricular Valves

As mentioned previously, each ventricle has its characteristic morphology (Figures 2 and 3A and B). The right ventricle is more ellipsoidal in shape, and its wall is thicker compared with the wall of the left ventricle. The difference in ventricular wall thickness is probably due to the higher resistance in the pulmonary circulation during fetal life. In contrast,

TABLE 4
Fetal Heart Structures Visible on Four-Chamber View

Left and right ventricle
Left and right atrium
Interventricular septum
Interatrial septum
Foramen ovale
Mitral and tricuspidal valve

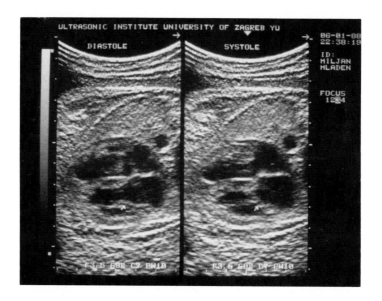

FIGURE 4.   Arrow points the lateral leaflet of tricuspidal valve; leaflet excursions during diastole (left) and systole (right) may be observed using high-resolution real-time equipment.

the left ventricle is oval or conical in shape (Figure 2). Precise examination of the inner ventricular morphology shows coarser trabeculation and moderator band inside the right ventricle.

Tricuspid and mitral valves can be clearly seen in the four-chamber view. In the last second trimester and during the third trimester, atrioventricular valve leaflets and their excursions may be observed (Figure 4), but for studying their function, real-time-directed M mode and color Doppler techniques may be used (see later). Papillary muscle architecture may be seen in the second and third trimesters using high-resolution ultrasound equipment, more prominence being seen in the right ventricle (Figure 5).

Interventricular and Interatrial Septa

Interventricular septum is visualized as an elongated V-shaped appearance, dividing the left from the right ventricle. It is thickest at the apex and narrows as it approaches the place of atrioventricular junction. Thus, if the interventricular septum is observed in the apical four-chamber view, with the ultrasound beam being parallel to the septum, occasionally its membranous part will not be visualized because of its thickness. It may be the source of misinterpretation and the false positive diagnosis of ventricular septal defect.

Interatrial septum is a thin, membranous-like structure, dividing the left from the right

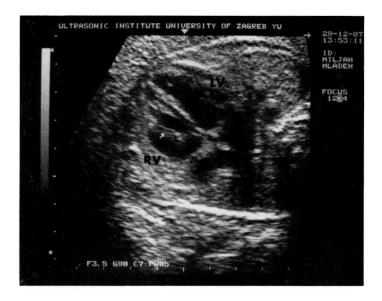

FIGURE 5.   Papillary muscle (arrow) within right ventricle. RV = right ventricle;
LV = left ventricle.

atrium (Figure 2). It is almost continuous with interventricular septum. In the middle portion
of interatrial septum, foramen ovale flap may be observed, exhibiting considerable movement
inside the left atrium.

Atria and Atrial Venous Connections

Each ventricle has its correspondent atrial chamber. Atria appear more spherical in
shape. Their walls are much thinner than ventricular (Figure 2). Left atrium may be identified
on the basis of pulmonary veins influencing it, as well as of the movement of foramen ovale
flap in it (Figure 6). The right atrium may be recognized on the basis of systemic vein
connections (vena cava inferior and superior).

Demonstration of the four-chamber view enables exclusion of the most frequent (interatrial and interventricular septal defects) as well as the most severe congenital heart defects
(ventricular hypoplasia, absence of normal atrioventricular connections, etc.). It is very easy
to obtain this section through the fetal heart, even for examiners who are not very experienced
in fetal echocardiography. Thus, it is our opinion that this echocardiographic plane has to
be used in routine work to explore fetal heart anatomy.

LONG AXIS THROUGH THE LEFT VENTRICLE

The purpose of this plane is to visualize the left ventricular outflow tract and ascending
aorta with its valve, but at the same time, additional data can be obtained about some heart
structures previously visualized on the four-chamber view (Table 5). This plane is achieved
by rotating the transducer into the longitudinal fetal axis and by tilting it more cranially,
toward the right shoulder. The origin of the aortic root from the left ventricle is clearly
visualized (Figure 7). It had to be stressed that the anterior wall of the aorta is seen to be
continuous with the interventricular septum, and the posterior wall with the anterior leaflets
of the mitral valve.

Using this echocardiographic plane, abnormalities of the aortic valve (stenosis, atresia,
etc.) and ascending part of the aorta (riding aorta, stenosis, poststenotic dilatation, etc.) may
be visualized, as well as some other abnormalities (ventricular septal defect, abnormalities
of the mitral valve).

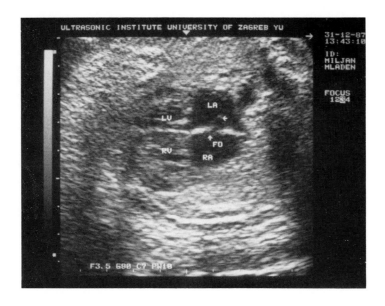

FIGURE 6. Interatrial septum with foramen ovale flap within the left atrium (arrow). LA = left atrium; RA = right atrium; FO = foramen ovale; LV = left ventricle; RV = right ventricle.

TABLE 5
Fetal Heart Structures Visible on the Long Axis through the Left Ventricle

Left ventricle (outflow tract)
Ascendent part of aorta
Aortic valve
Interventricular septum
Left atrium
Mitral valve
Right ventricle

SHORT AXIS THROUGH THE BASIS OF THE HEART

The purpose of this plane is to visualize the right outflow tract and pulmonary artery with its valve. This plane is achieved by rotating the probe to a semitransverse section (the ultrasound beam will be perpendicular to the four-chamber view) and by tilting it in a more cephalad direction. Fetal heart structures visible on the short axis at the level of the aortic and pulmonary valves are listed in Table 6.

At that level, the aorta is situated centrally, and it appears as a circle. It is surrounded by three chambers, the pulmonary artery partially wrapping around it (Figure 8). Thus, both aortic and pulmonary outflow tracts may be presented in the same plane. The visualized chambers are left and right atrium and right ventricle. The interatrial septum with foramen ovale flap separating the left from the right atria is noted. Adjacent to the right atrium lies the right ventricular inflow tract with tricuspid leaflets. Opposite to the atria, and nearer to the anterior chest wall, the right ventricular outflow tract is noted, with the pulmonary artery being adjacent to it. Excursions of the pulmonary valve leaflets may be observed. The pulmonary trunk may be followed to its branches (left and right pulmonary artery) (Figure 9), and via the ductus arteriosus to the descending aorta (Figure 10).

A normal appearance of the right outflow tract and pulmonary artery may help to eliminate some cardiac abnormalities, such as severe pulmonary stenosis and atresia, as well

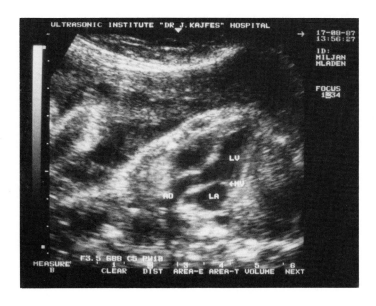

FIGURE 7. Long axis through the left ventricle. Left ventricular inflow and outflow tract and origin of ascendent aorta are seen. LV = left ventricle; AO = ascendent aorta; MV = mitral valve; LA = left atrium.

TABLE 6
Fetal Heart Structures Visible on the Short Axis at the Level of Aortic and Tricuspidal Valve

Right ventricle (outflow tract)
Pulmonary artery
Pulmonary valve
Tricuspidal valve
Right atrium
Interatrial septum
Left atrium
Aorta

as pulmonic poststenotic dilatation. In the same plane, some other abnormalities may be confirmed (atrial septal defect, transposition of the great vessels).

AORTIC ARCH

This view may be obtained by rotating the probe to the longitudinal section through the fetal trunk. The ascending aorta, aortic arch with vessels to the head and neck, as well as thoracic part of the descending aorta are noted (Figure 11). Visualization of this echocardiographic plane gives the opportunity in some cases to diagnose coarctation of the aorta and transposition of the great vessels.

ANTENATAL DETECTION OF CONGENITAL HEART DEFECTS

During the last decade, increasing attention has been paid to the prenatal diagnosis of fetal congenital heart defects using two-dimensional real-time ultrasound.[11,124-130] If the fetal heart is normal, there are no difficulties in estimation of position, heart axis, side of heart chambers, nor in examination of heart structures (described on the previous pages). The

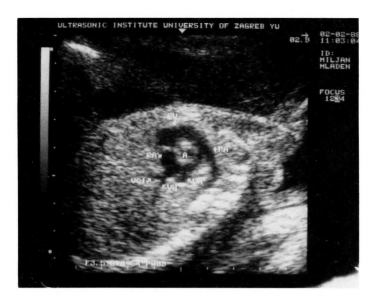

FIGURE 8. Short axis through the basis of the heart. Typical appearance of centrally situated aorta (A), surrounded with left atrium (LA), right atrium (RA), right ventricle (RV), and pulmonary artery (PA). VCI = inferior vena cava; VH = hepatic vein.

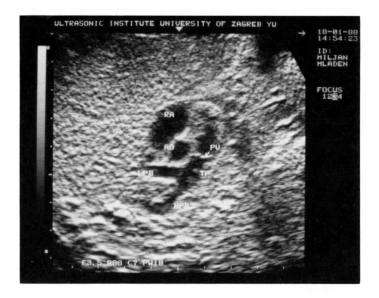

FIGURE 9. Branching of the pulmonary artery (TP) on the left (LPB) and right pulmonary branch (RPB). PV = pulmonary valve; AO = aorta; RA = right atrium.

problems arise when one is dealing with a malformed fetal heart. Often, if there is a complex heart malformation, it is quite impossible to make a diagnosis in a short time. In such cases, a step-by-step approach to cardiac diagnosis is recommended.

The appearance of particular congenital heart defects which may be diagnosed antenatally will not be described further here. We will try to point out just the main guidelines for their antenatal diagnosis. As it was mentioned before, the main echocardiographic plane for

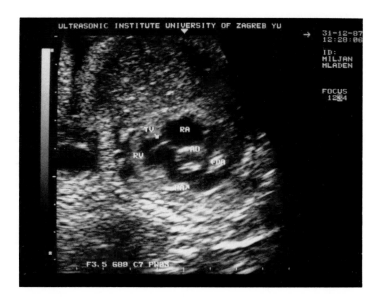

FIGURE 10.   Origin of ductus arteriosus (DA) from the pulmonary artery (PA). AO = aorta; RV = right ventricle; TV = tricuspidal valve; RA = right atrium.

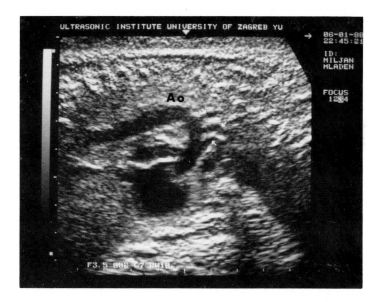

FIGURE 11.   Sagittal section through the fetal chest with ascendent aorta, aortic arch, and thoracic part of aorta. The vessels for head and arms, originating from aortic arch, are indicated with arrows. Ao = aorta.

evaluation of the fetal heart is the four-chamber view. There are two reasons for this opinion: (1) because it may be easily visualized and (2) because many congenital heart defects will be detectable in this echocardiographic plane or will produce some changes in the size and/or appearance of the cardiac structures obtainable in the four-chamber view.

Some of the simplest, most frequest heart defects, as atrial and ventricular septal defects, may be easily visualized in the four-chamber view (Figure 12). In cases of complex heart defects, normal intracardiac hemodynamics are disturbed. As a consequence, such complex

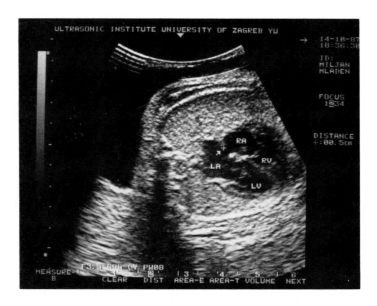

FIGURE 12.   Defect of interatrial septum (arrow) detectable on four-chamber view.
RA = right atrium; LA = left atrium; RV = right ventricle; LV = left ventricle.

heart abnormalities distort the normal anatomy of the four-chamber view, usually causing ventricular disproportion. Once abnormal anatomy or ventricular disproportion is noted during level I, or screening examination of the four-chamber view, attention should be directed to evaluation of ventricular size, the aortic and pulmonic outflow tracts, the arch of the aorta, and the ductus arteriosus. These examinations should be performed by an experienced fetal sonographer in collaboration with a pediatric cardiologist and constitute level II, or consultative examination.[11] Some illustrative cases of congenital heart defects are presented in Figures 12 to 17.

ESTIMATION OF FETAL HEART RATE AND RHYTHM

During the antepartum period, several methods are used to estimate fetal heart rate. The simplest and probably the oldest method to evaluate fetal heart rate is auscultation of fetal heart tones using a stethoscope. However, this does not provide recognition of the various types of fetal heart rate disturbances. When auscultation of the fetal heart rate reveals an abnormally slow, rapid, or irregular rate, the clinician is confronted with the dilemma of how to accurately diagnose the arrhythmia. For diagnosis of fetal heart rate and rhythm, fetal transabdominal electrocardiogram (ECG) can be used, but this technique is unfortunately of limited value due to its inability to demonstrate atrial depolarization (fetal P-waves, representing atrial systole are too small to be seen well and only the fetal QRS complex, representing ventricular systole, can be clearly visualized). The limitation of being able to record only ventricular systole has necessitated classification of arrhythmias by rhythm (regular or irregular) and rate (bradycardic or tachycardic). The external fetal heart rate monitor (CTG), widely used for antenatal care of fetal well-being, can also be used to estimate fetal heart rate, but while accurate for regular rhythm within the normal range, it may be inaccurate in the presence of fetal tachycardia.

The above-mentioned methods, traditionally used for estimation of fetal heart rate and/or rhythm, reflect primary ventricular rates, but not atrioventricular systolic timing relationships, which are a prerequisite for accurate diagnosis of fetal heart rhythm disturbances.

With the use of real-time-directed M mode echocardiography, both atrial and ventricular

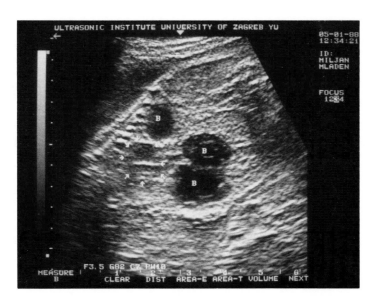

FIGURE 13. Sagittal section through the fetal chest demonstrating ectopia cordis in the case of diaphragmatic hernia. Fetal heart (indicated by arrows) is displaced from its normal place by intestinal loops protruding through the diaphragmatic aperture; it is situated cranially in thoracal cavity, just beneath the fetal neck.

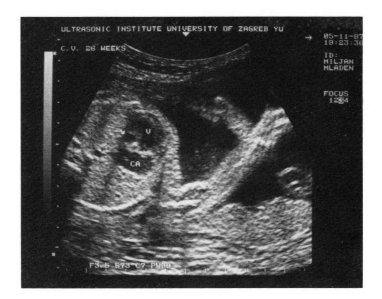

FIGURE 14. Cross-section through the fetal chest demonstrating hypoplastic left ventricle (indicated by arrow). Note the higher echogenicity of ventricular endocard, indicating the endocardial fibroelastosis. Interatrial septum was completely absent; thus, the common atrium (CA) was found. V = right ventricle.

systole can be recorded simultaneously. The basic limitation of this technique in the interpretation of fetal heart rate and rhythm is that only the mechanical effect of an electrical event can be observed. Despite this limitation, the technique has proven to be successful for defining all but very complex arrhythmias.[18]

In order to understand the M mode echocardiogram, the basic physiological events

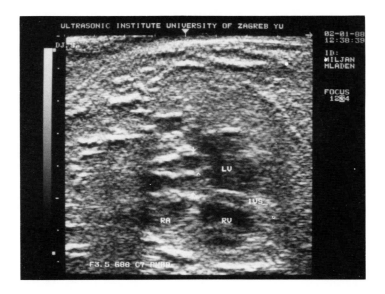

FIGURE 15.   Double-outlet left ventricle. Two great vessels (arrows) are found to originate from the left ventricle (LV). IVS = interventricular septum; RV = right ventricle; RA = right atrium.

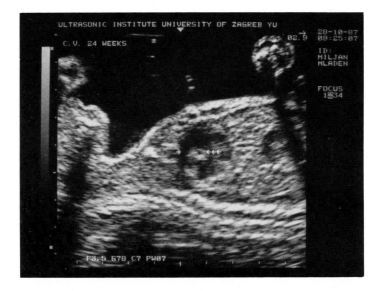

FIGURE 16.   Hypoplastic atretic pulmonary artery (indicated by three arrows) in a seriously malformed fetal heart (the same case as in Figures 14 and 17). Note the discrepancy of its size compared with the size of common truncus arteriosus (one arrow).

during the normal cardiac cycle has to be understood. The normal cardiac cycle begins by spontaneous depolarization of the sinoatrial node. The electrical impulse spreads through the right and left atria, resulting in atrial mechanical systole. Spreading through the atria, it reaches the atrioventricular node. As the conduction time in the atrioventricular node is longer than in atrial muscular bundles, the blood has enough time to pass through the

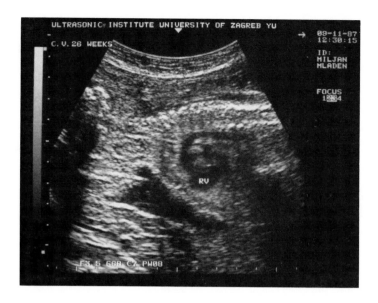

FIGURE 17. Common truncus arteriosus originating from the right ventricle (RV) in a fetus with complex heart malformations (see also Figures 14 and 16).

atrioventricular valves from the atria into the ventricles. The impulse then traverses the atrioventricular node and spreads through the ventricles using the His bundle and Purkinje network. Depolarization of the ventricles occurs, and it is manifested in ventricular mechanical systole. Electrical activation of the atria and ventricles, followed by mechanical contractions of the respective chambers, presupposes defining of the fetal heart rhythm by M mode echocardiography. Although there is a slight delay between the electrical impulse and changes in the specific points of motion selected from the echocardiogram, valve and wall motion represent the best indicators of the preceding electrical events.

Two standard M mode echocardiographic planes may be obtained for exact presentation of atrioventricular systolic timing relationships. The first one is obtained at the four-chamber view, when the M mode cursor is perpendicular to the interventricular septum at the level of the mitral and tricuspid valves (Figure 18). Atrial systole and diastole may be checked by atriventricular leaflets motion. Normally, the leaflets of both the tricuspidal and mitral valves demonstrate an M-shaped motion during ventricular diastole. At the onset of the rapid filling phase of ventricular diastole, the leaflets separate (D to E; Figure 19B) as blood crosses from the atria to the ventricles. Once completed, the leaflets begin to reapproximate as the volume of blood flow across the valves decreases (E to F). However, as a result of atrial systole, the leaflets rapidly open as more blood flows through the valvular orifice (F to A). Closure of the leaflets (A to C) completes atrial systole.[21] At the end of atrial systole (point C) ventricular systole begins. It may be recognized from the inward motion of the ventricular wall. Ventricular systole is completed at the end of onward motion of ventricular wall (Figure 19A).

The second M-mode echocardiographic plane in which precise estimation of atrial and ventricular systole may be obtained is left ventricular long axis. To obtain M mode echocardiogram in this plane, the M mode cursor has to pass through the aortic valve leaflets and the posterior atrial wall. As the aortic valve is clearly visualized, its leaflet motion may be used for estimation of the ventricular rate. At the onset of ventricular systole, the aortic leaflets separate as blood flows from left ventricular outflow tract to the ascending aorta (M to N; Figure 20B). During ventricular systole, the leaflets remain separated (N to P), forming a box-like structure on the M mode echocardiogram. As the intraventricular pressure drops

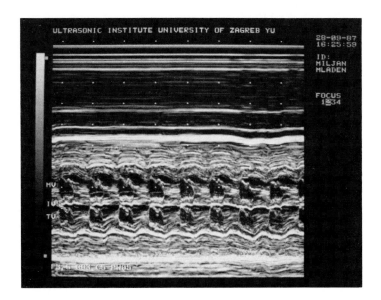

FIGURE 18.   Normal M mode echocardiogram in a case when the cursor is perpendicular to the interventricular septum, passing across the mitral and tricuspidal
valve. Typical M-like appearance of atrioventricular leaflet motions may be observed. MV = mitral valve; IVS = interventricular septum; TV = tricuspidal
valve.

at the end of ventricular systole, the aortic leaflets close (P to R) and remain closed during
the period of ventricular diastole (R to M). The onset of forward motion of the left atrial
posterior wall indicates the beginning of the atrial systole (Figure 20A). It is not always
possible to image atrial wall motion precisely because the amplitude of the atrial contraction
is small and its onset cannot always be located. In such cases, semilunar valve motion,
which is very similar to atrial wall motion, or the motion of aortic root can be helpful in
estimation of the onset of atrial systole.

Unlike in adult and pediatric echocardiography, where the exact places on the chest are
known to visualize each echocardiographic plane, in fetal echocardiography, many difficulties arise from the fact that the fetus is changing its position inside the uterine cavity.
Sometimes it is time consuming to visualize previously described planes and required heart
structures for M mode echocardiogram. Depending upon the position of the fetal heart in
relation to ultrasound beam, each plane in which the M mode cursor may be directed
simultaneously through atrial and ventricular wall may be used in routine work for M mode
echocardiographic examination. The onset of atrial and ventricular systole is determined on
the basis of the forward motion of the corresponding atrial and ventricular wall. Such
examination is less precise, but it takes less time. According to our experience, it may be
used routinely for screening of the fetuses with heart rhythm disturbances.

When the M mode echocardiogram is obtained, the fetal heart rate has to be estimated.
Silverman et al.[18] suggest construction of a standard ladder diagram to define atrial and
ventricular conduction sequence (Figures 19B and 20B). Because of the differing electro-
mechanical delays, it is important to use the same markers of atrial and ventricular contractions consistently.[18]

The normal fetal heart rate is found to be 140 ± 20 beats per min at around 20 weeks
of gestation, falling to 130 ± 20 beat per min towards term. Episodes of fetal bradycardia
lasting only a few seconds with heart rate of 70 to 100 beats per min are common, especially
in midtrimester pregnancies, often associated with fetal movement and decrease in frequency

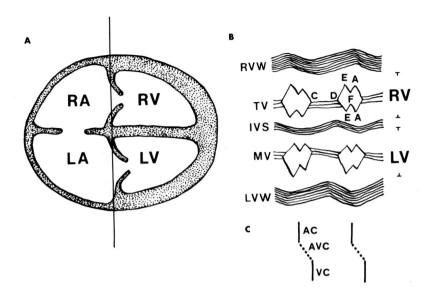

FIGURE 19.   (A) Schematic four-chamber view of the fetal heart from which M mode, presented on B, is recorded; cursor is perpendicular to the interventricular septum at the level of the mitral and tricuspid valves. RA = right atrium; LA = left atrium; RV = right ventricle; LV = left ventricle. (B) Schematic representation of the obtained M mode echocardiogram at the level presented in A (for detailed explanation, see text). RVW = right ventricular wall; TV = tricuspid valve; IVS = interventricular septum; MV = mitral valve; LVW = left ventricular wall; RV = right ventricular cavity; LV = left ventricular cavity. (C) Ladder diagram constructed to show interrelationship between atrial contraction (AC) and ventricular contraction (VC). The beginning of atrial contraction (AC) is defined by point F on atrioventricular valve motion representation, and the onset of ventricular contraction (VC) by point C from the atrioventricular valve and the beginning of forward motion of the ventricular wall. Diagonal line connecting the two vertical lines represents period of atrioventricular conduction (AVC).

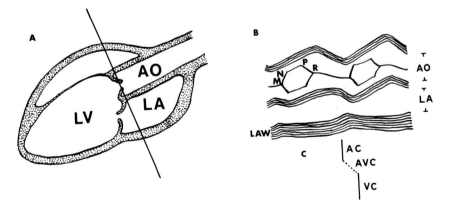

FIGURE 20.   (A) Schematic representation of the long axis through the left ventricle from which M mode echocardiogram, presented in B, is recorded. The cursor passes through the aortic valve leaflets and the left atrium. AO = aorta; LA = left atrium; LV = left ventricle. (B) Corresponding M mode echocardiogram obtained at the section presented in A (for detailed explanation, see text). AO = aorta; LA = left atrium; LAW = left atrial wall. (C) Corresponding ladder diagram shows the interrelationship between atrial contraction (AC) and ventricular contraction (VC), as well as the period of atrioventricular conduction (AVC). Atrial contraction (AC) is defined by the forward motion of the left atrial wall, and ventricular contraction (VC) by the onset of aortic valve opening (point M).

with advancing gestational age. Episodes of accleration of fetal heart rate to 160 to 180 beats per min also occur, especially toward the end of pregnancy.[18] Thus, one may conclude that a fetal heart rate ranging between 100 and 180 beats per min may be presumed as normal. Each persistent deviation of fetal heart rate above 180 beats per min or below 100 beats per min has to be considered as an abnormality in fetal heart rate. As it is seen in Figures 18, 19A, and 20A, normally each atrial systole (contraction) has to be followed by a corresponding ventricular systole (contraction). Absence of a temporal interrelationship between atrial and ventricular activation indicates some type of heart rhythm irregularity.

DETECTION OF FETAL HEART RATE END RHYTHM DISTURBANCES

During the past 3 decades, numerous papers have been published about the intrauterine diagnosis of fetal heart arrhythmias using the fetal ECG.[22,131-140] However, as mentioned before, good results are obtained only when the fetal membranes are interrupted and the scalp electrode is placed on the fetal head. Transabdominal electrodes may be used too, but the obtained results are not as good as during intrapartum use. As the fetal vernix caseosa partially eliminates conduction of the electrical impulses, only the QRS complex is obtained during the second and the beginning of the third trimester. Better results in transabdominal ECG are obtained during the last 3 to 4 weeks of pregnancy, when the vernix is eliminated from the fetal skin. As the transabdominal ECG usually does not permit visualization of the atrial depolarization during the second trimester, it is not useful in this period of pregnancy for detection of fetal heart rate end rhythm disturbances. The only method which enables the study of the atrioventricular systolic time relationship is M mode echocardiography.

Fetal arrhythmias are always due to abnormal electrical events in the fetal heart. They may be caused by (1) abnormal electrical triggering (when some emitter other than sinoatrial node appears) or by (2) abnormal conduction of electrical impulses between atria and ventricles.

Generally speaking, disturbances of fetal heart rate and rhythm may be divided into three main groups: (1) isolated premature contractions, (2) tachyarrhythmias, and (3) bradyarrhythmias.

ISOLATED PREMATURE CONTRACTIONS

Isolated premature beats may be supraventricular or ventricular. The pathogenesis of ectopic beats is very complex, and the emitting center of ectopic impulses may be situated anywhere inside the atrium or ventricle. Using M mode echocardiography, one is not always able to discover the appropriate origin of ectopic beats. The only conclusion that may be estimated is that the ectopic impulses are of ventricular or supraventricular origin.

Premature Atrial Contractions

According to Silverman et al.,[18] isolated premature atrial contractions are the most common rhythm disturbance in fetal life. Among 35 fetuses with heart rhythm disturbances, 19 were found to have premature atrial contractions. In such cases, basically the sinoatrial node emits regular impulses causing normal atrial depolarization. The electrical impulse passes through the atrioventricular node, and probably at some point other than the sinoatrial node, additional electrical impulses arise. As the frequency of these ectopic beats is different compared with the emitting frequency of the sinoatrial node, their appearance will produce a disturbance in fetal heart rhythm. After producing atrial activation, ectopic electrical impulses cross over the atrioventricular node and enter the ventricles, producing ventricular depolarization. Sometimes, the ectopic electrical impulse may be blocked at the level of the atrioventricular node, so that consequent ventricular depolarization does not occur.

In the M mode echocardiogram, a normal sequence of atrioventricular systole is noted

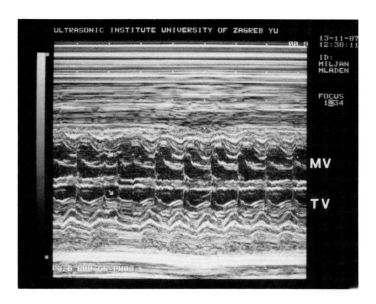

FIGURE 21. M mode echocardiogram obtained at the level of atrioventricular valves when the cursor was perpendicular to the interventricular septum in the case of premature atrial contraction. Premature atrial contraction (oblique arrows) is followed by ventricular contraction (vertical arrow). MV = mitral valve; TV = tricuspidal valve.

to occur prior to the premature atrial contraction. If the premature electrical impulse is not blocked at some level between the atria and ventricles, premature ventricular systole follows the premature atrial contraction (Figure 21). In the cases of blocked premature atrial impulses, premature atrial contraction is not followed with a consequent ventricular contraction. Instead of that, an incomplete compensatory pause occurs, and no evidence of ventricular contraction may be seen.

Premature atrial contractions are not uncommon either in childhood or in fetal life. Most reports suggest that these rhythms are benign,[25,129,141] although there are some reports that fetuses with premature atrial contractions subsequently developed atrial tachycardia.[18] It has been also shown that the great majority of fetuses with this rhythm disturbance do not show any structural heart abnormality, but Wladimiroff et al.[7] found associated cardiac structural abnormalities in 2 out of 16 fetuses with premature atrial ectopics (one of them died during intrauterine life). Thus, one may conclude that despite the fact that almost all the pregnancies with fetuses showing premature atrial contractions will develop uneventfully and will result in the delivery of a healthy infant, detailed structural analysis of the heart should be performed. No treatment is necessary, and normal delivery should be possible; but if the premature atrial contractions are diagnosed early enough in pregnancy, repeated echocardiographic examinations and evaluation of heart rate end rhythm are recommended. It has been shown that in 6 out of the 13 fetuses having this rhythm disturbance, abnormal beats disappeared in serial echocardiographic studies.[18]

Premature Ventricular Contractions

This type of ectopia originates some place in the ventricle. Appearing somewhere in the ventricle, ectopic electrical impulses produce the ventricular depolarization, e.g., its contraction. As the frequency of ectopic impulses is different from the frequency of impulses originating from the atrioventricular node, the ectopic beat will occur prematurely, producing an early ventricular activation. Probably sinus node discharge is occurring at the expected time, and atrial depolarization is occurring during ventricular systole. The forward atrial contraction is blocked in the region of the atrioventricular node, and the sinus node is not reset.[18] The next sinus beat arises at the expected time, and the normal atrioventricular timing relationship is not observed until the following ventricular ectopia occurs.

In the M mode echocardiogram, when the M mode cursor is directed through the atrioventricular valves perpendicular to the interventricular septum, premature ventricular contraction demonstrates the following characteristics: (1) excursion of the initial opening of the valve leaflets is decreased as a result of premature ventricular systole; (2) no A-wave; (3) incomplete relaxation of the ventricular wall during diastole; (4) a ventricular compensatory pause; and (5) enhanced diastolic filling of the subsequent cardiac cycle. When the cursor is directed through the aortic valve and atrial wall, a premature ventricular contraction is reflected by premature opening of the aortic leaflets without a preceding atrial contraction. Because of the inadequate filling of the ventricular chamber during diastole, the duration of the aortic valve opening is often decreased when compared to the previous normal cycle.[21] Usually, premature ventricular contractions do not persist into the neonatal period. Vaginal delivery of such fetuses is recommended, and no therapy during intrauterine life is necessary.

TACHYARRHYTHMIA

A fetal tachycardia exceeding 200 beats per minute without any variability or conduction abnormality is suggestive of supraventricular tachycardia.[23]

The commercially available cardiotachographs do not register fetal heart frequencies exceeding 220 beats per minute. The values that go beyond the preprogrammed parameters are eliminated. A fetal abdominal ECG would give a correct diagnosis. Although some authors obtained a reliable abdominal ECG,[142] an exact definition of the P-wave and QRS complex is not always possible. This is due to the low voltage of the fetal ECG (25 mV), the background noise (10 mV), and the interface of the maternal ECG (220 mV).[23] The only method which allows accurate antenatal diagnosis and follow-up of fetal tachycardia, even in midtrimester pregnancies, is M mode echocardiography.

It was found that short periods of fetal tachycardia can be seen in 0.4 to 0.6% of all pregnancies, without any clinical significance.[143] The duration of these periods of tachycardia varies greatly. Although they may last for 30 to 90 s, periods of up to several weeks are described.[138] Experience postnatally with neonatal supraventricular tachycardia suggests that the most commonly encountered electrophysiologic mechanism for this arrhythmia is atrioventricular reentry.[144] The reentrant basis for the arrhythmia, according to Kleinman et al.,[145] may be interpreted when M mode or pulsed Doppler fetal echocardiography demonstrates sudden onset and termination of tachycardia with induction of the arrhythmia by extrasystoles.[145] Onset and termination of arrhythmia may not be noted until after a therapeutic trial of antiarrhythmic medication is begun. If antiarrhythmic therapy results in second-degree atrioventricular block without termination of the arrhythmia, as has been observed in one case described in Kleinman's series, one can rule out atrioventricular reentry as the mechanism of the arrhythmia, and further attempts at therapy should be based on this information.[145]

According to Bergmans et al.,[23] fetal tachycardia may be due to

1. Sinus tachycardia: a frequency of more than 180 beats per minute, normal conduction, and a variability of 5 to 15 beats per minute. Most of the time, this form of fetal tachycardia is secondary to causes such as maternal anxiety, amnionitis, maternal fever, congenital infection, or drug administration. In this case, the underlying cause should be treated.[146] In the postterm fetus, it might be a symptom of severe fetal distress.[147]

2. Atrial flutter/fibrillation: an atrial rate of 300 to 460 beats per minute with a variable degree of A-V block, resulting in a ventricular rate of 60 to 200 beats per minute,

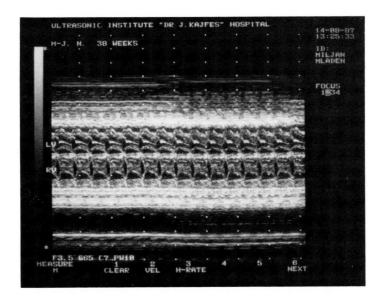

FIGURE 22.   M mode echocardiogram obtained at lateral four-chamber view with the cursor passing through the atrioventricular valves in a case of supraventricular tachycardia. LV = left ventricle; RV = right ventricle.

usually irregular, yet regular in case of a fixed A-V block. This condition is rarely diagnosed antenatally. In about 20% of the cases there is a concomitant congenital heart defect. In that case, fetal mortality is high.[146]

3.   Supraventricular tachycardia: a frequency often exceeding 200 beats per minute, normal conduction, and almost no variability (Figure 22). The P-waves on the fetal ECG are hardly recognizable. This is the most frequent form of fetal tachycardia. Short periods are probably of no clinical significance.[143] Persisting fetal supraventricular tachycardia, however, can lead to a high output failure of the heart, a serious, sometimes lethal complication.

Analyzing their 59 fetuses with intrauterine-diagnosed tachycardia, Bergmans et al.[23] found that 63% of fetuses had an Apgar score of less than 6 after 1 min. In 41% of cases, symptoms of congenital congestive heart failure were found, such as ascites and/or hydrothorax, diagnosed antenatally by echoscopy, or an enlarged liver and edema after birth. Another nine children (15.3%) had no signs of congestive heart failure at birth, but developed it within a few hours, which is probably secondary to the changing hemodynamic conditions immediately after birth. *In utero,* the right and the left ventricle keep up their cardiac output by working in parallel. After birth, they do so in series. This significant change, along with other factors, creates the need for a tripled increase in the output of each ventricle, this in spite of elimination of the placenta from fetal circulation. In nine cases (15.3%), the supraventricular tachycardia was secondary to a Wolf-Parkinson-White syndrome, and in four cases (6.8%), it was altered by atrial flutter/fibrillation.

The rate of congenital heart defects among the fetuses with tachycardia is different in various studies. In Bergmans' series,[23] 4 of the children (6.8%) had various types of congenital heart malformation, while Kleinman et al.[145] did not find any congenital heart defects among 18 fetuses with tachyarrhythmia.

If tachycardia lasts for a longer time, signs of congestive heart failure will develop: fetal ascites, hydrothorax, fetal edema, pericardial effusion, and maternal polyhydramnios. Kleinman et al.[145] found fetal edema, ascites, and maternal polyhydramnios in 16 out of 18 (88.8%) fetuses with tachycardia.

Treatment of Fetal Tachycardia

If there are no contraindications such as fetal immaturity, the pregnancy should be terminated by inducing labor or by primary cesarean section to treat the neonate properly. However, if the fetus is immature and its prolonged stay *in utero* is recommended, intrauterine therapy of tachycardia has to be attempted. For antepartum treatment of the fetus, different kinds of drugs can be used.[23,145,148-153]

Digitalis

Placental passage was first proved by Rogers et al.[154] The drug concentration in fetal cord blood was demonstrated to be approximately equal to maternal levels (cord level 90 to 100% maternal level). No teratogenic effects are ascribed to its use,[137] and successful cardioversion of the fetus was described.[24,148,150,155] A starting dose of 0.5 mg orally, to be repeated after 3 and 11 h, is recommended. Therapy can be continued by giving daily 0.25 mg orally from then on.[150] While it has been suggested that neonates may tolerate and even require higher serum levels of digoxin than adults,[154] the dose of digoxin given to the mother for transplacental therapy is limited by maternal tolerance. Administration of digoxin for treatment of supraventricular tachycardia of infancy is a policy undergoing reexamination in many centers. This reassessment is due to the high incidence of Wolff-Parkinson-White syndrome that has been found in infants with supraventricular tachycardia, and to the documentation of digitalis-induced shortening of the effective refractory period within the accessory conduction pathways of some of these children. The latter has been implicated as the underlying cause of the sporadic reports of sudden death in children with Wolf-Parkinson-White syndrome who are maintained on digitalis therapy. However, among 14 fetuses with supraventricular tachycardia, Kleinman et al.[145] have not documented evidence of preexcitation.

Propranolol

Propranolol is a drug from the group of beta blockers. These agents rapidly pass the placenta, although the degree of transfer has been disputed.[156] It might, however, hamper maternal uterine circulation, since recent reports have indicated that propranolol puts the neonate at risk for IUGR, depressed Apgar score, hypoglycemia, and bradycardia.[20,156] Sometimes, it was added to digoxin, but only limited success of this combination is found.[145]

Verapamil

Verapamil is an agent which belongs to the group of calcium antagonists. As a drug that blocks slow inward calcium and sodium currents, it is a potent agent for blocking atrioventricular nodal conduction.[157] Verapamil is, therefore, useful for treatment of reentrant tachycardias involving atrioventricular node conduction (either antegrade or retrograde) at one limb of the reentrant circuit.[145] These drugs also rapidly pass the placenta, and successful fetal cardioversion has been described.[151,158] A dose of 80 mg of verapamil three times daily is recommended. Over the past decade, this drug was extensively given to the pregnant women as a means of prophylaxis against the cardiovascular side effects of the beta agonists used for control of uterine contractions in the cases of imminent premature labor. Thus, enough experience has been documented about its safety in the second half of pregnancy. Studies of verapamil action on the normal heart suggest that despite the potential for a negative inotropic effect associated with calcium channel blockade, the drug is well tolerated by the normal heart. Cardiac output has remained in the normal range, the negative inotropic effects apparently countered by the afterload reduction related to vasodilation induced by the medication.[159] According to Kleinman et al.,[145] caution is necessary when considering verapamil administration, due to the possibility of precipitating severe bradycardia and depression of cardiac function when this drug is adminstered in a setting of severe cardiac failure. In the presence of severe fetal heart failure in the last second or early third trimester, with associated pulmonary immaturity, they believe that risk/benefit considerations indicate a role for verapamil treatment. Informed parental consent may have to be obtained before such treatment is instituted, and continuous hemodynamic monitoring of mother and fetus is essential.[145] These authors recommend verapamil therapy after initial administration of digoxin before considering administration of propranolol. One must be aware of the potential for digoxin accumulation due to impaired excretion when verapamil therapy is started, even after a digoxin steady state has been reached.[145]

Procainamide

Procainamide is also one of the antiarrhythmic drugs, used for cardioversion of fetal tachycardia into the normal heart rhythm. It belongs to a group of "Type I" antiarrhythmic drugs. The mechanism is based on the blocking of the sodium current responsible for the rapid phase 0 of the action potential. As a consequence, a decrease of the conduction velocity in atrial, ventricular, His-Purkinje, and accessory conduction tissue is noted. It also prolongs action potential duration and refractory periods of these tissues and may, therefore, be used for therapy of reentrant tachycardias mediated by conduction through these tissues. It has not been useful for treatment of supraventricular tachycardia due to abnormal automaticity. This medication is considered one of the drugs of choice for control of rapid ventricular response to atrial fibrillation/flutter in the presence of an atrioventricular bypass tract and should be considered for early inclusion in the treatment protocol when M mode echocardiography demonstrated atrial flutter or fibrillation. In this setting, digoxin, propranolol, or verapamil should be administered first, in order to prevent the rapid ventricular response that may occur if the atrial refractory period is increased. When reentrant supraventricular tachycardia is suspected, Kleinman et al.[145] recommend the use of this agent only if digoxin and/or verapamil have been unsuccessful and if the hydrops remains unchanged or appears to worsen. Caution should be exercised in the administration of procainamide to the pregnant woman, due to the potential for fetal and neonatal toxicity secondary to accumulation of drug and active metabolite in the fetus and the slow rate of elimination of these compounds by the neonate.

Bergmans et al.[23] have treated nine children antepartum. Of the five cases where digitalis was the only treatment, this was unsuccessful in three, but there was a slow-down of the fetal heart rate in one case; in fact, in only one case was a fetal cardioversion reached. So, from these scarce data, it might be deduced that a combination of a calcium antagonist and digitalis might lead to the best clinical results.[23] On the contrary, Kleinman et al.[145] reported a very high success rate in 14 fetuses with supraventricular tachycardia. Of the 14 fetuses, 13 had successful *in utero* conversion of supraventricular tachycardia to normal sinus rhythm; six patients responded to maternal digoxin administration, one to combined maternal digoxin and propranolol therapy, and six to a combination of digoxin and verapamil administration.[145]

It is interesting that in seven cases the heart rhythm changed during parturition, probably because of vagal stimulation secondary to pressure on the fetal head.[23] Martin et al.[160] reported one case of fetal supraventricular tachycardia in which cardioversion was achieved by compression of the fetal shoulder on the umbilical cord, which mimics the mechanism by which carotid sinus pressure or the Valsalva maneuver interrupts a supraventricular tachycardia.

Postpartum treatment possibilities are digitalis, diuretics, beta blockade, verapamil, electrocardioversion, or combinations of them.

According to Bergmans et al.,[23] about 60% of the children will be hypoxic at birth and need neonatal care, about 40% will be decompensated at birth, and another 15% will develop acute heart decompensation neonatally. Only 19% of the children are in good physical health at birth. After achieving cardioversion, about 18% of the children will have paroxysmal supraventricular tachycardia. For that reason, continuation of digitalis therapy at least during the first 6 months of life is recommended. In a group of fetuses with supraventricular tachycardia followed up for 1 year or longer, Kleinman et al.[145] did not find recurrence of tachycardia, and there was no mortality. None of their patients had evidence of Wolff-Parkinson-White syndrome on postnatal electrocardiograms. Prognosis is less promising in cases of atrial flutter or fibrillation.[145]

Of 59 cases, only 15 neonates (25.4%) had no signs of fetal distress, i.e., congenital or neonatal congestive heart failure or asphyxia, during or shortly after birth. This figure illustrates that persistent supraventricular tachycardia is indeed a threat to the fetus.[23] It is therefore important that all cases of fetal tachycardia be properly evaluated. Bergmans et al.[23] reported that in one child's heart, the rhythm changed during suctioning, which might also be caused by strong vagal stimulation.[23] In two cases, cardioversion was achieved by bilateral sinus carotid pressure, which is also a vagus effect.[23] Five children in which cardioversion was not achieved even during postnatal life died. However, in this series, three of five children had congenital heart malformation.[29]

In conclusion, it is clear that supraventricular tachycardia is a serious threat to the fetus, especially since it might lead to congestive heart failure. Therefore, treatment should begin as soon as the diagnosis is established.[23] Antepartum, some of the antiarrhythmic drug has to be given to the mother to achieve cardioversion. If the fetal supraventricular tachycardia and/or congestive heart failure perists and the condition for extrauterine life is not favorable, pregnancy termination is indicated. The timing and method of delivery are determined by the following factors: (1) presence or absence of fetal lung maturity, (2) response to pharmacologic therapy, (3) evidence of worsening hydrops, and/or (4) IUGR.[21] Sometimes, delivery itself causes cardioversion because of vagal stimulation; if not, the neonate can be treated.

BRADYARRHYTHMIA

When the fetal heart rate is under 100 beats per minute, fetal bradycardia is present. It is generally believed to be benign and associated with fetal movement[18,25,141] and occurs more commonly in the midtrimester.[141] A much more serious type of fetal bradyarrhythmia is congenital heart block, which will be described on the following pages.

Congenital Heart Block

Congenital complete heart block (third-degree A-V block) is reported with a frequency of 1 per 20,000 live births.[161] Fetal heart block is present either in association with collagen disease, structural congenital heart defects, or viral infection. It is thought that about 30% of fetuses with congenital heart block have congenital heart defect. Surveying the literature, Shenker[162] found 41 cases detected before delivery. Of the mothers of the affected babies, 30% are known to have or to develop connective tissue disease, especially systemic lupus erythematosus. Scott et al.[163] have demonstrated maternal antibodies to ribonucleoprotein (anti-RO(SS-A)) in affected babies before the age of 3 months, but not later.[163] Thus, the hypothesis of an etiological relationship between these antibodies and the destruction of the bundle of His has been postulated.[163-165] It is important to know that there is increasing evidence to suggest that subclinical collagen vascular disease may be present in at least some "healthy" mothers at the time they give birth to the affected child. Several retrospective reviews have noted the subsequent development of systemic lupus erythematosus in previously healthy mothers who gave birth to children with complete congenital heart block.[166-169] Therefore, complete congenital heart block in the offspring should be regarded as an indicator to investigate the mother for evidence of connective tissue disease and to provide satisfactory follow-up for her.[167]

In the M mode echocardiogram, congenital heart block may be diagnosed when discordance between opening and closing of the atrioventricular valves and the corresponding ventricular response is found.[21] As a result of altered cardiovascular dynamics, the fetus with congenital heart block is at increased risk for developing IUGR and/or hydrops.[170]

In complete atrioventricular block and other situations in which there is a slow heart rate, oscillation of the atrioventricular valves occurs. These oscillations should not be interpreted as being due to multiple atrial contractions.[18]

If the congenital heart block is not recognized antenatally, maternal welfare may be unnecessarily compromised during labor and delivery. Fetal bradycardia when unrecognized prior to the onset of labor has frequently been misconstrued as a sign of fetal asphyxia, and as a result, the mother has been subjected to hasty and unnecessary cesarean section.[171]

Generally speaking, fetuses of the mothers with collagen disease have a better prognosis than those with structural heart defects. The prognosis depends on any underlying anomalies and of the ventricular rate. The lower the rate, the worse the prognosis. If the ventricular rate is so low that the increased stroke volume and ventricular hypertrophy are inadequate to maintain cardiac output, congestive heart failure may develop. The prognosis for infants with congenital heart block, provided there is no other congenital malformation, is good, with a 95% 20-year survival for the affected children.[164]

Delivery of fetuses with congenital heart block must be planned for, with ready preparatory measures for emergency pacemaker implantation at hand. Fetal well-being in labor can be monitored using scalp blood pH measurements; thus, vaginal delivery may often be safely achieved.

COLOR DOPPLER FETAL ECHOCARDIOGRAPHY

During the past decade, visualization of the anatomical feature of the normal heart in the midtrimester fetus became feasible using high-resolution ultrasound equipment, as well as antenatal detection of congenital heart abnormalities. Real-time-directed M mode enabled the antenatal measurement of particular heart structures and estimation of fetal heart rate and rhythm and their disturbances. One of the difficulties for the fetal sonographer, however, has been the identification and complete elucidation of structural defects that are associated with intracardiac or great vessel flow disturbances. Following successful use in adults and pediatric echocardiography,[172-174] recently, the color Doppler was introduced in fetal echocardiography.[27-29]

BASIC ASPECTS

The name "color Doppler" is short for a mapping two-dimensional velocity measurement system which gives results equivalent to Doppler measurement, but operates on a slightly different principle. At this point, we shall, however, shortly describe the possibilities of measuring reflector velocities in the time domain, rather than in the pure frequency domain, as done in pure Doppler.

The simplest way to measure velocities in the time doman with an echoscope is the moving target identification (MTI) method. If we imagine two subsequent images made with sonar, we can see that in the two images all the dots which represent still targets stay put in the same position, while the moving targets appear in different places in the two images. In a way, it is similar to making two photographs of a street scene with a time lapse of, say, 1 s. The buildings and other still objects stay in the same position, but the streetwalkers will appear in slightly different places, depending on the direction and velocity of their movement. All that has to be done is to subtract the contents of the two images. In this procedure, the still objects vanish from the subtraction image and the moving "targets" show where they are and in which direction their movement is directed. This MTI method if feasible in situations where the single reflectors are prominent enough to be identified as separate entities. Airplanes on a radar image are such entities, but the human blood cells are too many, too small, and too densely packed to be measured correctly in this way. Therefore, after initial experiments, this method was not used for two-dimensional movement (flow) mapping.

However, a more complicated method, the autocorrelation method, which operates in the time domain could have been adopted for blood flow mapping, and a majority of the present color Doppler equipment operates in this way. The method is called the autocorrelation analysis. The details of the method are fairly complicated, but the underlying principles can be explained in a simple way.

The basic principle of calculation of an autocorrelation function of some time function is to multiply the time function itself at different time lapses. If the time function is totally random, its values after some time delay will bear little or no relation to its previous values. If, however, the time process has some memory or regularity, the previous values influence the later behavior of the process. Thus, in the process which changes in some regular way, the previously mentioned product — the autocorrelation function — will extract the information about the change of the time process with time. The time process in the case of blood flow measurement is the whole of the echoes from a moving blood stream. The calculation of the autocorrelation function may be done automatically and fast enough to measure the blood flow in the human body. Not surprisingly, the limitation turns out to be the same as in a pulsed Doppler system. The color code has to indicate the velocity, the direction, and the uncertainty (variance) of the measurement. The direction is coded in two different colors: red and blue. The velocity is coded for by the brightness, and the variance is coded for by adding a proportional part of yellow to red or cyan to blue. The result is a semiquantitative map of velocities, directions, and turbulences which bear much information to an educated eye.

CLINICAL APPLICATIONS

Visualization of the fetal intracardiac blood flow may be achieved using standard echocardiographic planes (e.g., four-chamber view, long axis through the left ventricle, short axis through the heart at the level of aortic and pulmonary valves, and sagittal section to visualize aortic arch) are used. The examination of the fetal heart starts with standard two-dimensional evaluation of fetal heart structures. When a high-contrast, noise-free B mode image is displayed, color Doppler flow is superimposed on a cross-sectional image to study blood flow patterns. As mentioned before, blood flow toward the transducer is coded in red, while the blue color designates flow going away from the transducer. Intensity of red and blue colors are brightness modulated, depending on the velocity of blood flow. Thus, semiquantitative data about the flow velocities may be obtained from two-dimensional Doppler presentation.

The best plane for study of atrioventricular blood flow is the four-chamber view. Optimal images are obtained when the flow direction is parallel with the ultrasound beam, e.g., in the apical or basal four-chamber view.

During diastole, blood flows from atria into the ventricles. When atria are nearer to the probe, blood flow is displayed in red-yellow color (Plate 1*), but if ventricles are nearer to the probe, blood flows in an opposite direction, and it is coded in blue color. If the M mode cursor is placed through the valves to be parallel with the flow direction, color M mode of the flow of the valves is obtained. It enables better visualization of the flow of the valves in relation to the particular parts of the cardiac cycle.

Entering the ventricles, blood flows along the interventricular septum toward the apex. At the same time, opposite color appears along the lateral ventricular walls, and it can be concluded that blood is flowing from the apex along the lateral ventricular walls in opposite direction. In ventricular systole, in the same echocardiographic plane, the aortic flow may be noted in the opposite color than previously seen for atrioventricular flow. Ventricular inflow and outflow may be visualized using the following two echocardiographic planes.

---

* Plates 1 to 5 appear following page 38.

Visualization of the left ventricular inflow and outflow tracts is possible when the left axis through the left ventricle is used. In this section, flow through the mitral valve during diastole is visualized, and during systole, flow through the aortic valve is observed in the opposite color (Plate 2). To study inflow and outflow of the right ventricle, the short axis through the fetal heart at the level of the aortic and pulmonary valve has to be obtained. The best results in pulmonary color flow mapping are obtained when the fetus is lying on its back. In such cases, blood which flows from the right ventricle into the pulmonary artery flows away from the probe; thus, it is coded in blue color. At the same time, aortic flow may be detected, but its direction is opposite with the direction of pulmonary flow. It is, therefore, coded in red-orange color (Plate 3). Visualization of blood flow through the aortic arch and descending aorta is possible when the longitudinal scan through the fetal trunk is obtained. In the cases when the fetal spine is oriented anteriorly, which represents, according to our experience, the best position, flow through the aortic arch is coded in red-orange color. One must be careful in coding flow through the descendent aorta. If the Doppler beam is perpendicular to the descendent aorta, no flow can be detected. Therefore, the examiner has to decline the probe slightly cranially to get descendent aorta in oblique position. In such a case, descendent aorta flow is coded in an opposite color than the flow in aortic arch, e.g., blue color.

When one becomes familiar with color Doppler flow mapping in the normal fetal heart, there are no difficulties in detecting abnormal flow such as appears in congenital heart defects.

In our ultrasonic institute, a total number of 357 echographic examinations were performed using color Doppler. The gestational age of examined fetuses varied from 16 to 40 weeks. According to our experience, the optimal gestational age for color Doppler examination was found to be between 20 and 24 weeks. In this time, fetal heart structures are big enough that their clear visualization may be achieved. One must bear in mind that the frame rate of presently available color Doppler equipment is lower than that of two-dimensional echocardiographic imaging systems alone at similar depths of imaging, as there is an inherent trade-off between the number of successive pulses, the line density per sector, and the depth. The other limiting factors for color Doppler echocardiography are found to be similar as for two-dimensional fetal echocardiography, e.g., maternal obesity, oligo- or polyhydramnios, anteriorly inserted hydropic placenta, and excessive fetal movements.

According to our experience, color Doppler technique reveals, in comparison with currently used echocardiographic techniques, at least four new possibilities in evaluation of the normal fetal heart: (1) intracardiac blood flow visualization, (2) fast, semiquantitative analysis of intracardiac blood flow velocities, (3) estimation of intracardiac flow direction, and (4) spatial orientation of flow jets which might allow precise quantitative intracardiac velocity measurements by conventional Doppler methods. Obtained data might be helpful in the study of fetal cardiac physiology, prenatal examination of cardiac valve function, and, of course, in prenatal detection of congenital heart defects.

The usefulness of the color Doppler technique was tested in seven cases of congenital heart defects. According to obtained experience, color Doppler was found to be helpful in diagnosis of some congenital heart defects unobtainable by standard two-dimensional echocardiographic methods. For example, we have diagnosed insufficiency of the tricuspid valve in two cases on the basis of the blood regurgitation observed during ventricular systole.[27,28] One of them is presented in Plate 4.

In some other congenital heart defects, color Doppler helps to establish a more accurate, definite diagnosis. In Plate 5, a case of atrial septal defect is presented. Although large atrial septal defects may be detected using two-dimensional fetal echocardiography, small defects may escape the diagnosis. Using color Doppler, left-to-right shunt may be detected, even when the small atrial defect is present, located in the middle of interatrial septum, in the area of foramen ovale.

According to our results, as well as the results published by other authors, there is no doubt that color Doppler represents a useful innovation in fetal echocardiography. It will not replace currently used echocardiographic techniques. It seems that two-dimensional echocardiography will retain its position in fetal cardiac structure visualization, M mode in visualization of cardiac structure movements, while color Doppler provides an important way to study physiology and pathophysiology of intracardiac blood flow, allowing a better understanding of normal and pathological events in the fetal heart.

Further investigations and more experience in this new field is mandatory, but preliminary results are indeed very encouraging.

REFERENCES

1. **Winsberg, F.,** Echocardiography of the fetal and newborn heart, *Invest. Radiol.,* 7, 152, 1972.
2. **Robinson, H. P.,** Detection of fetal heart movement in the first trimester of pregnancy using pulsed ultrasound, *Br. Med. J.,* 4, 466, 1978.
3. **Egeblad, H., Bang, J., and Northeved, A.,** Ultrasonic identification and examination of fetal heart structures, *J. Clin. Ultrasound,* 3, 95, 1975.
4. **Garrett, W. J. and Robinson, D. E.,** Fetal heart size measured in vivo by ultrasound, *Pediatrics,* 46, 25, 1970.
5. **Yamaguchi, D. T. and Lee, F. Y. L.,** Ultrasonic evaluation of the heart. A report of experience and anatomic correlation, *Am. J. Obstet. Gynecol.,* 134, 422, 1979.
6. **Nimrod, C., Nicholson, S., Machin, G., and Harder, J.,** In utero evaluation of fetal cardiac structure: a preliminary report, *Am. J. Obstet. Gynecol.,* 148, 516, 1984.
7. **Wladimiroff, J. W., Stewart, P. A., and Tonge, H. M.,** Ultrasonic assessment of fetal cardiovascular anatomy and functions: its significance in the prenatal diagnosis of cardiac structural defects, in *The Fetus as a Patient,* Kurjak, A., Ed., Elsevier, Amsterdam, 1985, 231.
8. **DeVore, G. R., Donnerstein, R. L., Kleinman, C. S., Platt, L. D., and Hobbins, J. C.,** Fetal echocardiography. I. Normal anatomy as determined by real-time-directed M-mode ultrasound, *Am. J. Obstet. Gynecol.,* 144, 249, 1982.
9. **Lange, L. W., Sahn, D. J., Allen, H. D., Goldberg, S. J., Anderson, C., and Giles, H.,** Qualitative real-time cross-sectional echocardiographic imaging of the human fetus during the second half of pregnancy, *Circulation,* 62, 799, 1980.
10. **Wladimiroff, J. W., Stewart, P. A., and Vosters, R. P. L.,** Fetal cardiac structure and function as studied by ultrasound, *Clin. Cardiol.,* 7, 239, 1984.
11. **DeVore, G. R.,** The prenatal diagnosis of congenital heart disease — practical approach for the fetal sonographer, *J. Clin. Ultrasound,* 13, 229, 1985.
12. **St. John Sutton, M. G., Gewitz, M. H., Shah, B., Cohen, A., Reichek, N., Gabbe, S., and Huff, D. S.,** Quantitative assessment of growth and function of the cardiac chambers in the normal fetus: a prospective longitudinal echocardiographic study, *Circulation,* 69, 645, 1984.
13. **Wladimiroff, J. W.,** Ultraschalluntersuchung des fetalen und neonatalen Herzens und des kardiovasculaeren Systems, *Ultraschall,* 2, 4, 1981.
14. **Shime, J., Gresser, C. D., and Rakowski, H.,** Quantitative two-dimensional echocardiographic assessment of fetal cardiac growth, *Am. J. Obstet. Gynecol.,* 154, 294, 1986.
15. **Sahn, D. J., Lahge, L. W., Allen, H. D., Goldberg, S. J., Anderson, C., Giles, H., and Haber, K.,** Quantitative real-time cross-sectional echocardiography in the developing normal human fetus and newborn, *Circulation,* 62, 588, 1980.
16. **Roge, C. L. L., Silverman, N. H., Hart, P. A., and Ray, R. M.,** Cardiac structure growth pattern determined by echocardiography, *Circulation,* 57, 285, 1977.
17. **DeVore, G. R., Siassi, B., and Platt, L. D.,** Fetal echocardiography. IV. M-mode assessment of ventricular size and contractility during the second and third trimesters of pregnancy in the normal fetus, *Am. J. Obstet. Gynecol.,* 150, 981, 1984.
18. **Silverman, N. H., Enderlein, M. A., Stanger, P., Teitel, D. F., Heyman, M. A., and Golbus, M. S.,** Recognition of fetal arrhythmias by echocardiography, *J. Clin. Ultrasound,* 13, 255, 1985.
19. **Allan, L. D., Crawford, D. C., Anderson, R. H., and Tynan, M.,** Evaluation and treatment of fetal arrhythmias, *Clin. Cardiol.,* 7, 467, 1984.

20. **Cottrill, C. M., McAllister, R. G., Gettes, L., and Noonan, J. A.,** Propranolol therapy during pregnancy, labor, and delivery: evidence for transplacental drug transfer and impaired neonatal drug disposition, *J. Pediatr.,* 91, 812, 1977.

21. **DeVore, G. R., Siassi, B., and Platt, L. D.,** Fetal echocardiography. III. The diagnosis of cardiac arrhythmias using real-time-directed M-mode ultrasound, *Am. J. Obstet. Gynecol.,* 146, 792, 1983.

22. **Hawrylyshyn, P. A., Miskin, M., Gilbert, B. W., Duncan, W. J., and Valtchev, K. L.,** The role of echocardiography in fetal cardiac arrhythmias, *Am. J. Obstet. Gynecol.,* 141, 223, 1981.

23. **Bergmans, M. G. M., Jonker, G. J., and Kock, H. C. L. V.,** Fetal supraventricular tachycardia. Review of the literature, *Obstet. Gynecol. Surv.,* 40, 61, 1985.

24. **Losure, T. A. and Roberts, N. S.,** In utero diagnosis of atrial flutter by means of real-time-directed M-mode echocardiography, *Am. J. Obstet. Gynecol.,* 149, 903, 1984.

25. **Kleinman, C. S., Donnerstein, R. L., Jaffe, C. C., DeVore, G. R., Weinstein, E. M., Lynch, D. C., Talner, N. S., Berkowitz, R. L., and Hobbins, J. C.,** Fetal echocardiography. A tool for evaluation of in utero cardiac arrhythmias and monitoring of in utero therapy: analysis of 71 patients, *Am. J. Cardiol.,* 51, 237, 1983.

26. **Inversen, O. E., Lossius, P., Lovset, T., and Finnem, P. H.,** Complete fetal heart block diagnosed by ultrasound, *Acta Obstet. Gynecol. Scand.,* 64, 533, 1985.

27. **Kurjak, A., Breyer, B., Jurkovic, D., Alfirevic, Z., and Miljan, M.,** Color flow mapping in obstetrics, *J. Perinat. Med.,* 15, 271, 1987.

28. **Kurjak, A., Alfirevic, Z., and Miljan, M.,** Conventional and color Doppler in the assessment of fetal and maternal circulation, *Ultrasound Med. Biol.,* accepted for publication.

29. **DeVore, G. R., Horenstein, J., Siassi, B., and Platt, L. D.,** Fetal echocardiography. VII. Doppler color flow mapping: new technique for the diagnosis of congenital heart disease, *Am. J. Obstet. Gynecol.,* 156, 1054, 1987.

30. **Nora, J. J. and Nora, A. H.,** *Genetics and Counseling in Cardiovascular Diseases,* Charles C Thomas, Springfield, IL, 1978.

31. **Polani, P. E.,** Chromosomal abnormalities and congenital heart disease, *Guy's Hosp. Rep.,* 117, 323, 1968.

32. **Copel, J. A., Pilu, G., and Kleinman, C. S.,** Congenital heart disease and extracardiac anomalies: associations and indications for fetal echocardiography, *Am. J. Obstet. Gynecol.,* 154, 1121, 1986.

33. **Wladimiroff, J. W., Stewart, P. A., Sachs, E. S., and Niermeijer, M. F.,** Prenatal diagnosis and management of congenital heart defects: significance of associated fetal anomalies and prenatal chromosome studies, *Am. J. Med. Genet.,* 21, 285, 1985.

34. **Bergsma, D., Ed.,** *Birth Defects Compendium,* 2nd ed., Alan R. Liss, New York, 1979.

35. **Nora, J. J., Lortcher, R. H., and Spangler, R. D.,** Echocardiographic studies of left ventricular disease in Ullrich-Noonan syndrome, *Am. J. Dis. Child.,* 129, 1417, 1975.

36. **Nora, J. J., Nora, A. H., Sinha, A. K., Spangler, R. D., and Lubs, H. A.,** The Ullrich-Noonan syndrome (Turner phenotype), *Am. J. Dis. Child.,* 127, 48, 1974.

37. **Nora, J. J. and Nora, A. H.,** The environmental contribution to congenital heart disease, in *Congenital Heart Disease: Causes and Processes,* Nora, J. J. and Takao, A., Eds., Futura, Mt. Kisco, NY, 1984, 15.

38. **Simpson, J. L., Golbus, M. S., and Martin, A. O.,** *Genetics in Obstetrics and Gynecology,* Grune & Stratton, New York, 1982.

39. **Jones, K. L., Smith, D. W., Ulleland, C. N., and Streissguth, A.,** Pattern of malformation in offspring of alcoholic mothers, *Lancet,* 1, 7815, 1973.

40. **Zierler, S.,** Maternal drugs and congenital heart disease, *Obstet. Gynecol.,* 65, 155, 1985.

41. **Monson, R. R., Rosenberg, L., Hartz, S. C., Shapiro, S., Heinonen, O. P., and Slone, D.,** Diphenylhydantoin and selected congenital malformations, *N. Engl. J. Med.,* 289, 1048, 1973.

42. **South, J.,** Teratogenic effects of anticonvulsants, *Lancet,* 2, 1154, 1972.

43. **Lowe, C. R.,** Congenital malformations among infants born to epileptic women, *Lancet,* 1, 9, 1973.

44. **Annegers, J. F., Elveback, L. R., Hauser, W. A., and Kurland, L. T.,** Do anticonvulsants have a teratogenic effect?, *Arch. Neurol.,* 31, 364, 1974.

45. **German, J., Kowal, A., and Ehlers, K. H.,** Trimethadione and human teratogenesis, *Teratology,* 3, 349, 1970.

46. **Zackai, E., Mellman, M. J., Neiderer, B., and Hanson, J. W.,** The fetal trimethadione syndrome, *J. Pediatr.,* 87, 280, 1975.

47. **Schou, M., Goldfield, M. D., and Weinstein, M. R.,** Lithium and pregnancy. I. Report from the register of lithium babies, *Br. Med. J.,* 2, 135, 1973.

48. **Weinstein, M. R. and Goldfield, M. D.,** Cardiovascular malformations with lithium use during pregnancy, *Am. J. Psychiatry,* 132, 529, 1975.

49. **Nora, J. J. and Nora, A. H.,** Genetic epidemiology of congenital heart diseases, in *Progress in Medical Genetics,* Vol. 5, Steinberg, A. G., Bearn, A. G., Motulsky, A. G., and Childs, R., Eds., W. B. Saunders, Philadelphia, 1983, 91.

50. **Nora, J. J. and Nora, A. H.,** Birth defects and oral contraceptives, *Lancet,* 1, 941, 1973.
51. **Nora, J. J., Nora, A. H., Perinchief, A. G., Ingram, J. W., and Fountain, A. K.,** Congenital abnormalities and first-trimester exposure to progestagen/oestrogen, *Lancet,* 1, 313, 1976.
52. **Harlap, S., Prywes, R., and Davies, A. M.,** Birth defects and oestrogens and progesterones in pregnancy, *Lancet,* 1, 682, 1975.
53. **Levy, E. P., Cohen, A., and Fraser, F. C.,** Hormone treatment during pregnancy and congenital heart defects, *Lancet,* 1, 611, 1973.
54. **Heinonen, O. P., Slone, D., and Monson, R. R.,** Cardiovascular birth defects and antenatal exposure to female sex hormones, *N. Engl. J. Med.,* 296, 67, 1977.
55. **Rothman, K. J., Fyler, D. C., Goldblatt, A., and Kreidberg, M. B.,** Exogenous hormones and other drug exposure of children with congenital heart disease, *Am. J. Epidemiol.,* 109, 433, 1979.
56. **Nora, J. J., Nora, A. H., Blu, J., Fountain, A., Peterson, M., Lortscher, R. H., and Kimberling, W. J.,** Exogenous progestogen and estrogen implicated in birth defects, *JAMA,* 240, 837, 1978.
57. **Stern, R. S., Rosa, F., and Baum, C.,** Isotertinoin and pregnancy, *J. Am. Acad. Dermatol.,* 10, 851, 1984.
58. **Penn, I., Makowski, E., and Droegemueller, W.,** Parenthood in renal homograft patients, *JAMA,* 216, 1755, 1971.
59. **Gregg, N. M.,** Congenital cataract following German measles in mother, *Trans. Ophthalmol. Soc. Aust.,* 3, 35, 1942.
60. **Manson, M. M., Logan, W. P. D., and Loy, R. M.,** Rubella and other virus infections during pregnancy, *Public Health Rep. Med. Sub.,* 101, 1960.
61. **Sheridan, M. D.,** Final report of a prospective study of children whose mothers had rubella in early pregnancy, *Br. Med. J.,* 2, 536, 1964.
62. **Tartakow, I. J.,** The teratogenicity of maternal rubella, *J. Pediatr.,* 66, 380, 1965.
63. **Campbell, M.,** Place of maternal rubella in the aetiology of congenital heart disease, *Br. Med. J.,* 1, 691, 1961.
64. **Rustein, D. D., Nickerson, R. J., and Herald, F. P.,** Season incidence of patent ductus arteriosus and maternal rubella, *Am. J. Dis. Child.,* 84, 199, 1952.
65. **Gibson, S. and Lewis, K.,** Congenital heart disease following maternal rubella during pregnancy, *Am. J. Dis. Child.,* 83, 317, 1952.
66. **Jackson, A. V.,** in *Studies in Pathology,* King, E. S. J., Lowe, T. E., and Cox, L. B., Eds., Melbourne University Press, Melbourne, 1950.
67. **Pitt, D. B.,** Congenital malformations and maternal rubella, *Med. J. Aust.,* 1, 233, 1957.
68. **Campbell, M.,** Causes of malformations of the heart, *Br. Med. J.,* 2, 895, 1965.
69. **Heiner, D. C. and Nadas, A. S.,** Patent ductus arteriosus in association with pulmonic stenosis, *Circulation,* 17, 232, 1958.
70. **Rowe, R. D.,** Maternal rubella and pulmonary artery stenosis. Report of 11 cases, *Pediatrics,* 32, 180, 1963.
71. **Venables, A. W.,** The syndrome of pulmonary stenosis complicating maternal rubella, *Br. Med. J.,* 27, 49, 1965.
72. **Emmanouilides, G. C., Linde, L. M., and Crittenden, I. H.,** Pulmonary artery stenosis associated with ductus arteriosus following maternal rubella, *Circulation,* 29, 514, 1964.
73. **Hastreiter, A. R., Joorabchi, B., Pujatti, G., van der Horse, R. L., Patacsil, G., and Sever, J. L.,** Cardiovascular lesions associated with congenital rubella, *J. Pediatr.,* 71, 59, 1967.
74. **Williams, H. J., and Carey, L. S.,** Rubella embriopathy. Roentgenologic features, *Am. J. Roentgenol.,* 47, 92, 1966.
75. **Nora, J. J. and Nora, A. H.,** The evolution of specific genetic and environmental counseling in congenital heart diseases, *Circulation,* 57, 205, 1978.
76. **Sever, J.,** Viruses and embryos, in *Congenital Malformations,* Fraser, F. C. and McKusick, V. A., Eds., Excerpta Medica, Amsterdam, 1970.
77. **Warkany, J.,** Etiology of congenital malformations, in *Advances in Pediatrics,* Vol. 2, Levine, S. Z., Ed., Interscience, New York, 1947, 1.
78. **Malmberg, N., Strener, G., and Lundmark, C.,** Asymptomatic maternal rubella as a probable cause of embryopathy, *Ann. Paediatr. Fenn.,* 3, 437, 1957.
79. **Swan, C., Tostevin, A. L., Moore, B., Mayo, H., and Black, G. H. B.,** Congenital defects in infants following infectious diseases during pregnancy, with special reference to relationship between German Measles and cataract, deaf-mutism, heart disease, and microcephaly and to period of pregnancy in which occurrence of rubella is followed by congenital abnormalities, *Med. J. Aust.,* 2, 201, 1943.
80. **Beswick, R. C., Warner, R., and Warkany, J.,** Congenital anomalies following maternal rubella, *Am. J. Dis. Child.,* 78, 334, 1949.
81. **Bolognese, R. J., Corson, S. L., Fuccillo, D. A., Sever, J. K., and Traub, R.,** Evaluation of possible transplacental infection with rubella vaccination during pregnancy, *Am. J. Obstet. Gynecol.,* 117, 939, 1973.

82. **Prebuld, S. R.,** Some current issues relating to rubella vaccine, *JAMA*, 254, 253, 1985.
83. **Potter, E. L.,** Placental transmission of viruses, with special reference to the intrauterine origin of cytomegalic inclusion body disease, *Am. J. Obstet. Gynecol.*, 74, 505, 1957.
84. **Brown, G. C. and Karunas, R. S.,** Relationship of congenital anomalies and maternal infection with selected enteroviruses, *Am. J. Epidemiol.*, 95, 207, 1972.
85. **Benirsche, K. and Pendelton, M. E.,** Coxsackie virus infection, an important complication of pregnancy, *Obstet. Gynecol. Surv.*, 12, 305, 1958.
86. **Javett, S. N., Heynemann, S., Mundel, B., Pepler, W. J., Lurie, H. I., Gear, J., Measroch, V., and Kirsch, Z.,** Myocarditis in the newborn infant, *J. Pediatr.*, 48, 1, 1956.
87. **Noren, G. R., Adams, P., and Anderson, R. C.,** Positive skin reactivity to mumps virus antigen in endocardial fibroelastosis, *J. Pediatr.*, 62, 604, 1963.
88. **St. Geme, J. W., Jr., Noren, G. R., and Adams, P., Jr.,** Proposed embryopathic relation between mumps virus and primary endocardial fibroelastosis, *N. Engl. J. Med.*, 275, 339, 1966.
89. **Rowland, T. W., Hubbell, J. P., and Nadas, A. S.,** Congenital heart disease in infants of diabetic mothers, *J. Pediatr.*, 83, 815, 1973.
90. **Gutgesell, H. P., Mullins, E. C., and Gillette, P. C.,** Transient hypertrophic subaortic atenosis in infants of diabetic mothers, *J. Pediatr.*, 89, 120, 1976.
91. **Miller, E., Hare, J. W., Cloherty, J. P., Dunn, P. J., Gleason, R. E., Soeldner, J. S., and Kitzmejller, J. L.,** Elevated maternal hemoglobin A1c in early pregnancy and major congenital anomalies in infants of diabetic mothers, *N. Engl. J. Med.*, 304, 1331, 1981.
92. **Levy, H. L., and Waisbren, S. E.,** Effects of untreated maternal phenylketonuria and hyperphenylalaninemia on the fetus, *N. Engl. J. Med.*, 309, 1269, 1983.
93. **Lenke, R. L. and Levy, H. L.,** Maternal phenylketonuria and hyperphenylalaninemia: an international survey of the outcome of untreated and treated pregnancies, *N. Engl. J. Med.*, 303, 1202, 1980.
94. **Stevenson, R. E. and Huntlet, C. C.,** Congenital malformations in offspring of phenylketonuric mothers, *Pediatrics*, 40, 33, 1967.
95. **Fisch, R. O., Doeden, D., and Lansky, L. L.,** Maternal phenylketonuria, *Am. J. Dis. Child.*, 118, 847, 1969.
96. **Reder, R. F. and Rosen, M. R.,** Basic electrophysiologic principles: application to treatment of dysrhythmias, in *Pediatric Cardiac Dysrhythmias*, Gilette, P. C. and Garson, A., Eds., Grune & Stratton, New York, 1981.
97. **Crawford, C. S.,** Antenatal diagnosis of fetal cardiac abnormalities, *Ann. Clin. Lab. Sci.*, 12, 99, 1982.
98. **Edwards, J. H.,** Familial predisposition in man, *Br. Med. Bull.*, 25, 58, 1969.
99. **Nora, J. J., McGill, C. W., and McNamara, D. G.,** Empiric recurrence risk in common and uncommon congenital heart lesions, *Teratology*, 3, 325, 1970.
100. **Whittemore, R., Hobbins, J. C., and Engle, M. A.,** Pregnancy and its outcome in women with and without surgical treatment of congenital heart disease, *Am. J. Cardiol.*, 50, 641, 1982.
101. **Rose, V., Gold, R. J. M., Lindsey, G., and Allen, M. A.,** A possible increase in the incidence of congenital heart defects among the offspring of affected parents, *J. Am. Coll. Cardiol.*, 6, 376, 1985.
102. **Nora, J. J.,** Multifactorial inheritance hypothesis for the etiology of congenital heart diseases: the genetic-environmental interaction, *Circulation*, 38, 604, 1968.
103. **Fuhrmann, W. and Vogel, F.,** *Genetic Counseling*, Springer-Verlag, New York, 1969.
104. **Nora, J. J.,** Etiologic factors in congenital heart diseases, *Pediatr. Clin. North Am.*, 18, 1059, 1971.
105. **Fraser, F. C. and Hunter, A. D. W.,** Etiologic relations among categories of congenital heart malformations, *Am. J. Cardiol.*, 36, 793, 1975.
106. **Warkany, J.,** *Congenital Malformations. Notes and Comments,* Year Book Medical Publishing, Chicago, 1971, chap. 48.
107. **Anderson, R. C.,** Congenital cardiac malformations in 109 sets of twins and triplets, *Am. J. Cardiol.*, 39, 1045, 1977.
108. **Schnitzel, A. A. G. L., Smith, D. W., and Miller, J. R.,** Monozygotic twining and structural defects, *J. Pediatr.*, 95, 921, 1979.
109. **Myrianthopulos, N. C.,** Congenital malformations in twins: epidemiology survey, *Birth Defects Orig. Artic. Ser.*, 11 (8), 1, 1975.
110. **Hutchison, A. A., Yu, V. Y., and Fortune, D. W.,** Nonimmunologic hydrops fetalis: a review of 61 cases, *Obstet. Gynecol.*, 59, 347, 1982.
111. **Etches, P. C. and Lemons, J. A.,** Non-immune hydrops fetalis. Report of 22 cases including three siblings, *Pediatrics*, 64, 326, 1979.
112. **Beischer, N. A., Fortune, D. W., and Macafee, C. A. J.,** Non-immunologic hydrops fetalis and congenital abnormalities, *Obstet. Gynecol.*, 38, 86, 1971.
113. **Allan, L. D., Crawford, D. C., Sheridan, R., and Chapman, M. G.,** Aetiology of non-immune hydrops: the value of echocardiography, *Br. J. Obstet. Gynaecol.*, 93, 223, 1986.

114. **Feldt, R. H., Strickler, G. B., and Weidman, W. H.,** Growth of children with congenital heart disease, *Am. J. Dis. Child.,* 117, 573, 1969.
115. **Kleinman, C. S., Hobbins, J. C., Lynch, D. C., Talner, N. S., and Jaffe, C. C.,** Prenatal echocardiography, *Hosp. Pract.,* 15, 81, 1980.
116. **McDonald, R. and Goldschmidt, B.,** Pancytopenia with congenital defects (Fanconi's anemia), *Arch. Dis. Child,* 35, 367, 1965.
117. **Stewart, P. A., Wladimiroff, J. W., and Essed, C. E.,** Prenatal ultrasound diagnosis of congenital heart disease associated with intrauterine growth retardation. A report of 2 cases, *Prenat. Diagn.,* 3, 279, 1983.
118. **Kleinman, C. S. and Santulli, T. V.,** Ultrasonic evaluation of the human fetal heart, *Semin. Perinatol.,* 7, 90, 1983.
119. **Silverman, N. H. and Golbus, M. S.,** Echocardiographic techniques for assessing normal and abnormal fetal cardiac anatomy, *J. Am. Coll. Cardiol.,* 5, 20S, 1985.
120. **Greenwood, R. D., Rosenthal, A., Parisi, L., Fyler, D. C., and Nadas, A. S.,** Extracardiac abnormalities in infants with congenital heart disease, *Pediatrics,* 55, 485, 1975.
121. **Wallgren, E. I., Landtman, B., and Rapola, J.,** Extracardiac malformations associated with congenital heart disease, *Eur. J. Cardiol.,* 7, 15, 1978.
122. **Gallo, P., Nardi, F., and Marinozzi, V.,** Congenital extracardiac malformations accompanying congenital heart disease, *G. Ital. Cardiol.,* 6, 450, 1976.
123. **Comstock, C. H.,** Normal fetal heart axis and position, *Obstet. Gynecol.,* 70, 255, 1987.
124. **Wladimiroff, J. W., Stewart, P. A., and Tonge, H. M.,** The role of diagnostic ultrasound in the study of fetal cardiac abnormalities, *Ultrasound Med. Biol.,* 10, 457, 1984.
125. **Allan, L. D., Tynan, M., Campbell, S., and Anderson, R. H.,** Identification of congenital cardiac malformations by echocardiography in midtrimester fetus, *Br. Heart J.,* 46, 358, 1981.
126. **Allan, L. D., Crawford, D. C., Anderson, R. H., and Tynan, M. J.,** Echocardiographic and anatomical correlations in fetal congenital heart disease, *Br. Heart J.,* 52, 542, 1984.
127. **Bovicelli, L., Picchio, F. M., Pilu, G., Baccarani, G., Orsini, L. F., Rizzo, N., Alampi, G., Benenati, P. M., and Hobbins, J. C.,** Prenatal diagnosis of endocardial fibroelastosis, *Prenat. Diagn.,* 4, 67, 1984.
128. **Gresser, C. D., Shime, J., Rakowski, H., Smallhorn, J. F., Hui, A., and Berg, J. J.,** Fetal cardiac tumor: a prenatal echocardiographic marker for tuberous sclerosis, *Am. J. Obstet. Gynecol.,* 156, 689, 1987.
129. **Kleinman, C. S., Donnerstein, R. L., DeVore, G. R., Jaffe, C. C., Lynch, D. C., Berkowtiz, R. L., Talner, N. S., and Hobbins, J. C.,** Fetal echocardiography for evaluation of in utero congestive heart failure, *N. Engl. J. Med.,* 306, 568, 1982.
130. **Ben-Ami, M., Shalev, E., Romano, S., and Zuckerman, H.,** Midtrimester diagnosis of endocardial fibroelastosis and atrial septal defect: a case report, *Am. J. Obstet. Gynecol.,* 155, 662, 1986.
131. **Young, B. K., Katz, M., and Klein, S. A.,** Intrapartum fetal cardiac arrhythmias, *Obstet. Gynecol.,* 54, 427, 1979.
132. **Hughey, M. and Elesh, R.,** Profound atrial tachycardia in utero, *Am. J. Obstet. Gynecol.,* 128, 463, 1977.
133. **Berube, S., Lister, G., Toews, W. H., Creasy, R. K., and Heyman, M. A.,** Congenital heart block and maternal lupus erythematosus, *Am. J. Obstet. Gynecol.,* 130, 595, 1978.
134. **Kendall, B.,** Abnormal fetal heart rates and rhythms prior to labor, *Am. J. Obstet. Gynecol.,* 99, 71, 1967.
135. **Lingman, G., Lundstrom, N.-R., Marsal, K., and Ohrlander, S.,** Fetal cardiac arrhythmia. Clinical outcome in 113 cases, *Acta Obstet. Gynecol. Scand.,* 65, 263, 1986.
136. **Sugarman, R. G., Rawlinson, K. F., and Schifrin, B. S.,** Fetal arrhythmia, *Obstet. Gynecol.,* 52, 301, 1978.
137. **Newburger, J. W. and Keane, J. F.,** Intrauterine supraventricular tachycardia, *J. Pediatr.,* 95, 780, 1979.
138. **Hedval, G.,** Congenital paroxismal tachycardia — a report of three cases, *Acta Paediatr. Scand.,* 62, 550, 1973.
139. **Chitkara, Y., Gergely, R. Z., Gleicher, N., Kerenyi, T. D., and Longhi, R.,** Persistant supraventricular tachycardia in utero, *Diagn. Gynecol. Obstet.,* 2, 291, 1980.
140. **Kamaromy, B., Gaal, J., Mihaly, G., Mocsary, P., Pohanka, O., and Suranyi, S.,** Data on the significance of fetal arrhythmia, *Am. J. Obstet. Gynecol.,* 99, 79, 1967.
141. **Allan, L. D., Anderson, R. H., Sullivan, I. D., Campbell, S., Holt, D. W., and Tynan, M.,** Evaluation of fetal arrhythmias by echocardiography, *Br. Heart J.,* 50, 240, 1983.
142. **Boos, R., Auer, L., Roettgers, H., and Kubli, F.,** A contribution to the monitoring of fetal arrhythmias, *J. Perinat. Med.,* 10, 85, 1982.
143. **Southhall, D. P., Richard, J., Hardwick, R. A., Shinebourne, E. A., Gibbons, G. L. D., Thelwall-Jones, H., De Swiet, M., and Johnston, P. G. B.,** Prospective study of fetal heart rate and rhythm patterns, *Arch. Dis. Child.,* 55, 506, 1980.
144. **Garson, A., Jr.,** Supraventricular tachycardia, in *Pediatric Cardiac Dysrrhythmias,* Gilette, P. C. and Garson, A., Eds., Grune & Stratton, New York, 1981, 77.

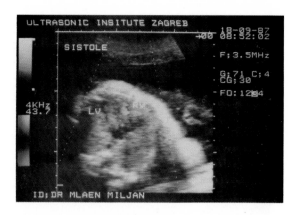

Plate 1.

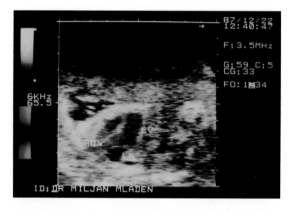

Plate 2.

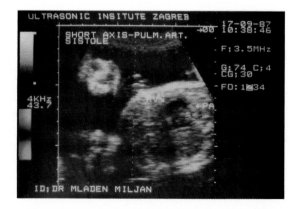

Plate 3.

Plate 1. Color-coded Doppler flow mapping of a normal atrioventricular flow obtained on apical four-chamber veiw during ventricular diastole. Atrioventricular flow is coded in reddish-yellow color. At the same time, blue color appears along the lateral ventricular walls. LV = left ventricle; RV = right ventricle. **Plate 2.** Long axis through the left ventricle (correspondent to the left parasternal view in adult echocardiography) during systole. Left ventricular outflow and flow through ascendent aorta is coded in blue color, as it flows away from the probe. LV = left ventricle; LA = left atrium; AO = ascendent aorta. **Plate 3.** Short axis at the level of pulmonary and aortic valve when a fetus is lying on its back. Pulmonary flow is coded in blue color. Centrally situated is the aorta; its flow is coded in reddish-yellow because it has opposite direction. PA = pulmonary artery; RV = right ventricle.

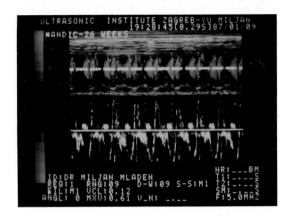

Plate 4.

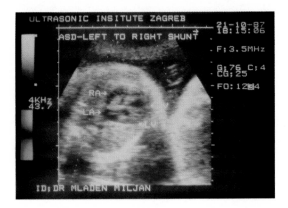

Plate 5.

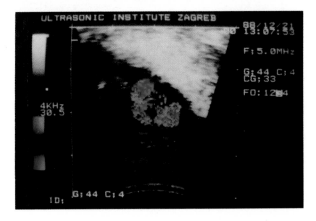

Plate 6.

Plate 4. Color-coded M mode in a case of tricuspidal leaflet agenesis (upper part of figure) obtained on apical four-chamber view, with cursor being parallel with interventricular septum and correspondent pulsed Doppler image (below). During diastole, normal flow through the tricuspidal valve is detected (reddish-yellow), but in systole, regurgitant flow is observed (blue). **Plate 5.** Lateral four-chamber view in a fetus with small atrial septal defect, located in the middle of the interatrial septum. Reddish-yellow color indicates flow from the left into the right atrium. On the basis of left-to-right shunt, diagnosis of atrial septal defect was established. LA = left atrium; RA = right atrium. **Plate 6.** Transvaginal color flow mapping of ovarian malignancy.

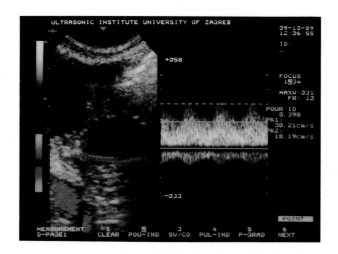

Plate 7.

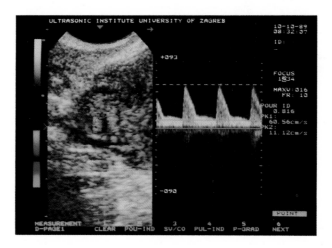

Plate 8.

Plate 7. Pulsed Doppler waveform from the septal part of the malignant tumor shows very low resistance and increased diastolic flow. **Plate 8.** Uterine fibroma with increased color flow on the border of the tumor. However, spectral Doppler analysis shows typical benign flow pattern with very high resistance and low diastolic flow.

145. **Kleinman, C. S., Copel, J. A., Weinstein, E. M., Santulli, T. V., and Hobbins, J. C.,** Treatment of fetal supraventricular tachyarrhythmias, *J. Clin. Ultrasound,* 13, 265, 1985.
146. **Shenker, L.,** Fetal cardiac arrhythmias, *Obstet. Gynecol. Surv.,* 34, 561, 1979.
147. **Ron, M., Adoni, A., Hochner-Celnikier, D., and Palti, Z.,** The significance of baseline tachycardia in the postterm fetus, *Int. J. Gynecol. Obstet.,* 18, 76, 1980.
148. **Kerenyi, T. D., Gleicher, N., Meller, J., Brown, E., Steinfeld, L., Chitkara, U., and Raucher, H.,** Transplacental cardioversion of intrauterine supraventricular tachycardia with digitalis, *Lancet,* 1, 393, 1980.
149. **Teucher, A., Bossi, E., Imhof, P., Erb, E., Stocker, F. P., and Weber, J. W.,** Effect of propranolol on fetal tachycardia in diabetic pregnancy, *Am. J. Cardiol.,* 42, 304, 1978.
150. **Harrigan, J. T., Kangos, J. J., Sikka, A., Spisso, K. R., Natarajan, N., Leiman, S., and Korn, D.,** Successful treatment of fetal congestive heart failure secondary to tachycardia, *N. Engl. J. Med.,* 304, 1527, 1981.
151. **Lingman, G., Ohrlander, S., and Ohlin, P.,** Intrauterine digoxin treatment of fetal paroxismal tachycardia, *Br. J. Obstet. Gynaecol.,* 87, 340, 1980.
152. **Wolf, F., Breukner, K. H., Schlensker, K. H., and Bolte, A.,** Prenatal diagnosis and therapy of fetal heart rate anomalies: with a contribution on the placental transfer for verapamil, *J. Perinat. Med.,* 8, 203, 1980.
153. **Dumesic, D. A., Silverman, N. H., Tobias, S., and Golbus, M. S.,** Transplacental cardioversion of fetal supraventricular tachycardia with procainamide, *N. Engl. J. Med.,* 307, 1128, 1982.
154. **Rogers, M. C., Willerson, J. T., Goldblat, A., and Smith, T. W.,** Serum digoxin concentration in the human fetus, neonate and infant, *N. Engl. J. Med.,* 287, 1010, 1972.
155. **Simpson, P. C. Trudinger, B. J., Walker, A., and Baird, P. J.,** The intrauterine treatment of fetal cardiac failure in a twin pregnancy with an acardiac, acephalic monster, *Am. J. Obstet. Gynecol.,* 147, 842, 1983.
156. **Habib, A. and McCarthy, J. S.,** Effects on the neonate of propranolol administered during pregnancy, *J. Pediatr.,* 91, 808, 1977.
157. **Antman, E. M., Stone, P. H., Muller, J. E., and Braunwald, E.,** Calcium channel blocking agents in the treatment of cardiovascular disorders. I. Basic and clinical electrophysiologic effects, *Ann. Intern. Med.,* 93, 875, 1980.
158. **Pringsheim, W., Windorfer, A., Jr., and Mross, F.,** Intrauterine Herzinsuffizienz und Hydrops congenitus, *Monatsschr. Kinderheilkd.,* 125, 453, 1977.
159. **Stone, P. H., Antman, E. M., Muller, J. E., and Braunwald, E.,** Calcium channel blocking agents in the treatment of cardiovascular disorder. II. Hemodynamic effects and clinical applications, *Ann. Intern. Med.,* 93, 886, 1980.
160. **Martin, C. B., Jr., Nijhuis, J. G., and Weijer, A. A.,** Correction of fetal supraventricular tachycardia by compression of the umbilical cord: report of a case, *Am. J. Obstet. Gynecol.,* 150, 324, 1984.
161. **Gochberg, S. H.,** Congenital heart block, *Am. J. Obstet. Gynecol.,* 88, 238, 1964.
162. **Shenker, L.,** Fetal cardiac arrhythmias, *Obstet. Gynecol. Surv.,* 34, 561, 1964.
163. **Scott, J. S., Maddison, P. J., Taylor, P. V., Esscher, E., Scott, O., and Skinner, R. P.,** Connective-tissue disease, antibodies to ribonucleoprotein, and congenital heart block, *N. Engl. J. Med.,* 309, 209, 1983.
164. **Vetter, L. V. and Rashkind, W. J.,** Congenital complete heart block and connective-tissue disease, *N. Engl. J. Med.,* 309, 236, 1983.
165. **Cobbe, S. M.,** Congenital complete heart block, *Br. Med. J.,* 286, 1769, 1983.
166. **Wright, R. B., Adams, P., and Anderson, R. C.,** Congenital atrioventricular dissociation due to complete or advanced atrioventricular heart block, *Am. J. Dis. Child.,* 98, 72, 1959.
167. **McCue, C. M., Mantakas, M. E., Tingelstad, J. B., and Ruddy, S.,** Congenital heart block in newborns of mothers with connective tissue disease, *Circulation,* 56, 82, 1977.
168. **Chameides, L., Truex, R. C., Vetter, V., Rashkind, W. J., Galioto, F. M., Jr., and Noonan, J. A.,** Association of maternal systemic lupus erythematosus with congenital complete heart block, *N. Engl. J. Med.,* 297, 1204, 1977.
169. **Hull, D., Binns, B. A. O., and Joyce, D.,** Congenital heart block and widespread fibrosis due to maternal lupus erythematosus, *Arch. Dis. Child.,* 41, 688, 1966.
170. **Hardy, J. D., Solomon, S., Banwell, G. S., Beach, R., Wright, V., and Howard, F. M.,** Congenital complete heart block in the newborn associated with maternal systemic lupus erythematosus and other connective tissue disorders, *Arch. Dis. Child.,* 54, 7, 1979.
171. **Reid, R. L., Pancham, S. R., Kean, W. P., and Ford, P. M.,** Maternal and neonatal implications of congenital complete heart block in the fetus, *Obstet. Gynecol.,* 54, 470, 1979.
172. **Switzer, D. F. and Nanda, N. C.,** Doppler color flow mapping, *Ultrasound Med. Biol.,* 11, 403, 1985.

173. **Bommer, W. J. and Miller, L.,** Real-time two-dimensional color-flow Doppler: enhanced Doppler flow imaging in the diagnosis of cardiovascular disease, *Am. J. Cardiol.,* 49, 944, 1982.
174. **Miyatake, K., Omoto, M., Kinoshita, N., Izumi, S., Owa, M., Takao, S., Sakakibara, H., and Nimura, Y.,** Clinical applications of a new type of real-time two-dimensional Doppler flow imaging system, *Am. J. Cardiol.,* 54, 857, 1984.

Chapter 2

INVASIVE DIAGNOSTIC PROCEDURES IN OBSTETRICS

Asim Kurjak and Zarko Alfirevic

INTRODUCTION

The assessment of fetal growth, gestational age, and detection of fetal malformations are still the main goals of ultrasound examination in obstetrics. However, in the last few years, a variety of other ultrasound techniques have been introduced in order to improve prenatal care. The two most important ones are Doppler ultrasound assessment of fetal and maternal circulation (described in a separate chapter) and ultrasonically guided fetal tissue biopsy.

For centuries the human fetus was felt, palpated, and listened to, but actually remained unapproachable. The introduction of ultrasound has dramatically changed perinatal care, enabling examination of the fetus and its environment. Besides bringing the fetus into sight, its major breakthrough is correct timing and safe execution of numerous antenatal intrauterine diagnostic procedures.

We believe that ultrasound should be used prior to any obstetrical procedure for diagnosis of multiple gestation, verification of fetal viability, confirmation of gestational age, and detection of fetal malformations. The optimal site for instrument insertion should be selected by means of ultrasound, taking into account placental location, fetal position, and amniotic fluid distribution, in order to reach the desired tissue.

Nowadays, the interventions are performed by using small hand-held real-time transducers with excellent image quality. In the majority of procedures, the continuous instrument tip visualization is simply achieved, thus effectively preventing fetal damage due to an uncontrolled instrument movement, as when the procedure is carried out blindly.

With the introduction of ultrasonically guided interventions, it has been possible to extend the simple amniocentesis to more complicated intrauterine procedures such as chorion biopsy and fetal blood sampling, bringing a virtual revolution in perinatal medicine.

SECOND-TRIMESTER AMNIOCENTESIS

In the majority of perinatal centers, the amniocentesis for prenatal diagnosis is performed at 16 weeks of gestation. However, the amniocentesis performed at 15 or 20 weeks of gestation can hardly be considered as an exception.[1-4] What are the reasons for such timing which seems to be so uniform, regardless of technique or laboratory? They can be summarized as follows:

1. The greatest ratio of viable to nonviable cells
2. Adequate volume of amniotic fluid
3. Enough time to repeat procedure if necessary and for therapeutic abortion[1,4,5]

The origin of amniotic fluid cells from the fetal skin has not been disputed, although the change from fetal periderm to epidermis at about 17 to 20 weeks of gestation and subsequent epidermal differentiation leads to changes in the cell structure.[5] The cell viability, judged by means of their ability to exclude vital stains (trypan blue, for example) or by cell sorting, is usually around 20% or less.[1,6] The total number of cells rises steadily from 12 weeks onward, reaching a plateau at 22 weeks.[5]

The unfavorable viable to nonviable cell ratio prior to 16 weeks of gestation has been one of the major reasons for the proposed timing.

Despite many classifications, at least two categories of amniotic fluid cells can be recognized: (1) large cells with irregular borders and small nuclei and (2) small, round, macrophagic-like cells.[6] The detailed description of amniotic fluid cell types and techniques of cell culturing can be found elsewhere.[6]

There have been several quite confusing reports on the average amniotic fluid volume in relation to the gestational age. Milunsky[7] summarized the estimates made from intact gestational sacs at hysterotomy, using dye dilution or isotopic methods, showing variations of the amniotic fluid volume in relation to the gestational age (207 ± 92 ml, 258 ± 97 ml, 365 ± 88 ml at 16, 18, and 20 weeks of gestation, respectively). According to Abramovich,[8] the volume virtually doubles between 14 and 16 weeks of gestation. Nevertheless, it seems that the optimal ratio between fetal volume and amniotic fluid volume, as far as accessibility of amniotic fluid is concerned, is between 16 and 18 weeks of gestation.

The time between the procedure and the obtained finding (long-term cell culture) is usually 3 weeks. With the advanced technology it can be shortened considerably. The shortest reported average time for specimen preparation has been 8.7 d.[4] Nevertheless, if the procedure is performed at 16 weeks of gestation, there is enough time to repeat it if the culture fails to grow, or to perform safe termination of pregnancy in cases of severe karyotype defect.

INDICATIONS

In the vast majority of cases, the second-trimester amniocentesis is performed with the purpose of karyotyping the fetus. Once the method was proved to be safe and accurate, its use and indications increased exponentially all over the world.

It is our policy that the procedure should be advocated only after genetic counseling and ultrasound examination in which fetal viability, absence of gross fetal malformation, and gestational age have been confirmed.

The most common indication is advanced maternal age. We have adopted 35 years as the "cut-off" age, although 37, 38, and 40 years have been also proposed.[9] The age-specific risk for nondisjunction leading to trisomies rises from 0.9% at 35 to 36 years to 7.8% at 43 to 44 years.[10] It should be borne in mind that the cited incidence is higher than the incidence of neonatal trisomy. If the incidence of trisomies in the delivery ward is taken into account, the real incidence would be underestimated due to late abortions and stillbirths.

A history of a child with trisomy indicates the requirement for genetic counseling and amniocentesis. However, it should be emphasized that increased risk in subsequent gestation of these women has not been supported in recent studies.[1]

The indication for amniocentesis includes also pregnancies in which one of the parents is a carrier of balanced translocation.

Determination of fetal sex may be used when there is a risk of a seriously handicapping, X-linked recessive disorder. It can be achieved from the karyotype or, more rapidly, but less precisely, from the directly stained amniotic fluid cells.[11]

A significant number of inborn metabolic errors may be diagnosed prenatally from enzyme analysis of cultured cells or from biochemical analysis of the fluid itself.[1,12]

Besides the above mentioned, there are several other indications listed in Table 1. The vast majority of them are discussed in detail in the appropriate chapters (spontaneous abortion, blighted ovum, fetal malformation, polyhydramnios, oligohydramnios, symmetrical IUGR, etc.)

In certain countries, second-trimester amniocentesis plays an important role in the detection of neural tube defects (NTD). Since the two most important NTDs, anencephaly and spina bifida, are well established 28 d after conception,[13] the increased level of α-fetoprotein (AFP) should be present very early in pregnancy. It is a fetal glycoprotein (M_r 70,000)

TABLE 1
Indications and Number of Second-Trimester Amniocentesis Performed in a 5-Year Period (1980 to 1985)

Indication	Number	%
Mother's age >35	620	48.9
Aneuploidy in previous pregnancies	109	8.6
Aneuploidy in family	15	1.2
Parents — quiet translocation carriers	10	0.8
Malformations in previous pregnancies	162	12.8
Malformations in family	6	0.5
Ultrasonically detected malformation	55	4.3
Spontaneous abortions, blighted ovum in previous pregnancies	40	3.2
Polyhydramnios	51	4.0
Oligohydramnios	10	0.8
Symmetrical intrauterine growth retardation (IUGR)	4	0.3
Exposure to X-rays in early pregnancy	30	2.4
Miscellaneous	154	12.2
Total	1266	100.0

synthesized in the fetal liver, yolk sac, and in the gastrointestinal tract.[14] Normally it is secreted via the fetal urine. If NTD is present, direct contact of spinal and amniotic fluid will lead to the significant elevation of AFP levels both in amniotic fluid and maternal serum.[14]

It is not our policy to indicate second-trimester amniocentesis solely because there is an increased risk for NTD. There are two major reasons for it. First, we believe that thorough ultrasound examination is the diagnostic method of choice in such cases and should be performed regardless of AFP finding. Second, no pregnancy should be terminated because of elevated AFP without ultrasound confirmation of underlying pathology.

There are several reasons for increased AFP level apart from NTD (gastrointestinal defects, Meckel's syndrome, trisomies, Turner's syndrome, intrauterine fetal death, congenital nephrosis, sacrococcygeal teratoma, multiple pregnancy, wrong gestational age, contamination by bleeding, etc.).[1,14] Practically all of them should be antenatally recognized either by ultrasound examination or by karyotyping.

Determination of acetylcholinesterase in the amniotic fluid is also a useful and predictive parameter in the diagnosis of NTD. The test is considered to be a more specific and sensitive indicator for NTD than AFP.[14]

TECHNIQUE

As we already mentioned, the second-trimester amniocentesis is best performed between 16 and 18 weeks of gestation. At this time, the uterus is accessible transabdominally, there is a sufficient volume of amniotic fluid, and the ratio of viable to nonviable cells appears to be greatest.[5,15]

Initially, amniocentesis was performed without knowledge about the position of the intrauterine contents. With the advent of ultrasound, the ultrasonographer has been allowed to select a pocket of amniotic fluid away from vital parts and the placenta. Although some studies reported that ultrasonography did not reduce the failure rate, incidence of multiple needle insertion, or the proportion of the amniotic fluid samples containing blood,[16-19] the majority of reports have demonstrated increased efficacy and safety with this modality.[20-24]

The 20-gauge needle is mainly used for the procedure (Figure 1). According to the Canadian Medical Research Council study, needles of a size larger than 19 gauge seem to carry a greater risk of abortion than those of smaller caliber.[25] The needle with stylette should be used in order to minimize the chance of contamination by maternal cells.

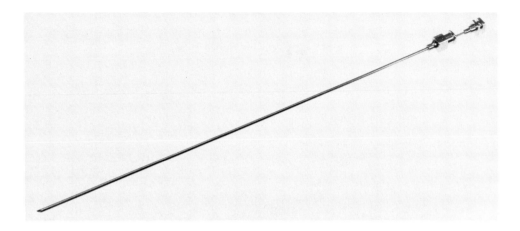

FIGURE 1.   A 20-gauge needle for amniocentesis.

We have performed more than 3000 amniocentesis in the last 10 years under ultrasound guidance, and in our opinion, it has an essential place in its safe and fast performance.

There are several ways to perform amniocentesis with the help of the ultrasound unit. They can be summarized in three groups.

1. Ultrasound examination is performed immediately before the free-hand puncture. The real-time transducer (linear, sector, or semiconvex) is stored in sterile solution, or sterile plastic bag, and the skin is painted with iodine. If there is enough amniotic fluid and placenta is posterior, the puncture is performed blindly, preferably in the median line. Although it is not actually an ''ultrasonically guided procedure'', fetal position and the optimal amniotic fluid pocket can be accurately assessed. The time between ultrasound examination and puncture should not exceed a few seconds. If there is any problem (dry tap, blood-stained fluid), needle position can be easily identified with the already sterile transducer.

2. There are several situations in which amniocentesis is often troublesome, as, for example, in cases of anterior placenta, oligohydramnios, large myoma, multiple pregnancy, etc. In such conditions, real ultrasonically guided procedure should be performed. The procedure is the same as previously described, apart from transducer used. Numerous types of transducers with needle guides and puncture adaptors are available today (Figures 2 and 3). The main difference is not in the type of the transducer, but in the angle between needle path and the ultrasound image. In some reports, the angling of the needle was described as a dangerous procedure which ought to be avoided.[26] If the needle path is parallel to the ultrasound beam, only the needle tip can be visualized (Figure 4). Furthermore, the ultrasound beam is not indefinitely thin. Very little unpurposeful angling of the needle will result in a false tip image, due to cross-sectioning of the needle and the ultrasound beam (Figure 5). Therefore, the angle between needle path and transducer should be at least 30° in order to allow clear visualization of the whole needle (Figure 6).

3. We have recently adopted an ultrasonically guided free-hand technique for some intrauterine procedures. It is especially feasible for fetal blood sampling and amniocentesis in selected difficult cases. The amniotic sac is visualized with a sterile semiconvex transducer held in one hand, while the uterus is punctured with the needle held in the other. The distance between the egde of the transducer and the puncture site should not exceed 3 cm. Once the needle is visualized on the screen, the transducer is moved

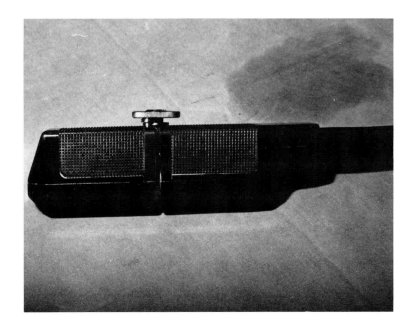

FIGURE 2.   Linear array puncture transducer.

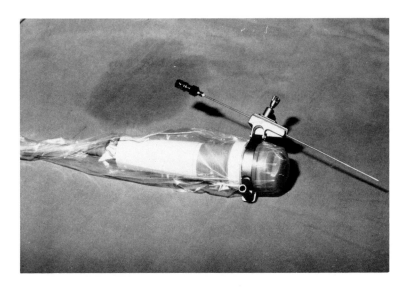

FIGURE 3.   Sector transducer with puncture adaptor. The transducer is placed in a sterile plastic bag.

away, keeping the needle in sight. The optimal image of the needle is obtained when the angle of needle path and ultrasound beams (both should be always in the same plane) approaches 90° (Figure 7).

Our preference is not to use local anesthesia. There is no uniform recommendation upon that matter,[4] and it is hard to find relevant scientific data to support a recommendation one way or another. We do not use local anesthetics because it causes delay in the performance of the procedure. Furthermore, according to Rodeck and Nicolaides,[15] the injection into the

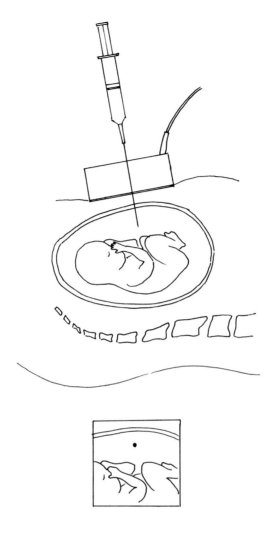

FIGURE 4.   Schematic drawing of the amniocentesis performed by means of linear array puncture transducer. Only needle tip is visualized due to unfavorable angle between the needle and ultrasound beams (practically 0°).

myometrium may result in a localized contraction, which can significantly alter the configuration of the uterus.

If the penetration of the placenta is necessary, it should be considered, once again, whether the benefit of the procedure outweighs the increased risk of spontaneous abortion in such cases.[27]

A recent study of Hanson et al.[28] has shown that amniocentesis can be safely performed even before 15 weeks of gestation. The samples contain fewer cells, but they seem to grow more vigorously. Although there is very limited experience with this technique, it deserves respect as a possible alternative to the chorion biopsy and second-trimester amniocentesis.

RISKS AND COMPLICATIONS

Properly performed, amniocentesis is a simple test, and the incidence of associated hazards is relatively low. The main hazard to the fetus is that of abortion, but fetal loss and morbidity later in pregnancy may also be a consequence. It appears simple to find out the complication rate of the procedure, but there are significant difficulties and biases. A patient

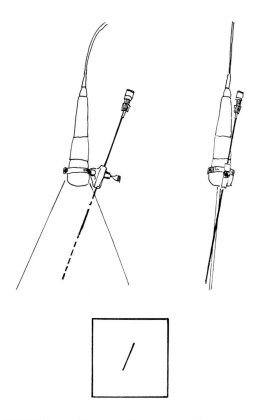

FIGURE 5.   Artifact caused by unpurposeful cross-sectioning of the needle and ultrasound beams. Middle part of the needle is visualized, which can be easily interpreted as the needle tip.

having the indication for the amniocentesis already carries an increased risk for complications, even before it is performed.[29]

Maternal complications such as infection, hemorrhage, and premature rupture of membranes are extremely rare and more a theoretical than a practical problem.[9] Rh isoimmunization could be a problem, especially if placenta is perforated or blood-stained fluid is obtained. Our policy is to give anti-D immunoglobulin only in these two cases, not to all nonsensitized Rhesus-negative women.

Only a few studies have been published which include a comparison group and are large enough to detect adverse fetal outcome possibly due to midtrimester amniocentesis.[25,30,31] A British collaborative study found an increase in the number of abortions following amniocentesis.[31] However, the control was inappropriate because it was selected late in gestation, when some potentially acceptable controls might have already aborted.

Fetal injuries and hemorrhage are not common complications. Recent reports have shown that the procedure does not appear to influence developmental and physical status.[32] Occasionally, needle marks can be seen after delivery.[32,33]

We have recently evaluated 300 ultrasonically monitored amniocenteses performed in our institution; 95% of the children were born alive, 2.66% of pregnancies were terminated, 0.66% were stillborn, and 5 (1.66%) women had a spontaneous abortion. Only one of them was thought to be the direct and only consequence of the procedure.[72]

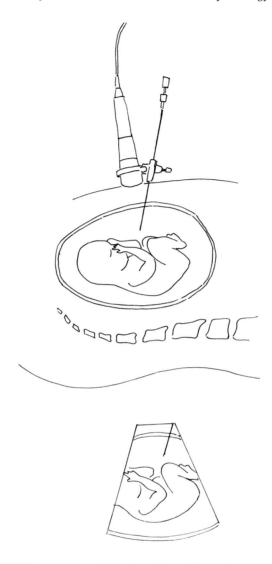

FIGURE 6.   Schematic drawing of the amniocentesis performed with the sector scanner with puncture transducer. Angle between needle and ultrasound beams of approximately 30° allows good visualization of the needle.

LATE AMNIOCENTESIS

The second-trimester "early" amniocentesis and third-trimester "late" amniocentesis are actually the same procedures. Only the indications are different. For the last amniocentesis, the two most frequent ones are Rh incompatibility and estimation of fetal lung maturity.

From the midcentury, the assessment and management of the condition have been based on the spectrophotometry and optical density difference recorded at 450 nm.[34,35] The procedure should be carefully performed because blood-stained taps make analysis inaccurate.

There are several tests for the assessment of fetal lung maturity.[36-38] For all of them, amniotic fluid obtained by means of amniocentesis is needed. The use of these procedures, once very popular, steady decreases with the increasing use of ultrasound and the accurate assessment of gestational age for the majority of the pregnant population. Even maternal diabetes mellitus, which has been a well-established indication for the maturity studies, is no longer an indication for late amniocentesis.

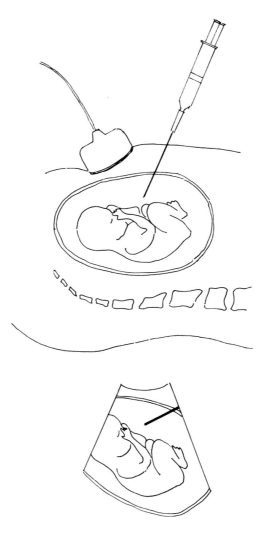

FIGURE 7.   Free-hand technique with the semiconvex scanner allows
optimal visualization of the whole procedure.

In the cases of significant polyhydramnios, the possibility of pain and dyspnoea relief by means of amniocentesis should always be considered.

The risk of spontaneous labor as a consequence of late amniocentesis is related to the proximity to term and increases from less than 1% in the middle of the third trimester to 10% after 38 weeks.[39] The reported rate of rupture of the membranes within 24 h is 3%, of blood taps 5%, and of fetal injury 1%.[40,41] It should be stressed that improvements in image quality and simultaneous ultrasonic monitoring of the procedure have reduced these figures.

CHORIONIC VILLUS SAMPLING

Starting in China in the 1970s, chorionic villus sampling (CVS) has spread worldwide in the past 6 years. At least 10,000 samples have been obtained early in pregnancy, and 3500 of the mothers have now delivered. Although CVS is widely practiced, only three centers (two in the U.S., one in Italy) have accomplished more than 700 antenatal diagnoses. Clinical experience has been insufficient to define the risks to fetus and mother that may be associated with CVS, and techniques are still being developed.

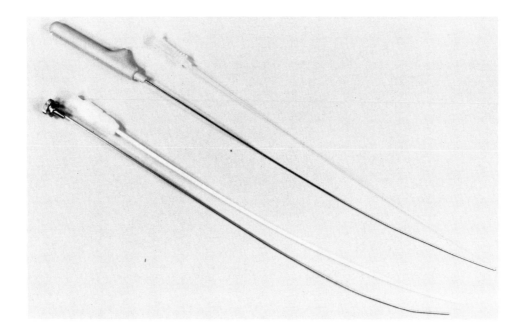

FIGURE 8.   Plastic catheter used for transcervical chorion biopsy.

The main disadvantages of this alternative (amniocentesis) are that, first, amniocentesis has to be carried out comparatively late in pregnancy (after 16 weeks, with the result not usually available before 20 weeks). This means that any necessary termination of pregnancy is more difficult and more upsetting for both the patient and her family, and for the medical and nursing staff. Second, only a few cells are obtained in amniotic fluid samples, and the laboratory testing can be done only after these cells have been grown and multiplied. This takes days, and if adequate growth is not obtained, it may be too late to repeat the procedure.

The separation of fetal lymphocytes[42] or deposited trophoblast[43] from maternal blood has limitations: (1) large volumes of maternal blood are required, (2) very few fetal cells are obtained after sorting, (3) there is a need for special genetic markers to be present, and (4) there is a very long survival of trophoblast in maternal circulation. It can survive for as long as 2 to 4 years.

Therefore, the technique which shows the greatest promise is that of chorionic villus sampling (CVS). The first published series on CVS came from China in 1975.[44] A metal cannula was inserted into the chorion, without ultrasound guidance, to obtain a sample of villi for fetal sexing. In their series of 100 patients, a sample was obtained in 99, with 4 fetal losses and 6 diagnostic errors.

Various techniques using ultrasound guidance have been developed since that time, involving either the transcervical or the transabdominal approach. The most popular method is the passage of a malleable catheter through the cervix into the chorion frondosum to aspirate a small sample of chorionic villi at 8 to 11 weeks of gestation (Figures 8 and 9). In addition to the use of expert ultrasound during the procedure, the success rate can be increased by microscopic examination of the sample to identify where sufficient villi have been obtained for diagnosis, so that if it is necessary, immediate repeat sampling can be performed. Although 10 mg of tissue is usually sufficient for cytogenetic analysis, more may be required for the diagnosis of biochemical disorders.

Once obtained, the sample is microscopically cleaned of decidua and blood to prevent contamination by maternal tissue. Cytogenetic examination can then be carried out by direct

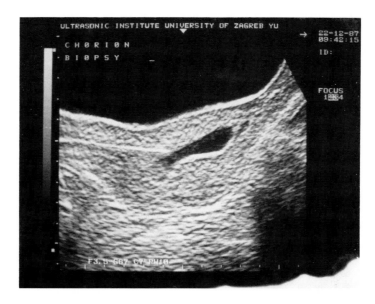

FIGURE 9.   Longitudinal ultrasound section of the uterus with the clearly visible inserted chorion biopsy catheter.

preparation technique which may yield results in a few hours, but which has the disadvantage of poor chromosomal spreads and banding. This difficulty may lead to inaccuracy in the diagnosis of small chromosomal rearrangements. The villi may also be cultured and better banding obtained, although contamination or overgrowth of maternal cells may occur. With increased laboratory experience and the development of new techniques, these difficulties should be overcome.

A further great potential advantage of CVS is that in addition to allowing chromosomal analysis, direct studies of DNA can be performed. DNA may be isolated from the tissue and analyzed for genetic defects using the technique of gene probes. This type of analysis is already in use in hemoglobinopathies, where the precise defects in the DNA are understood. It is hoped that soon there will be methods which allow detection of the gene defect in cases of X-linked conditions such as Duchenne muscular dystrophy and X-linked retinitis pigmentosa.

Various inborn errors of metabolism can also be diagnosed prenatally, although there are dangers in the use of uncultured cells because of the wide scatter values for the normal range, and for cultured cells because of the maternal cell contamination and occasional unusual cell types. Some conditions may now be amenable to more than one method of diagnosis, e.g., biochemically and with DNA probes.

Risks of CVS to the fetus are difficult to assess. To date, well over 4000 diagnostic procedures have been performed in the world,[45] with an overall loss rate of 4.1%, although in centers where at least 300 patients have been tested, the spontaneous abortion rate is only 2%.[46] The figure of 4.1% loss includes those centers with limited experience. The spontaneous abortion rate for ultrasonically viable pregnancies after 8 weeks of gestation is around 2%, suggesting a possible increased risk of CVS of 2%.[47] A paper by Jahoda et al.[48] has, in fact, suggested that overall, abortion rates for patients having CVS and amniocentesis are very similar.

The risks related to CVS must be clearly identified before it can be hailed as a successor to amniocentesis. Lippeman and co-workers[49] have shown that the abortion risk is the factor which influences most women in their choice between CVS or amniocentesis.

The best technique for CVS is not yet agreed upon. Most samples are at present obtained transcervically, and only 3% by the abdominal route. It seems likely, however, that a place will be found for each of these since some placentas are accessible to one, but not the other approach. The risks of either are not known. Transcervical CVS has a 1 to 3 per 1000 risk of producing severe maternal infection, which is possibly preventable, but more information is required about the organisms responsible and maternal risk factors. More frequent is abortion following CVS. With sampling at 9 to 11 weeks, this happens less often than before or after; the chance of it happening is increased if more than two samples are taken. The risk of spontaneous abortion increases with maternal age, so this is an important variable in assessing the risk of a procedure that may be indicated by the mother's age. There may be other unwanted effects during pregnancy or in the neonatal period, so randomized, controlled trials have been started in Canada, Denmark, and Finland to compare the known or suspected hazards of amniocentesis with those of CVS. A trial involving European and British centers has also started. Until the results of these are known, it will be difficult to counsel parents who contemplate antenatal diagnosis.

For a variety of reasons — medical, ethical, and economic — it is extremely important that new techniques are properly evaluated before they are accepted as routine services. Devoting resources to methods that are ineffective or unduly hazardous is not in the interests either of the patients concerned or of the community as a whole. This applies to CVS just as much as it does to other diagnostic methods or to new treatments.[50]

Any new method entering obstetric practice has public health implications. Amniocentesis, obstetric ultrasound, and periconceptional vitamin supplementation to avoid neural tube defects all entered regular practice without adequate initial evaluation, so that when legitimate queries are raised, especially about their possible long-term hazards, it is difficult to give satisfactory answers. The question is, will it be possible to avoid these difficulties in the case of CVS.[51]

The World Health Organization initiated an international effort at responsible evaluation at an early stage, pointing out that, "because of the high rate of spontaneous abortion in the first trimester of pregnancy, it could be difficult to define the obstetric risk unless large numbers are collected through international cooperation."[52] An informal WHO-sponsored International Registry was opened in 1983, and most CVS centers have filed information on case numbers, indications, fetal and neonatal losses, and diagnostic accuracy. By the end of 1984, 43 centers had reported over 3000 diagnostic cases. There was a 97% success rate in obtaining a satisfactory sample; about 10% of the pregnancies were terminated after diagnosis of an affected fetus; diagnosis had generally proved accurate (if maternal contamination was excluded); and 700 of the 2800 continuing pregnancies had already ended in the birth of a healthy child. The total fetal loss rate after CVS was 4.1%. This figure includes the early experience of all the groups: the average figure from the most experienced centers was 3.4%.

There are important questions to be answered before CVS becomes extensively used, possibly to replace amniocentesis.[53,54] What will be its impact on the number of abnormal children delivered? Should CVS be performed on a mother who has already threatened to abort, since the risk of abortion may well be increased by the procedure, but there is also an increased likelihood that the fetus is abnormal? How does the cost of CVS compare with that of amniocentesis? The answer to this is, in part, an exercise in accounting, but there is the incalculable factor of the number of couples who have avoided conception or antenatal diagnosis because they could not accept midtrimester termination, but who may find early diagnosis and termination acceptable. This has happened with thalassemia and may become more common as probes become available for cystic fibrosis and other diseases. Antenatal diagnosis from fetal cells in the maternal blood is still some distance away from clinical application.

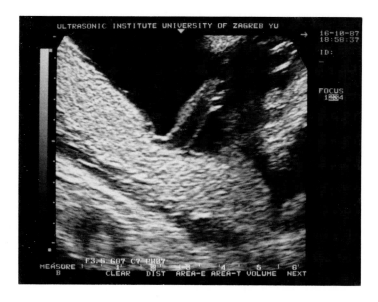

FIGURE 10. Placental insertion of the umbilical cord feasible for fetal blood sampling.

FETAL BLOOD SAMPLING

Fetal blood can be used for karyotyping, prenatal diagnosis of hemoglobinopathies, hemophilia, immunodeficiencies, inborn errors of metabolism, fetal viral infections, etc.[1,2]

The first method of obtaining pure fetal blood samples was by fetoscopy.[55] Today, it can be obtained in the second trimester from chorionic plate, umbilical cord vessel, or heart by fetoscopy or ultrasound-guided needling, and from fetal scalp in the third trimester.[56,57]

Initial attempts of blood sampling by fetoscopy were aimed at the blood vessels of the chorionic plate.[55] The difficulties of sampling anterior placenta, contamination of samples by maternal blood, disadvantage of heavy sedation, and relatively high incidence of amniotic fluid leakage have been overcome by cordocentesis.[58-61]

TECHNIQUE

Since fetoscopy carries a 2 to 7.5% risk of fetal loss, even in the most experienced hands,[1,56] it has precluded fetal blood sampling, except in special situations. An effort to overcome the limitations of fetal blood sampling by fetoscopy was direct fetal blood sampling from the umbilical vein with the needle under continuous real-time ultrasound guidance, as reported by Daffos et al. in 1983.[59]

The samples can be obtained by direct puncture of the umbilical vein near cord insertion on the placenta, or of the free part which flotates in the amniotic fluid (Figures 10 and 11). In cases where the placenta is anterior, a needle is introduced transplacentally (Figure 12). When the placenta is posterior, the needle is introduced transamniotically.

The technique is the same as for amniocentesis *(vide supra)*. Originally, a 20-gauge needle had been used. We have modified the technique by using an 18-gauge guide needle and a 22-gauge puncture needle. If the placenta lies anteriorly, the guide needle is inserted to the chorionic plate without passing it. When the placenta is posterior, the guide needle is inserted close to the umbilical vein. In both cases, the vessel is punctured with a 22-gauge needle. The main advantages of this procedure are the significantly smaller puncture sites and, consequently, the decreased possibility of significant fetal blood loss. The puncture area of a 22-gauge needle is 0.5 mm^2, and 0.8 mm^2 for a 20-gauge needle.

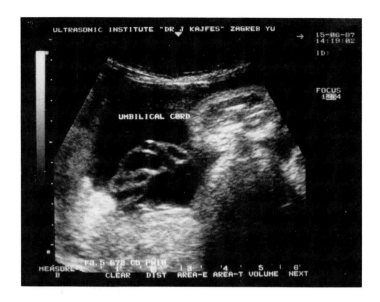

FIGURE 11.   Umbilical cord in the amniotic fluid. Zoomed image enables clear distinction of vein and arteries.

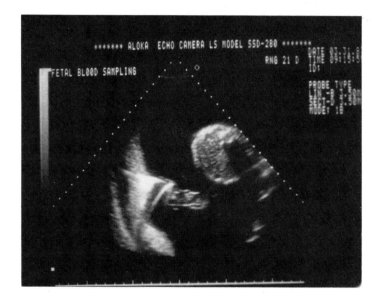

FIGURE 12.   Ultrasound monitoring of the transplacental fetal blood sampling.

The mother is given 10 mg of diazepam and 30 mg of pethidine 15 min before the procedure. Although the technique is often organized on the out-patient basis,[62] our patients are hospitalized for the time being.

In 1983, Bang[63] described a new method of fetal blood sampling from the fetal heart. Through the guide needle, a fine needle (0.6 mm outer diameter) is inserted into the lumen of the left ventricle and about 1 ml of pure fetal blood is aspirated. We have had much experience with the method,[57] but in spite of good preliminary results, cordocentesis, a much easier method for fetal blood sampling, has been adopted.

There have been several quite encouraging reports in which obtained fetal blood was used for assessment of fetal blood gases and acid-base status.[60,64,65] A significant correlation was found between the severity of fetal hypoxia and the degree of hypercapnia, acidosis, hyperlacticemia, hypoglycemia, and erythroblastosis. The hypoxic group of growth-retarded fetuses are those most at risk for intrauterine death or birth asphyxia. The most important fact is that traditional noninvasive methods for fetal monitoring, such as cardiotocography and ultrasound, usually fail to differentiate the subgroup of jeopardized fetuses from growth-retarded fetuses in good condition with normal P_{O_2} values. However, it seems that there is an excellent correlation between fetal acid-base status and Doppler blood flow studies.[66,67] If corroborative results would be obtained in larger, multicentric trial, noninvasive Doppler blood flow studies would be the method of choice for this purpose.

FETAL SKIN BIOPSY

Fetal skin may be used for the antenatal diagnosis of severe congenital disorders such as epidermolysis bullosa, ichthyosis congenita, epidermolytic hyperkeratosis, Ehlers-Danlos syndrome, oculocutaneous albinism, Sjoegren Larsson syndrome, etc. Fetal skin can be obtained at fetoscopy,[56,58,68,69] or by means of a biopsy instrument introduced transabdominally under continuous real-time ultrasonic guidance.[57,63]

We are using a Tru-cut needle which is introduced through the puncture transducer into the amniotic cavity (Figure 13A and B). The needle is opened and guided to the skin surface of the gluteal region (Figure 14). When the needle is closed, while pressed against the skin, biopsy is performed (Figure 15). The obtained skin specimen is stored in formaldehyde for light microscopy and in glutaraldehyde for electron microscope examination.

We have performed five ultrasonically guided skin biopsies using this technique. In all of them, the biopsy specimen was obtained and analysis performed. There were three pathological findings (epidermolysis bullosa). In two cases, fetal skin was normal, without cleavage in dermo-epidermal junction.[70]

FETAL TISSUE BIOPSY

Apart from amniotic fluid, blood, and skin, there are several other fetal tissues which can be obtained with an ultrasound-guided method and analyzed.

Some rare enzyme deficiencies can be diagnosed prenatally using fetal liver.[71] The prenatal diagnosis of type 3 cystic adenomatoid malformation has been reported.[56]

CONCLUSION

From all of these reports it is obvious that biopsy of any fetal organ or structure within gravid uterus can be performed easily. Continuous ultrasound monitoring of the biopsy procedure enables safe and precise placement of the instrument. The only potential problem of the ultrasonically guided procedure could be overestimation of their benefit. Therefore, the indications and cost effectiveness should be permanently evaluated.

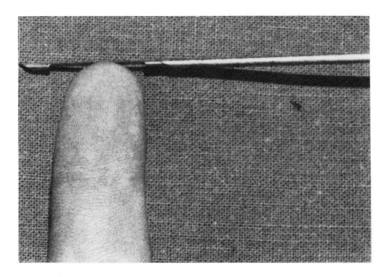

A

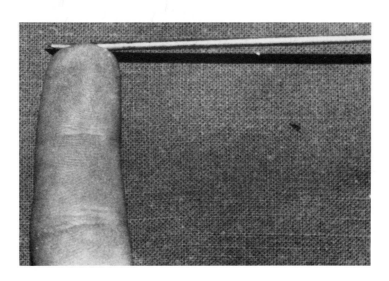

B

FIGURE 13.   Tru-cut needle for skin biopsy in the (A) open position and (B) closed position.

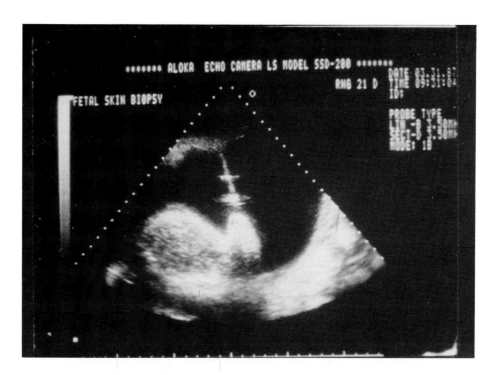

FIGURE 14. Open Tru-cut needle for skin biopsy inserted into the amniotic cavity.

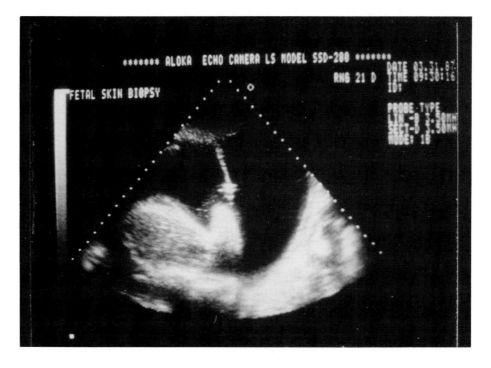

FIGURE 15. The skin biopsy has been performed. Tru-cut is closed and skin specimen obtained.

REFERENCES

1. **Harrison, M. R., Golbus, M. S., and Filly, R. A.**, *The Unborn Patient,* Grune & Stratton, New York, 1984, chap. 2.
2. **Rodeck, C. H.**, Obstetric techniques in prenatal diagnosis, in *Prenatal Diagnosis,* Proc. 11th Study Group of the RCOG, Rodeck, C. H. and Nicolaides, K. H., Eds., Royal College of Obstetrics and Gynecology, London, 1984, 15.
3. **Golbus, M. S.**, The role of ultrasound in prenatal diagnostic procedures, in *Ultrasonography in Obstetrics and Gynecology,* Callen, P. W., Ed., W. B. Saunders, Philadelphia, 1984, 169.
4. **Platt, L. D., Hill, L. M., and DeVore, G. R.**, Amniocentesis: current concepts and techniques, in *Principle and Practice of Ultrasonography in Obstetrics and Gynecology,* Sanders, R. C. and James, A. E., Eds., Appelton-Century-Crofts, New York, 1985, 375.
5. **Emery, A. E. H.**, Antenatal diagnosis of genetic disease, *Mod. Trends Hum. Genet.,* 1, 267, 1970.
6. **Gosden, M. C.**, Amniotic fluid cell types and culture, *Br. Med. Bull.,* 39, 248, 1983.
7. **Milunsky, A., Ed.**, *Genetic Disorders and the Fetus,* Plenum Press, New York, 1979, 322.
8. **Abramovich, D. R.**, Fetal factors influencing the volume and composition of liquor amnii, *J. Obstet. Gynaecol. Br. Commonw.,* 77, 865, 1970.
9. **Ritchie, J. W. K. and Thompson, W.**, A critical review of amniocentesis in clinical practice, in *Recent Advances in Obstetrics and Gynaecology,* Vol. 14, Bonnar, J., Ed., Churchill Livingstone, Edinburgh, 1982, 47.
10. **Simpson, J. L., Golbus, M. S., Martin, A. O., and Sarto, G. E.**, Genetics in obstetrics and gynecology, Grune & Stratton, New York, 1983, 1.
11. **Nadler, H. L.**, Indications for amniocentesis in the early prenatal detection of genetic disorders, *Birth Defects Orig. Artic. Ser.,* 7, 5, 1971.
12. **Patrick, A. D.**, Prenatal diagnosis of inherited metabolic diseases, in *Prenatal Diagnosis,* Proc. 11th Study Group of the RCOG, Rodeck, C. H. and Nicolaides, K. H., Eds., Royal College of Obstetrics and Gynecology, London, 1984, 121.
13. **Lemire, R. J., Leoser, J. D., and Leach, R. W.**, *Normal and Abnormal Development of the Human Nervous System,* Harper & Row, New York, 1975, 1.
14. **Hoffmann, G., Wellstein, R., Merz, E., Manz, B., Kreienberg, R., and Pollow, K.**, Relevance of biochemical parameters in the prenatal diagnosis of dysraphic malformations, in *Spina Bifida — Neural Tube Defects,* Voth, D. and Glees, P., Eds., Walter de Gruyter, Berlin, 1986, 131.
15. **Rodeck, C. H. and Nicolaides, K. H.**, Ultrasound guided invasive procedures in obstetrics, *Clin. Obstet. Gynecol.,* 10, 515, 1983.
16. **Hanson, F. W., Tennant, F. R., Zorn, E. M., and Samuels, S.**, Analysis of 2136 genetic amniocentesis: experience of a single physician, *Am. J. Obstet. Gynecol.,* 152, 436, 1985.
17. **Levine, S. C., Filly, R. A., and Golbus, M. S.**, Ultrasonography for guidance of amniocentesis in counselling, *Clin. Gen.,* 14, 133, 1977.
18. **Karp, L. E., Rothwell, R., and Conrad, S. H.**, Ultrasonic placental localization and blood taps in mid-trimester amniocentesis for prenatal genetic diagnosis, *Obstet. Gynecol.,* 50, 589, 1977.
19. **Golbus, M. S., Loughman, W. D., and Epstein, C. J.**, Prenatal genetic diagnosis in 3000 amniocentesis, *N. Engl. J. Med.,* 300, 157, 1979.
20. **Chandra, P., Nitowsky, H. M., and Marion, R.**, Experience with sonography as an adjunct to amniocentesis for prenatal diagnosis of fetal genetic disorders, *Am. J. Obstet. Gynecol.,* 133, 519, 1979.
21. **Crandon, A. J. and Peel, K. R.**, Amniocentesis with and without ultrasound guidance, *Br. J. Obstet. Gynecol.,* 86, 1, 1979.
22. **Benacerraf, B. R. and Frigoletto, F. D.**, Amniocentesis under continuous ultrasound guidance: a series of 232 cases, *Obstet. Gynecol.,* 65, 426, 1985.
23. **Defoort, P. and Thiery, M.**, Amniocentesis with the use of continuous real-time echography: experience with two hundred consecutive cases, *Am. J. Obstet. Gynecol.,* 147, 973, 1983.
24. **Kerenyi, T. D. and Walker, B.**, The preventability of "bloody taps" in second-trimester amniocentesis by ultrasound scanning, *Obstet. Gynecol.,* 50, 61, 1977.
25. **Canadian Medical Research Council**, Diagnosis of Genetic Disease by Amniocentesis during the Second Trimester of Pregnancy. A Canadian Study, Rep. No. 5, Supply Service, Canada, 1977.
26. **Jeanty, P., Rodesch, F., Romero, R., Venus, I., and Hobbins, J. C.**, How to improve your amniocentesis technique, *Am. J. Obstet. Gynecol.,* 146, 593, 1983.
27. **Kappel, B., Nielsen, J., Brogaard Hansen, K., Mikkelsen, M., and Therkelsen, A. A. J.**, Spontaneous abortion following mid-trimester amniocentesis. Clinical significance of placental perforation and blood-stained amniotic fluid, *Br. J. Obstet. Gynecol.,* 94, 50, 1987.
28. **Hanson, F. W., Zorn, E. M., Tennant, F. R., Marinos, S., and Samuels, S.**, Amniocentesis before 15 weeks' gestation: outcome, risks and technical problems, *Am. J. Obstet. Gynecol.,* 156, 1524, 1987.

29. **Turnbull, A. C. and MacKenzie, I. Z.**, Second-trimester amniocentesis and termination of pregnancy, *Br. Med. Bull.*, 39, 315, 1983.
30. **NICHD National Registry for Amniocentesis Study Group,** Midtrimester amniocentesis for prenatal diagnosis: safety and accuracy, *JAMA*, 236, 1471, 1976.
31. **Medical Research Committee,** Report on an assessment of the hazards of amniocentesis, *Br. J. Obstet. Gynecol.*, 85, 1, 1978.
32. **Finegan, J. K., Quarrington, B. J., Hughes, H. E., Rudd, N. L., Stevens, L. J., Weksberg, R., and Doran, T. A.,** Infant outcome following mid-trimester amniocentesis: development and physical status at age six months, *Br. J. Obstet. Gynecol.*, 92, 1015, 1985.
33. **Epley, S. L., Hanson, J. W., and Cruikshank, D. P.,** Fetal injury with midtrimester diagnostic amniocentesis, *Am. J. Obstet. Gynecol.*, 53, 77, 1979.
34. **Bevis, D. C. A.,** The composition of liquor amnii in haemolytic disease of the newborn, *J. Obstet. Gynaecol. Br. Emp.*, 60, 244, 1953.
35. **Liley, A. W.,** Liquor amnii analysis in management of pregnancy complicated by Rhesus sensitization, *Am. J. Obstet. Gynecol.*, 82, 1359, 1961.
36. **Clements, J. A., Platzker, A. C., Tierney, D. F., Hobel, C. J., Creasy, R. K., and Margolis, A. J.,** Assessment of the risk of the respiratory distress syndrome by a rapid test for surfactant in amniotic fluid, *N. Engl. J. Med.*, 286, 1077, 1972.
37. **Gluck, L. and Kulovich, M. V.,** Lecithin/sphingomyelin ratios in amniotic fluid in normal and abnormal pregnancy, *Am. J. Obstet. Gynecol.*, 115, 639, 1973.
38. **Whitfield, C. R.,** Prediction of fetal pulmonary maturity clinical application, in *Amniotic Fluid — Research and Clinical Application*, Fairweather, D. V. I. and Eskes, T. K. A. B., Eds., Excerpta Medica, Amsterdam, 1978, 393.
39. **Pedersen, J. F.,** Amniocentesis, late pregnancy, in *Interventional Ultrasound*, Holm, H. H. and Kristensen, J. K., Munsksgaard, Copenhagen, 1985, 129.
40. **Picker, R. H., Smith, D. H., Saunders, D. M., and Pennigton, J. C.,** A review of 2003 consecutive amniocentesis performed under ultrasonic control in late pregnancy, *Aust. N.Z. J. Obstet. Gynaecol.*, 19, 83, 1979.
41. **Galle, P. C. and Meis, P. J.,** Complications of amniocentesis, a review, *J. Reprod. Med.*, 27, 149, 1982.
42. **Walnowska, J., Conte, C. A., and Grumbach, M. M.,** Practical and theoretical implications of fetal/maternal lymphocyte transfer, *Lancet*, i, 1119, 1969.
43. **Covone, A. E., Mutton, D., Johnston, P. M., and Adinolfi, M.,** Trophoblast cells in peripheral blood from pregnant women, *Lancet*, ii, 841, 1984.
44. **Department of Obstetrics and Gynecology, Tietung Hospital of Anshan, Iron & Steel Company, Anshan,** Fetal sex prediction by sex chromatin of chorionic villi cells during early pregnancy, *China Med. J.*, 2, 117, 1975.
45. **C.V.S. Newsletter, February 1985,** c/o Dr. Laird Jackson, Division of Medical Genetics, Jefferson Medical College, Philadelphia.
46. **Jackson, L. G. and Warner, R. J.,** Fetal loss after chorionic villus sampling (C.V.S.) in small and large centres, *Prenat. Diagn.*, 5, 167, 1985.
47. **Wilson, L. J., Kendrick, J., Wittman, B. K., and McGillivary, B. C.,** Risk of spontaneous abortion in ultrasonically normal pregnancies, *Lancet*, ii, 920, 1984.
48. **Jahoda, M. G. J., Vosters, R. P. C., Sachs, E. S., and Galjaard, H.,** Safety of chorionic villus sampling, *Lancet*, ii, 941, 1985.
49. **Lippeman, A., Perry, T. B., and Cartier, L.,** Chorionic villus sampling: patient attitude, *Am. J. Hum. Genet.*, 36, 135, 1984.
50. **Maxwell, D., Lilford, R., Czepulkowski, B., and Heaton, D.,** Transabdominal chorionic villus sampling, *Lancet*, i, 123, 1986.
51. **Modell, B.,** Chorionic villus sampling, *Lancet*, i, 737, 1985.
52. **WHO Working Group,** Fetal diagnosis of hereditary disease, *Bull. WHO*, 62, 345, 1984.
53. **Jackson, L. G.,** Prenatal genetic diagnosis by chorionic villus sampling, in *Perinatal Genetics: Diagnosis and Treatment*, Porfer, I. H., Hatcher, H. N., and Willey, A. M., Eds., Academic Press, Orlando, FL, 1986, 95.
54. **Brambati, B., Oldrini, A., and Lanzani, A.,** Transabdominal chorionic villus sampling: a freehand ultrasound-guided technique, *Am. J. Obstet. Gynecol.*, 157, 134, 1987.
55. **Hobbins, J. C., Mahoney, M. J.,** In utero diagnosis of hemoglobinopathies: technique for obtaining fetal blood, *N. Engl. J. Med.*, 290, 1065, 1974.
56. **Soothill, P. W., Nicolaides, K. H., and Rodeck, C. H.,** Invasive techniques for prenatal diagnosis and therapy, *J. Perinat. Med.*, 15, 117, 1987.
57. **Kurjak, A., Alfirevic, Z., and Jurkovic, D.,** Ultrasonically guided fetal tissue biopsy, *Acta Obstet. Gynecol. Scand.*, 66, 523, 1987.

58. **Rodeck, C. H. and Campbell, S.,** Umbilical cord insertion as a source of pure fetal blood for prenatal diagnosis, *Lancet,* 146, 985, 1983.
59. **Daffos, F., Cappella-Pavlosky, M., and Forestier, F.,** Fetal blood sampling via the umbilical cord using a needled guided by ultrasound. Report of 66 cases, *Prenat. Diagn.,* 2, 271, 1983.
60. **Nicolaides, K. H., Soothill, P. W., Rodeck, C. H., and Campbell, S.,** Ultrasound-guided sampling of umbilical cord and placental blood to assess fetal wellbeing, *Lancet,* i, 1065, 1986.
61. **Daffos, F., Cappella-Pavlosky, M., and Forestier, F.,** Fetal blood sampling during pregnancy with the use of a needle guided by ultrasound: a study of 606 consecutive cases, *Am. J. Obstet. Gynecol.,* 153, 655, 1985.
62. **Bradley, R. J. and Nicolaides, K. H.,** Ultrasound guided procedures in small for gestation fetuses, in *Intrauterine Growth Retardation — Diagnosis and Treatment,* Kurjak, A. and Beazley, J., Eds., CRC Press, Boca Raton, FL, 1988, in press.
63. **Bang, J.,** Ultrasound in needle diagnosis and treatment of fetal diseases, in *The Fetus as a Patient,* Kurjak, A., Ed., Excerpta Medica, Amsterdam, 1985, 272.
64. **Soothill, P. W., Nicolaides, K. H., Rodeck, C. H., and Campbell, S.,** The effect of gestational age on blood gas and acid-base values in human pregnancy, *Fetal Ther.,* 1, 166, 1986.
65. **Soothill, P. W., Nicolaides, K. H., and Campbell, S.,** Prenatal asphyxia, hyperlacticaemia, and erythroblastosis in growth retarded fetuses, *Br. Med. J.,* 294, 1051, 1987.
66. **Soothill, P. W., Nicolaides, K. H., Bilardo, C., Hackett, G., and Campbell, S.,** Uteroplacental blood velocity resistance index and umbilical venous pO_2, pCO_2, pH, lactate, and erythroblast count in growth retarded fetus, *Fetal Ther.,* 1, 174, 1986.
67. **Soothill, P. W., Nicolaides, K. H., Bilardo, C. M., and Campbell, S.,** Relation of fetal hypoxia in growth retardation to mean blood velocity in the fetal aorta, *Lancet,* i, 1065, 1986.
68. **Golbus, M. S., Sagebiel, R. W., and Filly, R. A.,** Prenatal diagnosis of congenital bullous ichthyosiform erythroderma (epidermolytic hyperkeratosis) by fetal skin biopsy, *N. Engl. J. Med.,* 302, 93, 1980.
69. **Elias, S., Mazur, M., and Sabbagha, R.,** The prenatal diagnosis of harlequin ichthyosis congenita, *Clin. Genet.,* 17, 275, 1980.
70. **Eady, R. A. and Rodeck, C. H.,** Prenatal diagnosis of disorders of the skin, in *Prenatal Diagnosis,* Proc. 11th Study Group of the RCOG, Rodeck, C. H. and Nicolaides, K. H., Eds., Royal College of Obstetrics and Gynecology, London, 1984, 147.
71. **Rodeck, C. H., Patrick, A. D., Pembrey, M. F., Tzannatos, C., and Whitfield, A. E.,** Fetal liver biopsy for prenatal diagnosis of ornithine carbamyl transferase deficiency, *Lancet,* ii, 297, 1982.
72. **Ermin, M.,** Unpublished data.

Chapter 3

FETAL THERAPY — APPROACHES AND PROBLEMS

Wolfgang Holzgreve and Wolfram Niedner

INTRODUCTION

Over the last 15 years, there have been substantial advances in the field of prenatal diagnosis through improved techniques of genetic analyses and, at the same time, the developments in high-resolution dynamic ultrasound imaging. Ever since real-time ultrasound was used for the first time in obstetrics in the late 1960s at the Westf. Wilhelms-University Muenster,[1] the image quality has progressed very fast, and the application of this noninvasive monitoring technique has expanded up to a point where, e.g., every pregnant woman in the Federal Republic of Germany now is offered two routine ultrasound screening examinations during the course of her pregnancy.[2]

The ultimate goal of prenatal medicine, however, is not the ability to diagnose severe and untreatable fetal disorders so that termination of pregnancy can be offered early in gestation, but the development of techniques for effective fetal treatment to prevent the manifestation of irreversible damage *in utero*.

The concept of the fetus as a patient was first introduced by the tremendous breakthrough in the prenatal treatment of Rhesus incompatibility through blood transfusions *in utero*.[3] Recently, there have been the first reports of successful surgery in the fetus,[4,5] which is a dramatic type of intervention requiring enormous preparation and proper selection of suitable cases. There has also been some progress in the nonsurgical treatment of fetal disorders, e.g., the pharmacologic suppression of the fetal adrenal gland by maternal replacement doses of dexamethasone following prenatal diagnosis of 21-hydroxylase deficiency.[6] Additionally, there are initial attempts to correct genetic diseases permanently by early transplantation of normal hematopoietic cells into a preimmune fetal recipient.[7,8]

This chapter attempts to summarize the current achievements up to the middle of 1988 in these areas, but also the problems which have been recognized during this time as well as some ethical and legal aspects of fetal therapy.

GENERAL CONSIDERATIONS FOR APPROACHING THE FETUS AS A PATIENT

The first prerequisite prior to fetal therapy is an accurate diagnosis of the congenital abnormalities of the fetus, which must be based on a clear understanding of the pathophysiology and natural history of the disorder.

It has been shown in a number of series over the last few years that the rate of chromosomal abnormalities is considerably high depending on the specific malformation in fetuses with congenital abnormalities. For example, in obstructive uropathies, the rate of chromosomal aneuploidies is 23%, in hydrocephalus 22%, and in exomphalos 67%;[9] in fetuses with cystic hygroma, this rate can be even higher.[10] Trisomies 13 and 18 are especially associated with characteristic fetal abnormalities which can be detected prenatally by ultrasound.[11]

Fortunately, there are techniques available now for rapid karyotyping, so that the decisions about the perinatal management or prenatal intervention don't have to wait for the results of lengthy amniotic fluid cultures any more. The so-called pipette method[12] and lymphocyte cultures from fetoscopically obtained fetal blood[13] allow karyotypes to be obtained in 3 to 5 d, and cytogenetic analyses can be performed even faster using the newly developed technique of placental biopsy and chorionic villi direct preparation.[14] This latter technique is especially feasible in cases of oligo- or polyhydramnios, where fetal blood sampling can be difficult.

Because often these associated anomalies determine the ultimately fatal outcome independently from *in utero* intervention for isolated fetal anomalies, they should be looked for very carefully before contemplating prenatal intervention.[15] Already in 1982,[16] it has been suggested by a panel of experts in the field of fetal treatment that when considering a particular case for *in utero* treatment, the fetus should be known to be a singleton with no associated anomalies based on an evaluation by level II ultrasound and amniocentesis for karyotype, α-fetoprotein (AFP) concentration, and viral cultures. The panel also demanded that the family has to be fully informed about the risks and benefits of the treatment proposed and should agree to all aspects of this therapy, including long-term follow-up.

Another prerequisite for fetal therapy is a multidisciplinary team which should include at least a specialized sonographer and obstetrician with good experience in prenatal interventions, a pediatric surgeon, a neonatologist, and the availability of appropriate bioethical and psychosocial counseling. *In utero* surgery should not be performed after a time in gestation when the fetus can be safely delivered and more definitive postnatal diagnosis and therapy is possible. Since fetal therapy is new and in many areas still very experimental, all cases should be carefully documented and openly discussed.

ALTERNATIVES TO FETAL SURGERY IN APPROACHING THE FETUS WITH CONGENITAL ANOMALIES

First, there are sonographically diagnosable conditions which at the present time cannot be corrected *in utero* and probably will not be approachable therapeutically within the foreseeable future. These include, for example, achondrogenesis, campomelia, thanatophoric dwarfism, bilateral renal agenesis, holoprosencephaly (Figure 1), or severe forms of cloacal malformation (Figure 2A and B). In these cases, termination of pregnancy can be offered to the parents if untreatable fetal malformations are diagnosed before the legal limit, e.g., in the Federal Republic of Germany, the 22nd week of gestation.

It was clearly shown by Modell et al.[17] that often only the availability of prenatal diagnosis encourages couples with a known recurrence risk to take a chance on further pregnancies after the birth of a baby with a genetic disease.

In cases of anencephaly which were missed by ultrasound screening and only diagnosed late in the third trimester, the only psychological relief that can be offered to the parents is to allow the organs of the anencephalic to be donated to patients waiting for transplantation.[18] Even though anencephalics can have residual brain stem activity after birth, the explantation of organs after cessation of spontaneous breathing, according to our opinion, does not seem to violate any interests of the anencephalics if it is done with proper safeguards, dignity, and upon request of the parents (Figure 3A and B).

In the case of many correctable fetal malformations, an early induction of delivery can be beneficial, for example, in some areas of obstructive hydronephrosis[19] with progressive oligohydramnios after the 32nd week of gestation (Figure 4A and B), in cases of sacrococcygeal teratomas[20] with secondary progressive consequences such as polyhydramnios and urinary obstruction (Figure 5), in congenital ileus with NIHF[21] due to midgut volvulus or meconium peritonitis (Figure 6), or in omphaloceles with progressive intestinal tract obstruction (Figure 7). In cases of progressive nonimmune hydrops fetalis with unknown etiology or due to twin-to-twin transfusion syndrome (Figure 8), sometimes early delivery can prevent *in utero* death from cardiac failure,[22] whereas ascites punctures are usually not successful because of rapid reaccumulation (Figure 9).

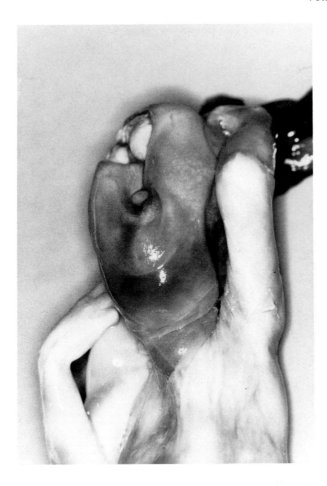

FIGURE 1. Holoprosencephaly. Lethal malformation which can be diagnosed easily by prenatal sonography.

Most prenatally diagnosable conditions, however, are best treated after a term delivery. In many instances, a delivery by Cesarean section (CS) is preferable, e.g., in fetal malformations which would cause dystocia, like a large teratoma of the neck, preventing the fetal head to flex in the birth canal (Figure 10), a giant sacrococcygeal teratoma type I (Figure 11), or a large omphalocele with liver content and a thin membrane (Figure 12A to C).

In many cases of prenatally diagnosed fetal malformations, not a CS, but only preparation for appropriate postnatal care is necessary, e.g., in uncomplicated omphaloceles, small meningomyeloceles or unilateral kidney dysplasias. In cases of duodenal atresia, which can be diagnosed sonographically from the presence of polyhydramnios and the double-bubble sign (Figure 13) as well as from the characteristic acetylcholinesterase without AFP increase in the amniotic fluid,[23] postnatal oral feeding should be avoided before proper evaluation and correction after normal delivery at term.

So far, there are only a few anatomic malformations in which *in utero* interventions could alleviate progressively damaging effects on fetal organ development: urinary tract obstruction, obstructive hydrocephalus, congenital diaphragmatic hernia, hydro/chylothorax, twin-to-twin transfusion syndrome, sacrococcygeal teratoma, and ovarian cysts.[24]

MEDICAL TREATMENT *IN UTERO*

Treatment of the fetus via maternal drug intake has been applied for many years, e.g.,

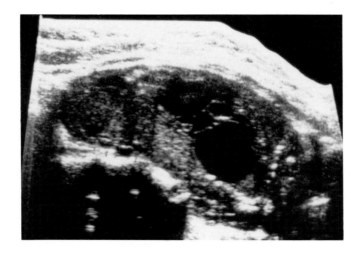

A

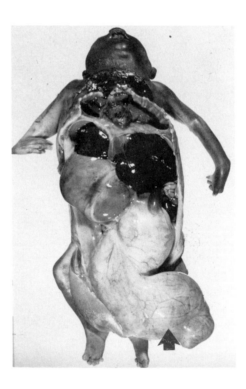

B

FIGURE 2.   Cloacal malformation in a fetus. (A) Prenatal sonogram showing characteristic cysts in the abdomen. (B) Fetus after termination of pregnancy. Open abdomen shows cloacal sac (arrow).

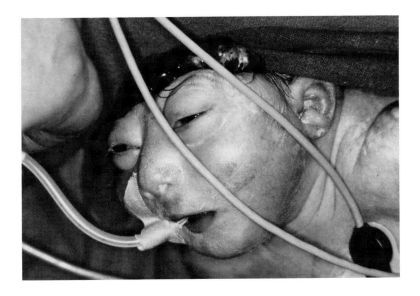

A

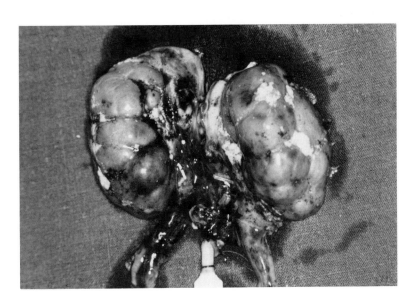

B

FIGURE 3.   Kidney transplantation from anencephalic donor in Muenster. (A) Anencephalic intubated immediately after cessation of spontaneous breathing. (B) Kidneys after en bloc explantation.

by giving glucocorticoids or thyroid hormone for acceleration of fetal lung maturation.[25] Combined pre- and postnatal phenobarbital application has been considered for prophylaxis of hyperbilirubinemia,[26] and even fluoride tablet supplementation during pregnancy for fetal caries immunity has been suggested.[27] Ampola et al.[28] reported the prenatal diagnosis and subsequent therapy of a fetus with a vitamin B_{12} responsive form of methylmalonic acidemia by high dose cyanocobalamin application to the mother. More recently, Rosenblatt et al.[29] used a similar approach with vitamin B_{12} therapy of a fetus with methylcobalamin deficiency

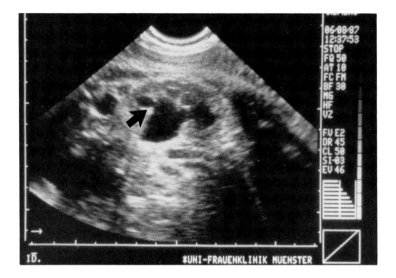

A

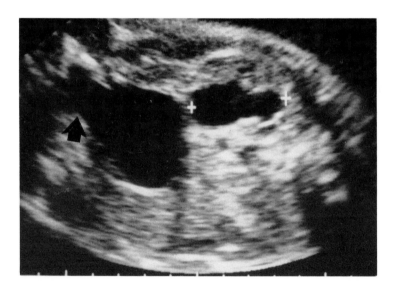

B

FIGURE 4.   Fetal hydronephrosis. (A) Mild degree of hydronephrosis with caliectasis
(arrow). (B) More progressed hydronephrosis next to a dilated bladder in a case with
urethral obstruction (arrow).

(cobalamin E disease). Packman et al.[30] gave high-dose biotin to the mother to treat a fetus
with prenatally diagnosed biotin-responsive multiple carboxylase deficiency. Even though
there was clinical and biochemical evidence of a therapeutic effect in these cases, it is
impossible to assess the benefits of this prenatal treatment unequivocally.[31]

Fetal endocrine disorders can be successfully approached by prenatal therapy, e.g.,
maternal dexamethasone administration after prenatal diagnosis of 21-hydroxylase deficiency
in a female fetus in order to prevent masculinization.[32] It has been suggested[33] that prenatal
treatment of hypothyroidism could be effective, but thyroid hormone has to be administered
intra-amniotically or into the umbilicus, because this hormone does not traverse the placenta.[34]

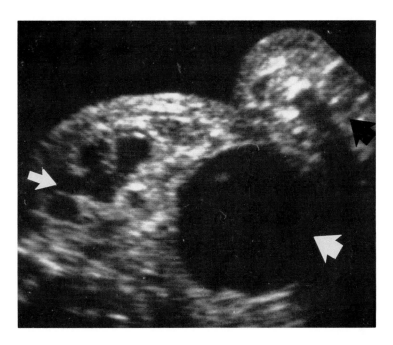

FIGURE 5.   Prenatal sonogram of a fetus with sacrococcygeal teratoma type I (black arrow) which has caused bladder dilatation (big white arrow) and hydronephrosis (small white arrow).

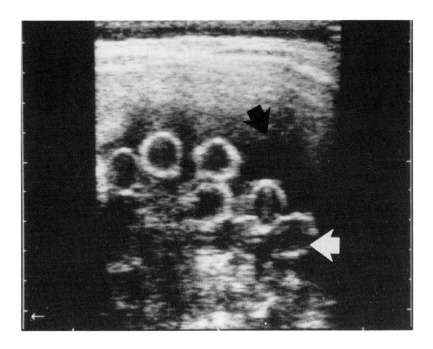

FIGURE 6.   Prenatal sonogram of a fetus with meconium peritonitis. The fluid-filled intestinal tract (white arrow) and the intra-abdominal ascites (black arrow) can be recognized.

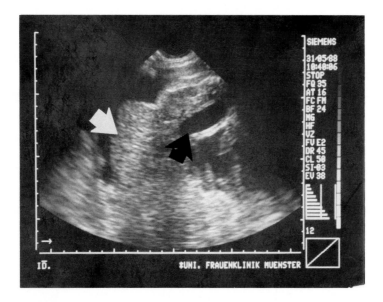

FIGURE 7.   Prenatal sonogram of fetal omphalocele (white arrow) with intestinal tract dilatation (black arrow).

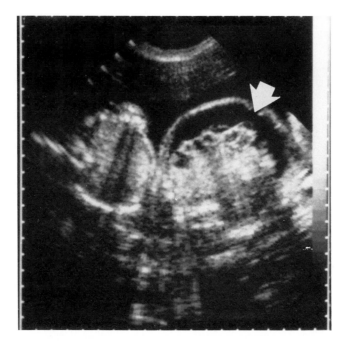

FIGURE 8.   Prenatal sonogram of twin-to-twin transfusion syndrome. Intra-abdominal ascites (white arrow) in the hydropic twin.

There have been numerous reports about attempts of prenatal cardioversion after sonographic diagnosis of fetal tachyarrhythmias by applying antiarrhythmic drugs such as digoxin, verapamil, propanolol, or quinidine to the mother.[35] It is very difficult, however, to monitor the drug levels without fetal blood sampling. Furthermore, endogenous digoxin-immunoreactive substances have been detected in the blood of pregnant women, amniotic

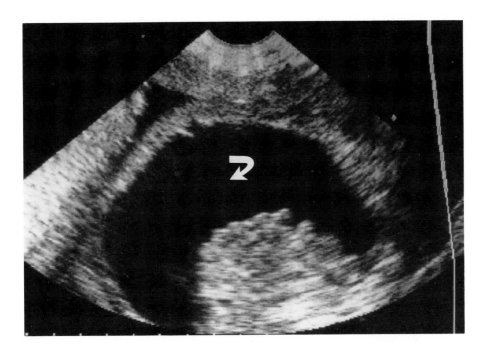

FIGURE 9. Fetal ascites 1 d after *in utero* drainage. Complete reaccumulation of the intra-abdominal fluid.

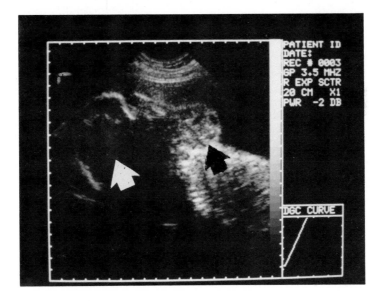

FIGURE 10. Sonogram of fetal neck teratoma. The tumor (black arrow) prevents flexion of the head (white arrow).

fluid, and cord blood, so that these baseline levels should be known before starting transplacental therapy.[36] In all cases of fetal cardiac tachyarrhythmias, congenital heart disease has to be excluded,[37] and the frequency of aneuploidy in prenatally diagnosed congenital heart disease is known to be in the range of 5 to 10%.[38]

The most successful and earliest attempt of intrauterine therapy is the treatment of severe

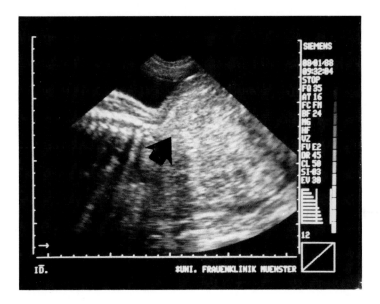

FIGURE 11.   Fetal sacrococcygeal teratoma type I (arrow) located at the caudal pole of the fetus.

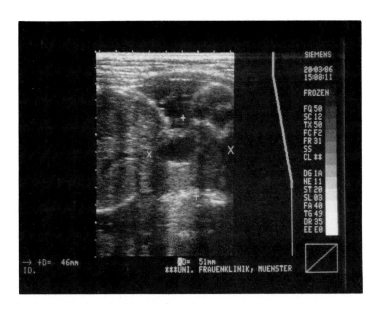

A

FIGURE 12.   Large fetal omphalocele. (A) Prenatal sonogram. Omphalocele is marked with the calliper. (B) Baby immediately after delivery at term. (C) Baby right after surgery where the defect was first closed with lyodura.

Rhesus incompatibility by intraperitoneal instillation of erythrocytes, as introduced by Liley.[3] Later, Rodeck et al. introduced intravascular blood transfusion by fetoscope,[39] and most recently, ultrasound-guided cordocentesis[40] for even *in utero* exchange transfusions.[41]

The ability to gain an early direct access to the fetal intravascular space by percutaneous cordocentesis offers not only potential for very specific diagnoses,[42] but also new modes of treatment besides treatment of erythroblastosis fetalis.

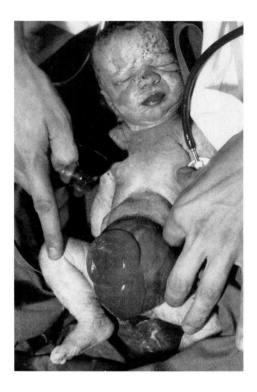

FIGURE 12B.

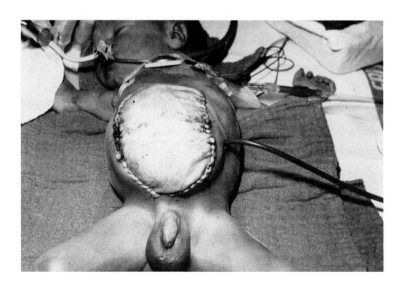

FIGURE 12C.

STRUCTURAL ANOMALIES OF THE FETUS POTENTIALLY AMENABLE TO TREATMENT *IN UTERO*

OBSTRUCTIVE HYDROCEPHALUS

Because congenital hydrocephalus is often associated with severe neurologic disability in surviving individuals, there has been considerable motivation not only to diagnose this

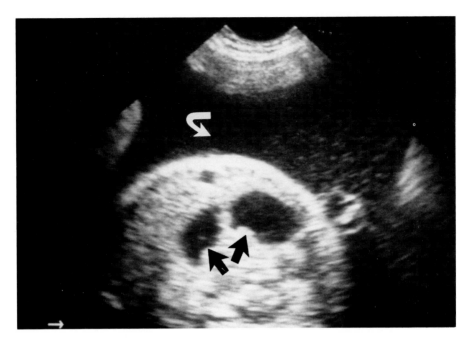

FIGURE 13. Prenatal sonogram of duodenal obstruction. Polyhydramnios (white arrow) and ''double-bubble'' sign (black arrows) caused by dilated stomach and proximal duodenum.

condition prenatally, but also to treat it before permanent damage has occured *in utero*.[43] The incidence of neonatal isolated hydrocephaly, without spina bifida, varies from 0.4 to 0.9 per 1000 births, about 30% of those diagnosed in children have a stenosis of the aqueduct of Sylvius.[44]

After the first reports of prenatal shunting of fetal hydrocephalus by serial percutaneous cephalocentesis,[45] a permanent ventriculoamniotic shunt (Figure 14) was introduced by Clewell et al.[5]

Fetal ventriculomegaly (Figure 15) can be clearly diagnosed with current high-resolution ultrasound and differentiated from lethal conditions such as hydranencephaly and holoprosencephaly (Figure 1). The natural history of fetal ventriculomegaly, however, was not very well studied until recently, and an enormous heterogeneity and high rate of associated anomalies has been documented in a number of recent studies.[46-48]

According to the report of the International Fetal Surgery Registry in July 1986,[15] 41 fetuses with hydrocephalus were treated by surgical decompression *in utero* up to that time. Of the treated fetuses, 17% died, which means a procedure-related mortality of 10%. In the group of patients with aqueduct stenosis, 50% had severe handicaps, and only 35% were assessed as normal at the time of reporting. Because there has not been any evidence of improved outcome in the prenatally treated cases with hydrocephaly so far, this type of fetal treatment has to be considered as highly experimental and probably not beneficial.[49] A key problem lies in the fact that we currently lack proper selection criteria for cases which might benefit from prenatal shunting. Large porencephalic cysts (Figure 16A and B), for instance, may be associated with normal neurologic status, whereas only mild and even ''normal pressure hydrocephalus'' can lead to severe dementia and moving disorders.[50]

Michejda et al.[51] attempted to treat hydrocephalus in rhesus monkeys through insertion of ventriculo-amniotic shunts into the fetal lateral ventricles via open uterotomy, but these authors also conclude from their studies that ''new shunting materials and better imaging technology will be necessary before intrauterine treatment can be objectively assessed and become standard, accepted medical practice.''[52]

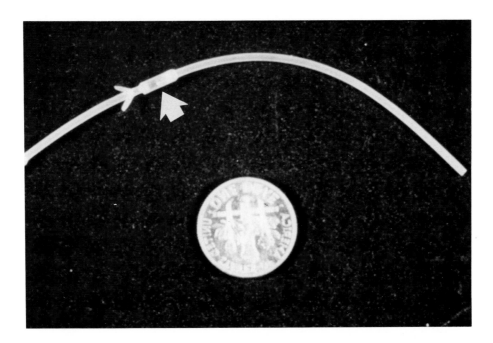

FIGURE 14. Ventriculo-amniotic ''Denver'' shunt for intrauterine drainage of hydrocephalus. One-way valve is marked by arrow.

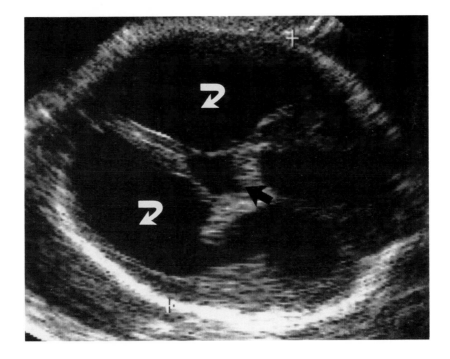

FIGURE 15. Fetal hydrocephalus. Increased biparietal diameter (marked by calliper), dilated lateral (white arrows) and third (black arrow) ventricles.

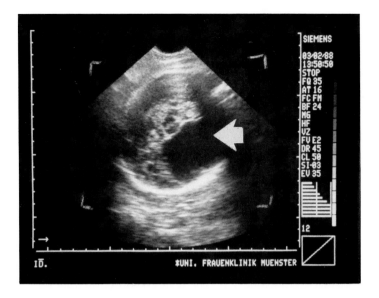

A

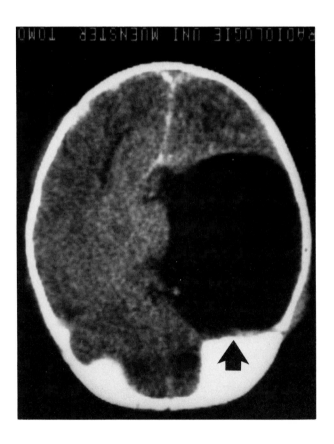

B

FIGURE 16.   Fetal porencephalic cyst (arrows). (A) Prenatal sonogram. (B) CAT scan after delivery of the neurologically normal baby.

OBSTRUCTIVE UROPATHIES

Fetal urinary tract obstructions with megacystis, megaureters, and/or hydronephrosis can be easily recognized prenatally by ultrasound.[53] The characteristic keyhole image of the fetal bladder appears on ultrasound in cases of urethral obstruction (Figure 17A to C). Diagnostic problems can occur in differentiating among multicystic dysplastic kidneys and ureteropelvic junction obstruction (Figure 18A) and dilatation due to reflux (Figure 18B) or obstruction.[54]

Ever since the first successful application of a fetal vesico-amniotic shunt in a case of fetal urethral obstruction (Figure 19A and B) was reported by Golbus et al.,[55] this type of "fetal surgery" became an area of great interest in the medical and lay population.[56] This procedure can be considered if the pregnancy is before 32 weeks of gestation, if sonographic evaluation has documented that a bilateral obstruction is not transient and that the quantity of amniotic fluid is decreasing critically.[4]

Unfortunately, sonography alone cannot determine whether severe fetal renal dysplasia is present, which would indicate that this particular fetus could not benefit from a drainage procedure, and, therefore, other criteria are required to select appropriate candidates for *in utero* therapy.[57] In a retrospective study of 20 cases, Glick et al.[58] found that fetal urinary sodium levels above 100 mmol/l, chloride above 90 mmol/l, and osmolarity above 210 mOsm were associated with insufficient tubular reabsorption capacity and, hence, irreversibly damaged renal function at birth. Lenz et al.[59] showed that concentrations of neutral aminoacids in the fetal urine similar to plasma values are also predictive of irreversibly destroyed kidneys because they reflect poor tubular capacity.

In our program, we have investigated 13 out of 112 pregnancies with fetal urinary tract obstruction using these reported biochemical parameters. In all but three cases, this urinalysis profile was able to predict correctly the renal function at birth. We therefore looked for additional prenatal kidney markers and investigated the usefulness of protein analysis as one of the currently most sensitive renal function tests applied in many nephrology and transplantation services. In the postnatal as well as the prenatal period, proteinuria in the course of renal disease is caused either by a pathologic process in the glomeruli and/or by a damage of the tubular reabsorption capacity. Because this pathogenetic difference is expressed by the molecular weight of urinary proteins,[60] the site and degree of underlying lesions in kidneys with pathologic proteinuria can be identified by separating urinary proteins on polyacrylamide gel electrophoresis with sodium dodecyl sulfate as detergent (SDS-PAGE).

We recently experienced a successful case of shunting in which bladder electrolytes and osmolarity were compatible with irreversible renal damage, but the addition of protein analysis by SDS-PAGE was more predictive of the ultimate good outcome. The patient was referred at 18 weeks with anhydramnios, fetal bilateral equally pronounced hydronephrosis/hydroureters, a large megacystis filling almost the whole abdominal cavity, and a dilated proximal urethra (Figure 20A). There were no other abnormalities, and the karyotype was 46, XY. The second biochemical test after spontaneous refilling of the fetal bladder following the first ultrasound-guided needling of the megacystis revealed a sodium level of 99.8 mmol/l, chloride of 94 mmol/l, osmolarity of 262 mOsm, and amino acid analysis, e.g., methionine 20.1 μmol/l and leucine 68.6 μmol/l, which was highly suggestive of already irreversible renal dysplasia. However, the protein content of the fetal urine was 4.0 mg/ml, and SDS-PAGE revealed only mild damage of the glomeruli as well as of the tubular reabsorption capacity. After extensive counseling and communication of the uncertainties about the conflicting biochemical results in the different fetal urinalysis parameters, the parents requested that everything possible should be done to allow for fetal pulmonary development and, hopefully, also recovery of the renal function. Therefore, at 19 weeks of gestation, a double reversed vesico-amniotic pigtail stent (Angiomed, Karlsruhe, Federal Republic of Germany) was placed under ultrasound guidance, which drained the bladder immediately and led to a fast reaccumulation of liquor (Figure 20B to E). The left hydro-

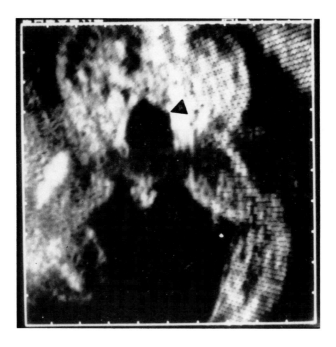

A

FIGURE 17.   Fetal obstructive uropathies. (A) Sonogram of normal bladder (arrow) in a male fetus. (B) "Key hole" bladder (arrow) in a male
fetus with urethral obstruction (arrow). Residual amount of amniotic fluid
(oligohydramnios). (C) "Key hole" bladder due to urethral obstruction.
No amniotic fluid left (ahydramnios).

nephrosis gradually disappeared, while the right hydronephrosis/hydroureter persisted to
some mild degree (Figure 20F). Repeat fetal bladder sampling at 29 weeks revealed a sodium
level of 51 mmol/l, chloride of 46 mmol/l, osmolarity of 259 mOsm, and only trace concentrations of most amino acids. Normal fetal amounts of amniotic fluid, fetal growth, and
intrauterine behavior were observed. At 36 weeks, a CS was performed because of fetal
distress during spontaneous onset of labor and a 2820-g boy was delivered who did not
require ventilation or supplementary oxygen except for a transient respiratory acidosis
(P_{CO_2} 40.5) after birth. Nephrologic investigations including transurethral cystoscopy and
radiologic exams revealed a narrow portion of the urethra at the level between pars prostatica
and membranacea, undescended testes, mildly dilated ureters, and some degree of hydronephrosis with 20% function of the right kidney and 80% of the left side. A suprapubic
catheter was placed and the baby was treated with antibiotics. The serum creatinine level
was 0.8 after birth, and the thriving baby could be discharged at 4 weeks of age with a
creatinine of 0.5 mg/dl.

This case demonstrates that the prediction of renal function by "diagnostic catheter"
placement can be improved by the SDS-PAGE protein analysis. Even though the vesicoam-
niotic shunt clearly and persistently increased the amount of liquor after placement and
pulmonary development was normal after the procedure, it is difficult to demonstrate con-
vincingly an improvement in renal function because urinary electrolytes show a steady
decrease over gestation in normal fetuses.[107]

It can also be argued that our case showed features of the Eagle-Barrett (prune belly)
or megacystis-megaureter (massive primary vesicoureteral reflux) syndrome which, according to Elder and colleagues,[61] probably do not benefit from *in utero* drainage. We do not,

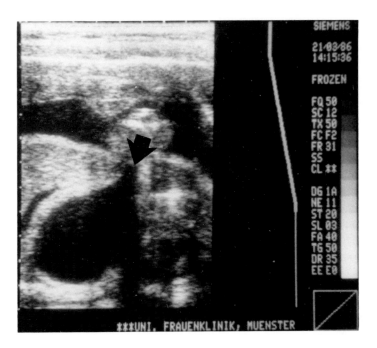

FIGURE 17B.

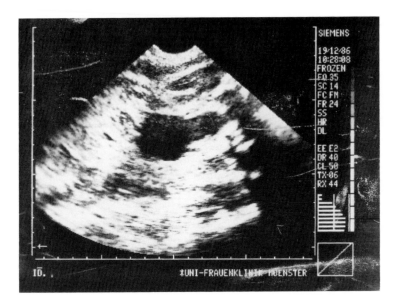

FIGURE 17C.

however, entirely agree with this opinion because in cases of persistent anhydramnios, independent from the etiology, sufficient pulmonary development will be impossible,[62] and the "prune belly" phenotype with abdominal distention can resolve if drainage of the megacystis is performed early enough.[63]

Nicolini et al.[64] have pointed out that the selection of fetuses for vesico-amniotic shunting by prenatal ultrasound-guided needling and analysis of fetal urine can be further improved by a serial sampling of each kidney separately.

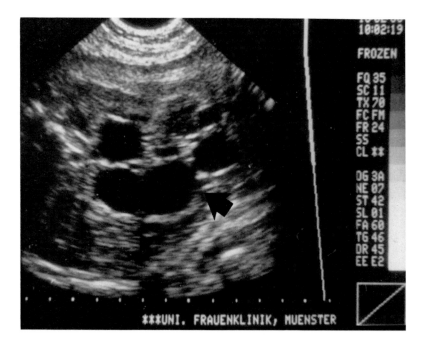

A

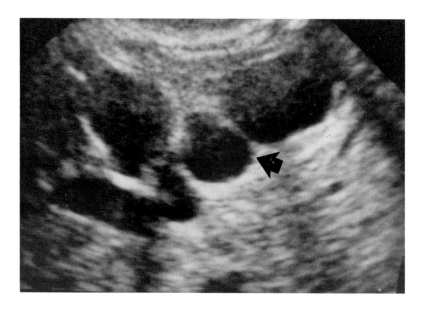

B

FIGURE 18.   Prenatal sonograms of dilated fetal ureter (A) due to ureteropelvic junction obstruction and (B) due to reflux.

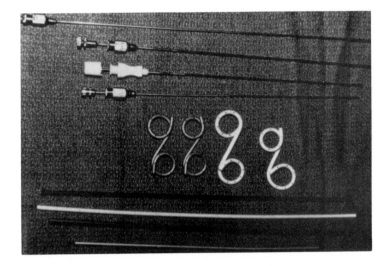

A

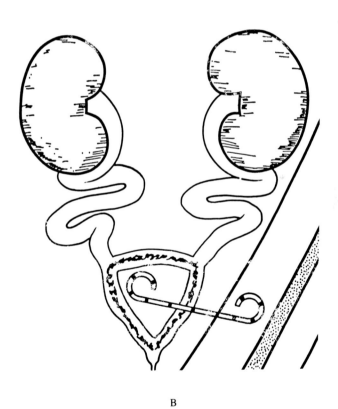

B

FIGURE 19.   Fetal vesico-amniotic shunt. (A) ''Harrison'' catheter set with introducer needle (top of the picture) and pusher (bottom of the picture). (B) Schematic picture of double pigtail catheter *in situ*.

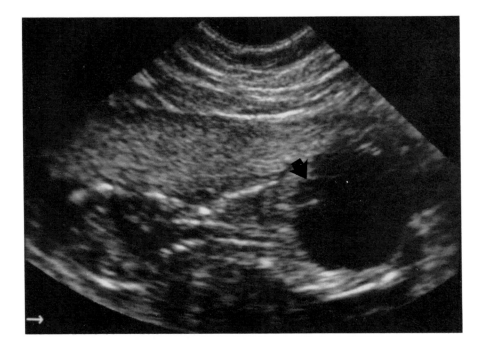

A

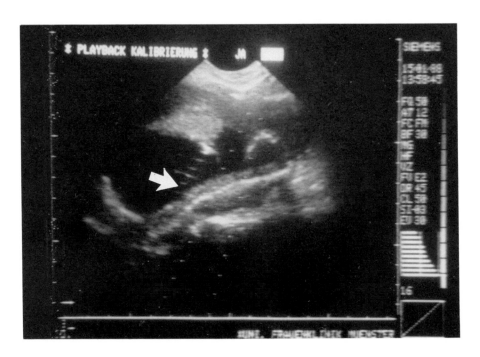

B

FIGURE 20.   Prenatal treatment of urinary tract obstruction. (A) Fetus with 18 weeks of gestation. Ahy-dramnion and megacystic (arrow). (B to D) Insertion of vesico-amniotic catheter (arrows) and well-functioning catheter. (E) A few hours after and (F) 7 weeks after placement of the double pigtail shunt.

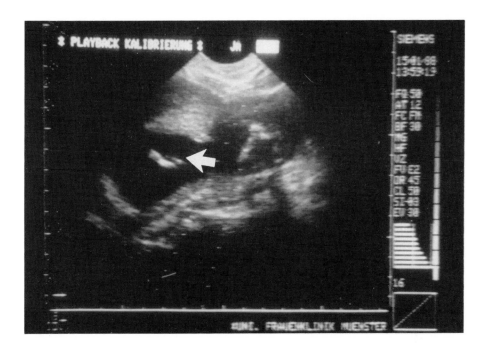

FIGURE 20C.

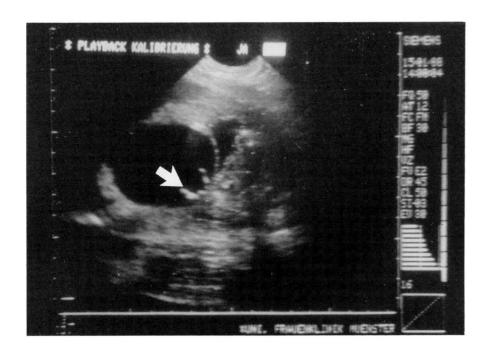

FIGURE 20D.

Further studies are required to improve the selection criteria for prenatal treatment of fetal obstructive uropathies. Analysis of fetal urine obtained with a diagnostic catheter clearly gives more information than analysis of microglobulins in amniotic fluid alone.[65]

Up to June 1987, there were 87 cases of fetal obstructive uropathies with percutaneous shunting reported to the Fetal Surgery Registry.[66] Death occurred in 52 cases, of which 25%

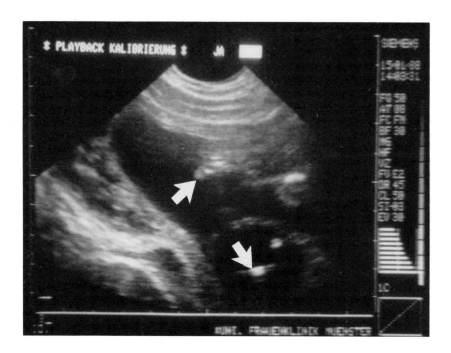

FIGURE 20E.

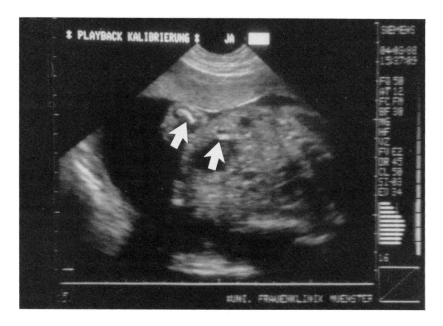

FIGURE 20F.

were due to elective termination, 2% due to associated anomalies, 7.7% related to the procedure, 63% due to pulmonary hypoplasia, and only 1.9% due to renal disease. The survival rates varied according to the underlying diagnosis from 100% in uretero-pelvic obstruction to only 17% in cases with urethral atresia.

A comparison of the results of shunt treatment *in utero* with the results in unmatched published series as controls suggests that prenatal therapy, at least in cases of posterior

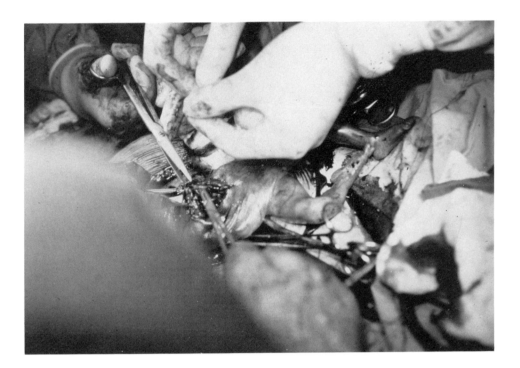

FIGURE 21.   "Open" surgery for continuous drainage of fetal obstructive uropathy at the University of California in San Francisco.

urethral valve syndrome, may increase survival rates and reduce rates of pulmonary hypoplasia and residual renal disease in survivors.[67]

With all percutaneous shunt applications, one of the major difficulties in the past has been the frequent need for multiple catheter placements because of the high incidence of the catheter becoming dislodged or obstructed, depending on the material and shape of the device. For this reason and because of the availability of tocolytic agents, "open" procedures have been investigated. The technique developed by Harrison et al.[4] involves a hysterotomy incision and marsupialization of the bladder for continuous drainage bypassing the obstruction of posterior urethral valves (Figure 21). Even though the first reported "open surgery" performed on a human fetus was not successful because the kidneys were already irreversibly damaged and there were no renal function studies available at that time, it showed that direct access to the fetus was possible without inducing premature labor and that a pregnancy can go on for weeks after such a procedure.

In the meantime, five cases of obstructive uropathies were treated with "open surgery", resulting in one death, which was probably unrelated to surgery, and three delivered children, i.e., one with renal insufficiency, one with questionable kidney function, and one with normal kidney function.[108]

In a large series of case observations, Harrison et al.[68] could show that prenatal intervention is not warranted in cases with unilateral fetal hydronephrosis (Figure 22) and/or dilated ureter (Figure 23A and B) with normal amniotic fluid volume. Also, in cases of bilateral urinary tract obstruction with normal amniotic fluid volume, expectant management with serial ultrasound examinations is justified.

With improvements in the resolution of ultrasound imaging, pure pressure hydronephrosis (Figure 24A) can be differentiated early from cystic dysplasia (Figure 24B), which is characteristic of Potter type IV degeneration in obstructive uropathies and which has always been associated with irreversible renal damage (Figure 24C and D), but before *in utero*

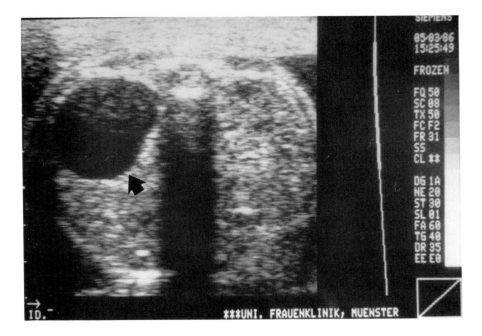

FIGURE 22.   Prenatal sonogram of unilateral hydronephrosis (arrow).

surgery is undertaken, with all its potential fetal and maternal risks, further and more invasive studies are required.

FETAL OVARIAN TUMORS

Ovarian cysts in newborns are rare events, and only a few have been diagnosed pre-natally.[69] An ovarian cyst can be suspected if a fluid-filled structure is visualized next to a fetal kidney (Figure 25A) and female external genitalia (Figure 25B) are recognizable. Kurjak et al.[70] were the first to point out that prenatal and postnatal observation using the improved diagnostic capacities of ultrasound may partly replace operative treatment schedules in the future, which is beneficial because even with microsurgical techniques, it can be difficult to preserve the very small ovaries if they are firmly attached to the cystic wall (Figure 25C).

We have experience with three cases of ovarian cysts where the size of the tumor was so enormous that secondary hydronephrosis because of upper urinary tract obstruction oc-curred (Figure 25D). In those cases, prenatal drainage of the cysts, which at the same time allows for steroid analysis of the cyst fluid and thus confirmation of the diagnosis, has permanently resolved the problem in two cases, in the other case, the cyst fluid rapidly accumulated.

Seeds et al.[71] reported a case with a large fetal abdominal cystic mass and subsequent hydramnios and maternal renal failure which resolved after percutaneous drainage of the fetal cyst. Rapid reaccumulation of the mass resulted in redrainage and placement of an indwelling cyst/amniotic diversion shunt which worked for 4 weeks until delivery.

In contrast to the relatively high incidence of 40% in adults, malignant tumors in neonates are very rare, and there is only one report of a bilateral malignant ovarian dysgerminoma in a fetus.[72] Ovarian teratomas are usually more solid (Figure 26) than benign ovarian cysts, which are characteristically completely filled with fluid and have a thin, smooth membrane. Benign cysts, as for instance, corpus luteum cysts, cystomas, and cystadenomas, form the majority of all ovarian cysts recognizable at the time of birth, and, therefore, after prenatal diagnosis of ovarian cysts conservative management is warranted.

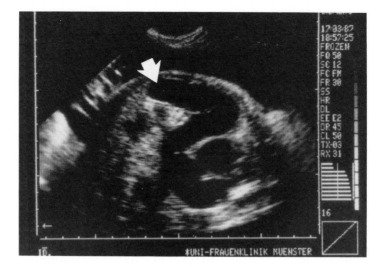

A

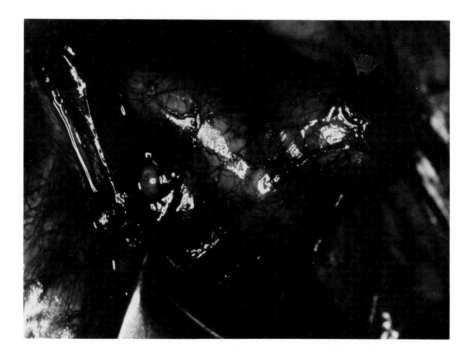

B

FIGURE 23.   Dilated ureter (arrows) without major renal involvement. (A) Prenatal sonogram shows normal amount of amniotic fluid. (B) Dilated ureter of the baby at the time of surgery after birth.

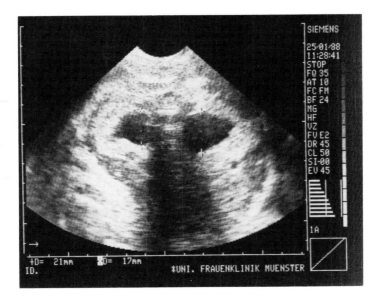

A

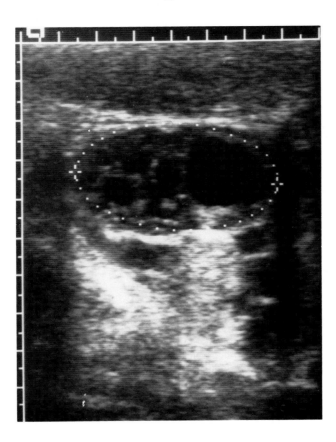

B

FIGURE 24.   Fetal uropathies. (A) Sonogram of a moderate bilateral hydronephrosis (marked by callipers). (B) Sonogram of dysplastic cystic degeneration in a Potter type IV kidney (marked by callipers). (C) Fetus immediately after delivery. Signs of Potter syndrome and macropenis are recognizable. (D) Pathologic specimen of the same fetus shows urethral obstructions along the penis and megacystic and dysplastic fetal kidneys (Potter type IV).

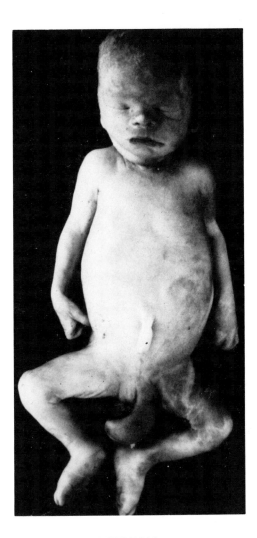

FIGURE 24C.

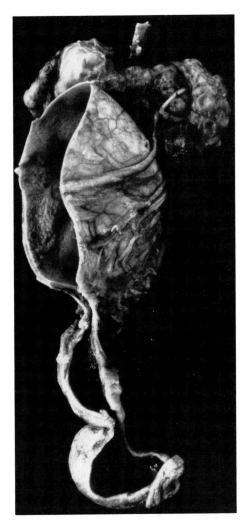

FIGURE 24D.

DIAPHRAGMATIC HERNIA

In an unselected series of congenital diaphragmatic hernias, the mortality is still 50 to 80%, even with greatly improved neonatal techniques and prenatal diagnosis in many cases.[73] Most of these deaths are due to pulmonary hypoplasia secondary to compression by herniated viscera.[74]

In order to improve the prognosis, Harrison et al. developed animal models for the correction of congenital diaphragmatic hernia *in utero*[75] and a successful surgical technique using abdominoplasty to avoid compromise of umbilical blood flow.[76] So far, only four cases of diaphragmatic hernia in human fetuses have been approached by the Fetal Treatment Group in San Francisco.[77] There were three intrauterine deaths, probably partly related to surgery, whereas in the fourth case, the hernia seemed to be successfully repaired *in utero*, even though the baby died 1 month post partum from unrelated complications.

The experience so far shows that even though much has been learned through the elegant studies conducted by Harrison and co-workers, many questions remain open about the risk/benefit evaluations concerning the mother and her unborn patient.

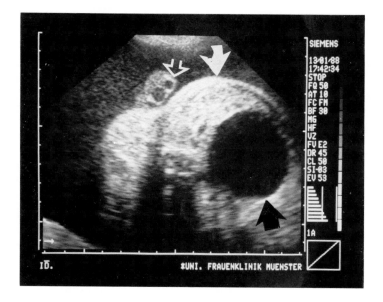

A

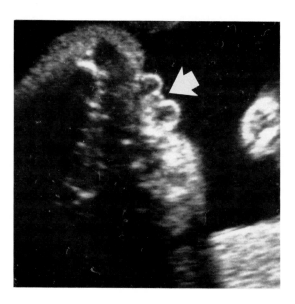

B

FIGURE 25.   Fetal ovarian cyst. (A) Prenatal sonogram. Ovarian cyst (black arrow) next to normal kidney (white arrow). Note that there is only one umbilical artery, which is always suspicious of fetal malformations. (B) Female external genitalia (arrow) visualized in a fetus with ovarian cyst. (C) Fetal ovarian cyst after surgery (diameter 12 cm). (D) Fetal ovarian cyst (white arrow) causing bilateral hydrone-phrosis (black arrows).

HYDRO-/CHYLOTHORAX AND NONIMMUNE HYDROPS FETALIS

Whereas drainage of fetal abdominal ascites in cases with nonimmune hydrops fetalis usually is not a successful therapy due to rapid recurrence,[78,79] prenatal drainage can lead to successful decompression of the lungs in cases of congenital bilateral chylothorax.[80]

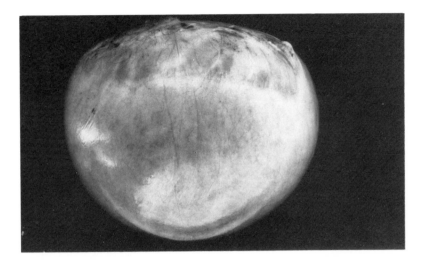

FIGURE 25C.

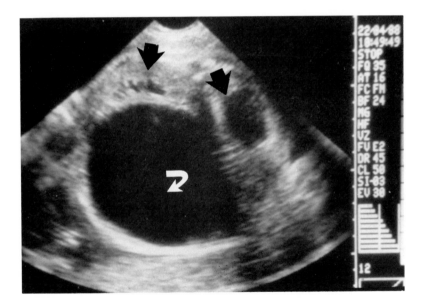

FIGURE 25D.

Shimokawa et al.[81] reported about fetal transfusions of albumin in cases of nonimmune hydrops fetalis and were able to raise the cord blood albumin levels to the normal range and to increase the fetal urine volume significantly. De Lia et al.[82] treated a pregnant woman with fetal twin-to-twin transfusion syndrome with digoxin and could demonstrate that the signs of cardiac failure were resolved before elective CS at 34 weeks. Because of the enormous heterogeneity of etiologies for nonimmune hydrops fetalis, only a few cases with severe ascites could be helped this way and the mortality of nonimmune hydrops will remain high.[79]

GROWTH RETARDATION

It was shown by Cetin et al.[83] that small-for-gestational-age fetuses have significantly lower concentrations of α-aminonitrogen in umbilical cord blood obtained at CS or by

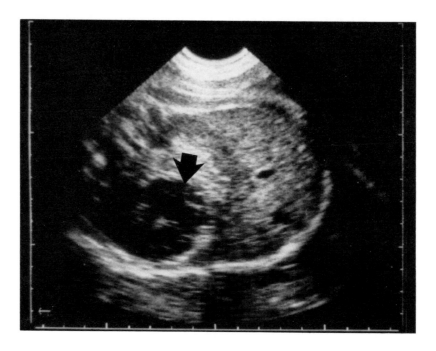

FIGURE 26.   Fetal malignant ovarian teratoma.

transabdominal cord sampling when compared to appropriate-for-gestational-age fetuses. Dudenhausen et al.[84] could demonstrate that amino acids can be absorbed from the amniotic fluid via the umbilical cord. Saling[85] reported a first attempt to transfer nutrients to a growth-retarded fetus through a transabdominal catheter. Nicolaides et al.[86] administered humidified oxygen (55%) continuously through a face mask to five pregnant women with severely growth-retarded fetuses and low mean blood velocity in the fetal thoracic aorta and could show an increase of the fetal P_{O_2} and the mean blood velocity in the fetal aorta.

Further cases, however, are awaited until these interesting approaches can be fully evaluated.

SELECTIVE FETOCIDE

Multiple gestation is a known complication of ovulation induction, causing increased maternal and fetal risks with a clear positive correlation to the number of fetuses (Figure 27). Therefore, some groups have performed selective first-trimester abortions in high multiple pregnancies.[87-89]

Dumez and Oury[87] first used the technique of transvaginal vacuum aspiration, but later they changed to the transabdominal method described by Kanhai et al.[88] In order to achieve a selective fetocide, the transabdominal technique was first applied for fetal trauma and exsanguination. We have used this method for intracardiac application of isotonic potassium chloride in the second trimester for selective fetocide (Figure 28) after prenatal diagnosis of trisomy 18 in one twin,[90] and after prenatal diagnosis of trisomy 21 in a triplet pregnancy, we had the impression that it is the safest, most reliable, and least invasive method for the patient.

Selective fetocide in a twin pregnancy after prenatal diagnosis of discordant findings with a severe, untreatable anomaly in only one twin does not seem substantially different from the termination of pregnancy in a singleton pregnancy. A reduction in a multiple pregnancy after ovulation induction, however, performed to significantly diminish the risks

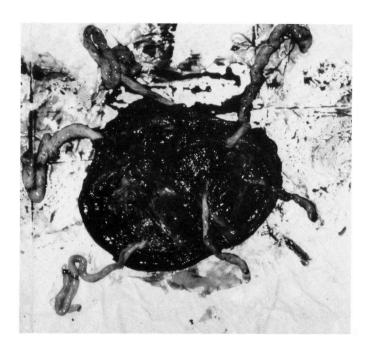

FIGURE 27. Placenta of a pregnancy with six fetuses which ended in a spontaneous abortion at 25 weeks of gestation. Note six umbilical cords coming out of the placenta.

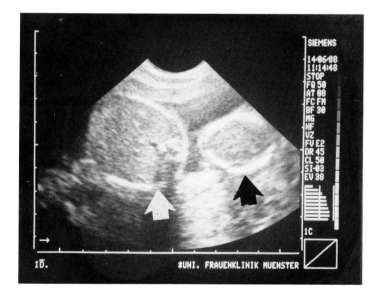

FIGURE 28. Prenatal sonogram taken after selective fetocide in a twin pregnancy. An abdominal cross-section of the healthy twin (white arrow) and the head of the aborted co-twin (black arrow) are recognizable.

for mother and increase the chances for a term delivery, principally represents a deviation from the Kantian philosophy widely shared in our society that no individual can be reduced to a mean in order to achieve a goal, no matter how good that goal may be.[91] On the other hand, there is a considerable majority of professionals in the fields of obstetrics and genetics who responded to a recent questionnaire compiled by Evans[92] that they would be in favor of, e.g., reducing quadruplets to twins in order to improve the chances of the pregnancy.

FUTURE THERAPY *IN UTERO*

From the first time that rhesus erythroblastosis was treated by intrauterine application of red blood cells, the fetus has become an unborn patient, and the goal is to find intervention procedures for more and more diseases which can be diagnosed prenatally.

Bone marrow transplantation has been attempted in children with known metabolic disorders to permanently replace the deficient cells, but problems including graft vs. host disease remain, and the success in getting the enzymes across the blood-brain barrier has been very limited.[93] The fetus, however, is more tolerant to foreign cells,[94] and in some animal models, *in utero* stem cell transplantation has already been successful.[95-97] Fetal liver cell suspension injected into the umbilical cord can be transferred to the fetal microcirculation[90] with permanent colonization.

Flake's group[7] reported in 1986 the successful creation of stable hematopoietic sheep chimeras by intraperitoneal injection of allogeneic fetal stem cells into normal fetal lambs. Because the fetuses usually seed their bone marrow with hematopoietic cells from the liver prior to the 20th week of gestation, this should be the optimal time for transplantation. Linch's group[8] was the first to apply this technique of corrective bone marrow transplantation in a human at 17 weeks of gestation, but there was failure of engraftment for unknown reasons, so that further studies in nonhuman primates have to be performed.

Another approach to early corrective fetal treatment would be somatic cell gene therapy resulting in the correction of a genetic disorder in the body cells of a patient, or germ line gene therapy resulting in the insertion of a gene into the reproductive tissue of a patient. Whereas somatic cell gene therapy should be possible within the near future, germ line cell therapy is still more unlikely in humans, but society must determine whether this option should be allowed.[99,100]

LEGAL AND ETHICAL ASPECTS OF FETAL THERAPY

Few approaches to fetal therapy have been established as safe and effective since the first surgical procedures on the fetus were performed some years ago.[101] Because of the advances in the area of *in utero* treatment, there is not only the choice of either doing nothing or having an abortion after prenatal diagnosis of fetal anomalies, but also how the choice of the parents to decide in favor or against a treatment that may benefit but also harm their child.[102] In all kinds of fetal therapy, the expected benefit must clearly exceed the results of exclusively postnatal procedures.[103]

If the fetus is considered as a patient, this further implies that concern has to be given also to questions like whether the fetus can experience pain from procedures *in utero*.[104]

If a physician wants to try an experimental *in utero* technique in order to help the fetus, the mother must be deferred to, and if she refuses her decision, it is not allowed to override her decision as might be if the therapy were established as safe and effective.[105] If the mother is competent and has been fully informed about the unproven status of experimental surgery, she is legally allowed to undergo some medical risks in order to improve the prognosis for her baby. If the physician is conducting research, approval of an institutional review board (ethics committee) is required.

A key legal issue that is not resolved yet is whether a mother can refuse an established prenatal therapy to protect her own bodily integrity.[102] Fletcher[106] stated that in a previable fetus, the woman's choice about abortion should be protected, but help for the fetus should not be blocked if the mother won't be physically harmed or abused by providing an access to help.

Addressing the issue whether saving fetuses with genetic diseases will preserve more harmful genes in the population, he concludes: "Genetic perfection does not exist and never can exist. We are under a moral obligation, which began with the advent of prenatal diagnosis, to learn, at a minimum, if effective therapy can be discovered for inherited disorders."

REFERENCES

1. **Hofmann, D., Holländer, H. J., and Weiser, P.,** The gynaecological and obstetrical importance of ultrasonic diagnosis, *Gynaecologia,* 164, 24, 1967.
2. **Mutterschafts-Richtlinien,** Beilage No. 4 zum Bundesanzeiger No. 22, 1980.
3. **Liley, A. W.,** Intrauterine transfusion of fetus in haemolytic disease, *Br. Med. J.,* 5365, 1107, 1963.
4. **Harrison, M. R., Golbus, M. S., Filly, R. A., Callen, P. W., Katz, M., de Lorimier, A. A., Rosen, M., and Jonsen, A.,** Fetal surgery for congenital hydronephrosis, *N. Engl. J. Med.,* 306, 591, 1982.
5. **Clewell, W. H., Johnson, M. L., Meier, P. R., Newkirk, J. B., Zide, S. L., Hendee, R. W., Bowes, A. W., Jr., Hecht, F., O'Keefe, D., Henry, G. P., and Shikes, R. H.,** A surgical approach to the treatment of fetal hydrocephalus, *N. Engl. J. Med.,* 306, 1320, 1982.
6. **Evans, M. I., and Schulman, J. D.,** Biochemical fetal therapy, *Clin. Obstet. Gynecol.,* 29, 523, 1986.
7. **Flake, A. W., Harrison, M. R., Adzick, S., and Zanjani, E. D.,** Transplantation of fetal hematopoietic stem cells in utero: the creation of hematopoietic chimeras, *Science,* 233, 776, 1986.
8. **Linch, D. C., Rodeck, C. H., Nicolaides, K., Jones, H. M., and Brent, L.,** Attempted bone-marrow transplantation in a 17-week fetus, *Lancet,* ii, 1453, 1986.
9. **Nicolaides, K. H., Rodeck, C. H., and Gosden, C. M.,** Rapid karyotyping in non-lethal fetal malformations, *Lancet,* i, 283, 1986.
10. **Williamson, R. A., Weiner, C. P., Patil, S., Benda, J., Varner, M. W., and Abu-Yousef, M. M.,** Abnormal pregnancy sonogram. Selective indication for fetal karyotype, *Obstet. Gynecol.,* 69, 15, 1987.
11. **Benacerraf, B. R., Miller, W. A., and Frigoletto, F. D.,** Sonographic detection of fetuses with trisomies 13 and 18: accuracy and limitations, *Am. J. Obstet. Gynecol.,* 158, 404, 1988.
12. **Claussen, U.,** The pipette method: a new rapid technique for chromosome analysis in prenatal diagnosis, *Hum. Genet.,* 54, 277, 1980.
13. **Daffos, E., Forestier, F., and Capella-Pavlovsky, M.,** Fetal blood sampling during the third trimester of pregnancy, *Br. J. Obstet. Gynaecol.,* 91, 118, 1984.
14. **Holzgreve, W., Miny, P., Basaran, S., Fuhrmann, W., and Beller, F. K.,** Safety of placental biopsy in the second and third trimester, *N. Engl. J. Med.,* 317, 1159, 1987.
15. **Manning, E., Harrison, M. R., Rodeck, C. H., and Members of the International Fetal Medicine and Surgery Society,** Catheter shunting for fetal hydronephrosis and hydrocephalus, *N. Engl. J. Med.,* 315, 336, 1986.
16. **Harrison, M. R., Filly, R. A., Golbus, M. S., et al.,** Fetal treatment 1982, *N. Engl. J. Med.,* 307, 1651, 1982.
17. **Modell, B., Ward, R. H. T., and Fairweather, D. V. I.,** Effects of introducing antenatal diagnosis on reproductive behaviour of families at risk for thalassemia major, *Br. Med. J.,* 280, 1347, 1980.
18. **Holzgreve, W., Beller, F. K., Buchholz, B., Hansmann, M., and Köhler, K.,** Kidney transplantation from anencephalic donors, *N. Engl. J. Med.,* 316, 1069, 1987.
19. **Adzick, N. S., Harrison, M. R., Glick, P. L., and Flake, A. W.,** Fetal urinary tract obstruction: experimental pathophysiology, *Semin. Perinatol.,* 9, 79, 1985.
20. **Holzgreve, W., Mahony, B. S., Glick, P. L., Filly, R. A., Harrison, M. R., DeLorimier, A. A., Holzgreve, A. C., Müller, K. M., Callen, P. W., Anderson, R. L., and Golbus, M. S.,** Sonographic demonstration of fetal sacrococcygeal teratoma, *Prenat. Diagn.,* 5, 245, 1985.
21. **Lyrenäs, S., Cnattingius, S., and Lindberg, B.,** Fetal jejunal atresia and intrauterine volvulus — a case report, *J. Perinat. Med.,* 10, 247, 1982.
22. **Holzgreve, W., Holzgreve, B., and Curry, C. J. R.,** Nonimmune hydrops fetalis: diagnosis and management, *Semin. Perinatol.,* 9, 52, 1985.

23. **Holzgreve, W. and Golbus, M. S.,** Aminotic fluid acetylcholinesterase as a prenatal diagnostic marker for upper gastrointestinal atresias, *Am. J. Obstet. Gynecol.,* 147, 837, 1983.

24. **Harrison, M. R., Golbus, M. S., and Filly, R. A., Eds.,** *The Unborn Patient. Prenatal Diagnosis and Treatment,* Grune & Stratton, New York, 1984.

25. **Ballard, P. L.,** Combined hormonal treatment and lung maturation, *Semin. Perinatol.,* 8, 283, 1984.

26. **Boreus, L. O., Jalling, B., and Wallin, A.,** Plasma concentrations of phenobarbital in mother and child after combined prenatal and postnatal administration for prophylaxis of hyperbilirubinaemia, *J. Pediatr.,* 93, 695, 1978.

27. **Glenn, F. B., Glenn, W. D., and Duncan, R. C.,** Fluoride tablet supplementation during pregnancy for caries immunity: a study of offspring produced, *Am. J. Obstet. Gynecol.,* 143, 560, 1982.

28. **Ampola, M. G., Mahoney, M. J., Nakamura, E., and Tanaka, K.,** Prenatal therapy of a patient with vitamin B12-responsive methylmalonic acidemia, *N. Engl. J. Med.,* 293, 313, 1975.

29. **Rosenblatt, D. S., Cooper, B. A., Schmutz, S. M., Zaleski, W. A., and Casey, R. E.,** Prenatal vitamin B12 therapy of a fetus with methylcobalamin deficiency (cobalamin E disease), *Lancet,* i, 1127, 1985.

30. **Packman, S., Cowan, M. J., Golbus, M. S., Caswell, N., Sweetman, L., Burri, B., Nyhan, W., and Baker, H.,** Prenatal treatment of biotin-responsive multiple carboxylase deficiency, *Lancet,* i, 1435, 1982.

31. **Schulman, J. D.,** prenatal treatment of biochemical disorders, *Semin. Perinatol.,* 9, 75, 1985.

32. **David, M. J. and Forest, M. G.,** Prenatal treatment of congenital adrenal hyperplasia resulting from 21-hydroxylase deficiency, *J. Pediatr.,* 105, 799, 1984.

33. **Weiner, S., Scharf, J., Bolognese, R., and Librizzi, R.,** Antenatal diagnosis and treatment of fetal goiter, *J. Reprod. Med.,* 24, 39, 1980.

34. **Prout, T. E.,** Thyroid disease in pregnancy, *Am. J. Obstet. Gynecol.,* 122, 669, 1975.

35. **Kleinman, C. S., Copel, J. A., Weinstein, E. M., Santulli, T. V., and Hobbins, J. C.,** In utero diagnosis and treatment of fetal supraventricular tachycardia, *Semin. Perinatol.,* 9, 113, 1985.

36. **Graves, S. W., Valdes, R., Brown, B. A., et al.,** Endogenous immunoreactive substances in human pregnancies, *J. Clin. Endocrinol. Metab.,* 58, 747, 1984.

37. **Stewart, P. A. and Wladimiroff, J. W.,** Cardiac tachyarrhythmia in the fetus: diagnosis, treatment and prognosis, *Fetal Ther.,* 2, 7, 1987.

38. **Copel, J. A., Cullen, M., Green, J. J., Mahoney, M. J., Hobbins, J. C., and Kleinman, C. S.,** The frequency of aneuploidy in prenatally diagnosed congenital heart disease: an indication for fetal karyotying, *Am. J. Obstet. Gynecol.,* 158, 409, 1988.

39. **Rodeck, C. H., Nicolaides, K. H., Warsof, S. L., Fysh, W. J., Gamsu, M. R., and Kemp, J. R.,** The management of severe rhesus isoimmunization by fetoscopic intravascular transfusion, *Am. J. Obstet. Gynecol.,* 150, 769, 1984.

40. **Berkowitz, R. L., Chitkara, Y., Goldberg, J. D., Wilkins, I., and Chervenak, F. A.,** Intravascular transfusion in utero: the percutaneous approach, *Am. J. Obstet. Gynecol.,* 154, 622, 1986.

41. **Grannum, P. A., Copel, J. A., Plaxe, S. C., Scoscia, A. C., and Hobbins, J. C.,** In utero exchange transfusion by direct intravascular injection in severe erythroblastosis fetalis, *N. Engl. J. Med.,* 314, 1431, 1986.

42. **Hogge, W. A., Thiagarajah, S., Brenbridge, A. N., and Harber, G. M.,** Fetal evaluation by percutaneous blood sampling, *Am. J. Obstet. Gynecol.,* 158, 132, 1988.

43. **Clewell, W. A., Manco-Johnson, M. L., and Manchester, D. K.,** Diagnosis and management of fetal hydrocephalus, *Clin. Obstet. Gynecol.,* 29, 514, 1986.

44. **Elridge, A. R.,** Treatment of obstructive lesions of the aqueduct of Sylvius and the fourth ventricle by interventriculostomy, *J. Neurosurg.,* 24, 11, 1966.

45. **Birnholz, J. C. and Frigoletto, F. D.,** Antenatal treatment of hydrocephalus, *N. Engl. J. Med.,* 304, 1021, 1981.

46. **Chervenak, F. A., Duncan, C., Ment, L. R., Hobbins, J. C., McClure, M., Scott, D., and Berkowitz, R. L.,** Outcome of fetal ventriculomegaly, *Lancet,* ii, 179, 1984.

47. **Williamson, R. A., Schauberger, C. W., Varner, M. W., and Aschenbrenner, C. A.,** Heterogeneity of prenatal onset hydrocephalus: management and counseling implications, *Am. J. Med. Genet.,* 17, 497, 1984.

48. **Clewell, W. H., Meier, P. R., Manchester, D. K., Manco-Johnson, M. L., Pretorius, D. H., and Hendee, R. W., Jr.,** Ventriculomegaly: evaluation and management, *Semin. Perinatol.,* 9, 98, 1985.

49. **Rodeck, C. H. and Members of the International Fetal Medicine and Surgery Society,** Intrauterine shunting for ventriculomegaly, *Lancet,* i, 92, 1986.

50. **Benson, D. F., LeMay, M., Patten, D. H., and Rubens, A. B.,** Diagnosis of normal-pressure hydrocephalus, *N. Engl. J. Med.,* 283, 609, 1970.

51. **Michejda, M. and Hodgen, G. D.,** In utero diagnosis and treatment of fetal skeletal anomalies. I. Hydrocephalus, *JAMA,* 246, 1093, 1981.

52. **Michejda, M.,** Intrauterine treatment of hydrocephalus, *Fetal Ther.,* 1, 75, 1986.

53. **Manning, F. A.,** Fetal surgery for obstructive uropathy: rational considerations, *Am. J. Kidney Dis.,* 10, 259, 1987.
54. **Avni, E. F., Rodesch, F., and Schulman, C. C.,** Fetal uropathies: diagnostic pitfalls and management, *J. Urol.,* 134, 921, 1985.
55. **Golbus, M. S., Harrison, M. R., Filly, R. A., Callen, P. W., and Katz, M.,** In utero treatment of urinary tract obstruction, *Am. J. Obstet. Gynecol.,* 142, 383, 1982.
56. **Blakeslee, S.,** Fetal surgery pioneered in California, *Int. Herald Tribune,* p. 8, October 9, 1986.
57. **Golbus, M. S., Filly, R. A., Callen, P. W., Glick, P. L., Harrison, M. R., and Anderson, R. L.,** Fetal urinary tract obstruction: management and selection for treatment, *Semin. Perinatol.,* 9, 91, 1985.
58. **Glick, P. L., Harrison, M. R., Golbus, M. S., et al.,** Management of the fetus with congenital hydronephrosis. II. Prognostic criteria and selection for treatment, *J. Pediatr. Surg.,* 20, 376, 1985.
59. **Lenz, S., Lund-Hansen, T., Bang, J., and Christensen, E.,** A possible prenatal evaluation of renal function by amino acid analysis on fetal urine, *Prenat. Diagn.,* 5, 259, 1985.
60. **Peterson, P. A., Errin, P. E., and Berggard, I.,** Differentiation of glomerular, tubular and normal proteinuria: determinations of urinary excretion of β-2-microglobulin, albumin and total protein, *J. Clin. Invest.,* 48, 1189, 1969.
61. **Elder, J. S., Duckett, J. W., and Snyder, H. M.,** Intervention for fetal obstructive uropathy: has it been effective?, *Lancet,* ii, 1009, 1987.
62. **Harrison, M. R., Nakayama, D. K., Noall, R., and DeLorimier, A. A.,** Correction of congenital hydronephrosis in utero. II. Decompression reverses the effects of obstruction on the fetal lung and urinary tract, *J. Pediatr. Surg.,* 17, 965, 1983.
63. **Nakayama, D. K., Harrison, M. R., Chin, D. H., and DeLorimier, A. A.,** The pathogenesis of prune belly, *Am. J. Dis. Child.,* 138, 834, 1984.
64. **Nicolini, U., Rodeck, C. H., and Fisk, N. M.,** Shunt treatment for fetal obstructive uropathy, *Lancet,* ii, 1338, 1987.
65. **Burghard, R., Leititis, J. U., Bald, R., and Brandis, M.,** Protein Analysis in Amniotic Fluid and Fetal Urine for the Assessment of Fetal Renal Function and Dysfunction, abstract at the 5th Annu. Meet. of the Int. Fetal Medicine and Surgery Soc. Bonn, June 1 to 4, 1988.
66. **Evans, M. I.,** Uropathies, *Int. Fetal Med. Surg. Soc. Newsl.,* p. 3, 1988.
67. **Manning, F. A., Lange, I. R., Harrison, I., and Harman, C.,** Treatment of the fetus in utero: evolving concepts, *Clin. Obstet. Gynecol.,* 27, 378, 1984.
68. **Harrison, M. R., Golbus, M. S., Filly, R. A., Nakayama, D. K., Callen, P. W., DeLorimier, A. A., and Hricak, H.,** Management of the fetus with congenital hydronephrosis, *J. Pediatr. Surg.,* 17, 728, 1982.
69. **Holzgreve, W., Winde, B., Willital, G. H., and Beller, F. K.,** Prenatal diagnosis and perinatal management of fetal ovarian cyst, *Prenat. Diagn.,* 5, 155, 1985.
70. **Kurjak, A., Latin, V., Mandruzzato, G., D'Addario, V., and Rajhvajn, B.,** Ultrasound diagnosis and perinatal management of fetal genito-urinary abnormalities, *J. Perinat. Med.,* 12, 291, 1984.
71. **Seeds, J. W., Cefalo, R. C., Herbert, W. N. P., and Bowes, W. A.,** Hydramnios and maternal renal failure: relief with fetal therapy, *Obstet. Gynecol.,* 64, 26S, 1984.
72. **Ziegler, E. E.,** Bilateral ovarian carcinoma in a 30 week fetus, *Arch. Pathol.,* 40, 279, 1945.
73. **Harrison, M. R., Adzick, N. S., Nakayama, D. K., and DeLorimier, A. A.,** Fetal diaphragmatic hernia: fatal but fixable, *Semin. Perinatol.,* 9, 103, 1985.
74. **Harrison, M. R. and DeLorimier, A. A.,** Congenital diaphragmatic hernia, *Surg. Clin. North Am.,* 61, 1023, 1981.
75. **Harrison, M. R., Jester, J. A., and Ross, N. A.,** Correction of congenital diaphragmatic hernia in utero. I. The model: intrathoracic balloon produces fatal pulmonary hypoplasia, *Surgery,* 88, 174, 1980.
76. **Harrison, M. R., Ross, N. A., and DeLorimier, A. A.,** Correction of congenital diaphragmatic hernia in utero. III. Development of a successful surgical technique using abdominoplasty to avoid compromise to umbilical blood flow, *J. Pediatr. Surg.,* 16, 934, 1981.
77. **Evans, M.,** Open fetal surgery, *Int. Fetal Med. Surg. Soc. Newsl.,* p. 4, 1988.
78. **Seeds, J. W., Herbert, W. N., Bowes, W. A., and Cefalo, R. C.,** Recurrent idiopathic fetal hydrops: results of prenatal therapy, *Obstet. Gynecol.,* 64, 30S, 1984.
79. **Holzgreve, W., Curry, C. J. R., Golbus, M. S., Callen, P. W., Filly, R. A., and Smith, J. C.,** Investigation of nonimmune hydrops fetalis, *Am. J. Obstet. Gynecol.,* 150, 805, 1984.
80. **Petres, R. E., Redwine, F. D., and Cruikshank, D. P.,** Congenital bilateral chylothorax: antepartum diagnosis and successful intrauterine surgical management, *JAMA,* 248, 1360, 1982.
81. **Shimokawa, H., Hara, K., Koyanagi, T., Hirakawa, T., Heri, E., Maed, H., and Nakano, H.,** Intrauterine treatment of nonimmunologic hydrops fetalis associated with pleural effusion, *Nippon Sanka Fujinka Gakkai Zasshi,* 37, 66, 1985.
82. **De Lia, J., Emery, M. G., Sheafer, S. A., and Jennison, T. A.,** Twin transfusion syndrome: successful in utero treatment with digoxin, *Int. J. Gynaecol. Obstet.,* 23, 197, 1985.

83. **Cetin, I., Marconi, A. M., Bozzetti, P., Sereni, L. P., Corbetta, C., Pardi, G., and Battaglia, F. C.,** Umbilical amino acid concentrations in appropriate and small for gestational age infants: a biochemical difference present in utero, *Am. J. Obstet. Gynecol.,* 158, 120, 1988.

84. **Dudenhausen, J. W., Kynast, G., and Saling, E.,** The absorption of aminoacids via the umbilical cord, in *Perinatal Medicine,* Bossard, H., Cruz, J. M., Huber, A., Prod'hom, L. S., and Sistek, J., Eds., Hans Huber, Bern, 1973.

85. **Saling, E.,** Report at the Int. Multidisciplinary Symp. in Ultrasound and Fetal Medicine, London, November 17 to 21, 1986.

86. **Nicolaides, K. H., Campbell, S., Bradley, R. J., Bilardo, C. M., Soothill, P. W., and Gibbs, D.,** Maternal oxygen therapy for intrauterine growth retardation, *Lancet,* i, 942, 1987.

87. **Dumez, Y. and Oury, J. F.,** Method for first trimester selective abortion in multiple pregnancy, *Contrib. Gynecol. Obstet.,* 15, 50, 1986.

88. **Kanhai, H. H., van Russel, E. J. C., and Meerman, R. J.,** Selective termination in quintuplet pregnancy during first semester, *Lancet,* ii, 1447, 1986.

89. **Farquharson, D. F., Wittman, B. K., Hansmann, M., Yuen, B. H., Baldwin, V. J., and Lindahl, S.,** Management of quintuplet pregnancy by selective embryocide, *Am. J. Obstet. Gynecol.,* 158, 413, 1988.

90. **Westendorp, A. K., Miny, P., Holzgreve, W., and Aydinly, K.,** Selective fetocide by direct intracardiac application of isotonic potassium chloride, *Arch. Gynecol.,* 1988, in press.

91. **Kant, I. (Paton, H. J., Transl.),** *Groundwork of the Metaphysics of Morals,* Harper & Row, New York, 1964.

92. **Evans, M.,** Ethical Attitudes Towards Selective Termination in First and Second Trimester, abstract presented at the 5th Annu. Meet. of the Int. Fetal Medicine and Surgery Soc., Bonn, June 1 to 4, 1988.

93. **Rappeport, J. M. and Ginns, E. I.,** Bone marrow transplantation in severe Gaucher's disease, *N. Engl. J. Med.,* 311, 84, 1984.

94. **Silverstein, A. M.,** Ontogeny of the immune response, *Science,* 144, 1423, 1964.

95. **Simpson, T. J. and Golbus, M. S.,** In utero fetal hematopoietic stem cell transplantation, *Semin. Perinatol.,* 9, 68, 1985.

96. **Seller, M. J.,** Transplantation of anemic mice of the w-series with haemopoietic tissue bearing marker chromosomes, *Nature (London),* 220, 300, 1968.

97. **Fleischman, R. A. and Mintz, B.,** Prevention of genetic anemias in mice by microinjection of normal hematopoietic stem cells into the fetal placenta, *Proc. Natl. Acad. Sci. U.S.A.,* 76, 5736, 1979.

98. **Gustavii, B., Löfberg, L., and Olofsson, T.,** Transfer of tissue cells to the fetus, *Acta Obstet. Gynecol. Scand.,* 61, 361, 1982.

99. **Anderson, W. F.,** Prospects for human gene therapy in the born and unborn patient, *Clin. Obstet. Gynecol.,* 29, 586, 1986.

100. **Doetschman, T., Gregg, R. G., Maeda, N., Hooper, M. L., Melton, D. W., Thompson, S., and Smithies, O.,** Targetted correction of a mutant HPRT gene in mouse embryonic stem cells, *Nature (London),* 330, 576, 1987.

101. **Robertson, J. A.,** Legal issues in prenatal therapy, *Clin. Obstet. Gynecol.,* 29, 603, 1986.

102. **Robertson, J. A.,** Legal considerations: the duties of mothers and physicians in fetal treatment, in *The Unborn Patient,* Harrison, M. R., Golbus, M. S., and Filly, R. A., Eds., Grune & Stratton, New York, 1984, 171.

103. **Arant, B. S.,** Prevention of hereditary nephropathies by antenatal interventions, *Pediatr. Nephrol.,* i, 553, 1987.

104. **Richards, T.,** Can a fetus feel pain?, *Br. Med. J.,* 291, 1220, 1985.

105. **Robertson, J. A.,** Legal issues in fetal therapy, *Semin. Perinatol.,* 9, 136, 1985.

106. **Fletcher, J. C.,** Ethical considerations in and beyond experimental fetal therapy, *Semin. Perinatol.,* 9, 130, 1985.

107. **Rodeck, C. H.,** Unpublished results presented at the 5th Annu. Meet. Int. Fetal Medicine and Surgery Soc., Bonn, June 1 to 4, 1988.

108. **Harrison, M. R.,** Unpublished data presented at the 5th Annu. Meet. Int. Fetal Medicine and Surgery Soc., Bonn, June 1 to 4, 1988.

Chapter 4

DOPPLER ULTRASOUND IN THE ASSESSMENT OF FETAL AND MATERNAL CIRCULATION

Asim Kurjak and Zarko Alfirevic

INTRODUCTION

The normal growth of the fetus during intrauterine life, its ability to withstand the stress of labor and delivery, and its healthy development during the neonatal period depend to a great extent upon the integrity of the fetoplacental circulatory system.

During intrauterine life, this system has the major responsibility of transporting the essential elements that are transferred from the mother across the placenta to the fetal tissues and of returning to the placenta fetal catabolic products to be eliminated. After birth, the circulatory system plays a major role in the adjustment of the newborn for an external environment and maintenance of normal development.[1,2]

HISTORY OF NONULTRASONIC BLOOD FLOW MEASUREMENT

Interest in the circulation was expressed as early as the 5th century B.C. Pre-Hippocrates philosophers, Diogenes of Apolonia and, later, Diokles of Canisto, spoke about the so-called cotyledons or acetabula of the uterine inner surface from which the fetus feeds, sucking, preparing itself for the postnatal breast feeding.[3] The continuing research can be followed through writings of Da Vinci, Harvey, Sabatier, and others.[3,4]

Volume flow measurements were already carried out in 1884 by Cohnstein and Zuntz,[5] but systematic measurements of the fetal blood flow began to emerge from the 1930s onward. Barcroft and associates performed radiographic studies on the fetal goat and lamb to establish fetal circulation.[6,7] The first reasonably successful technique was developed by Cooper and Greenfield,[8] who immersed a fetal lamb in a bath of warm saline and used a plethysmograph to measure the umbilical blood flow. They reported flows in near-term lambs of 500 ml/min. The method has even been applied to the human fetus by Greenfield et al.[9] It was only applicable after the preparation had been subjected to surgery and anesthesia; thus, results obtained by directly invasive methods such as these should only be interpreted to be representative of fetuses in relatively poor physiological condition.[10]

Dawes and Mott[11] published the results of a series of experiments in which the umbilical blood flow in near-term lambs was measured directly with an electromagnetic flowmeter. They reported the umbilical blood flow to be 170 ml/min/kg. With an average fetal weight of 4.22 kg, the absolute umbilical blood flow was 717 ml/min, which, as Dawes predicted, is higher than the values obtained by plethysmography. In a similar experiment, Kirschbaum et al.[12] reported the mean umbilical flow in the near-term fetal lamb to be 138 ml/min/kg. Meschia et al.[13] measured the umbilical blood flow using the Fick principle with urea as the test substance. They reported that the umbilical blood flow in fetuses above 3 kg was 178 ml/min/kg. This led them to develop a method for the simultaneous measurement of umbilical and uterine blood flows, which has been successfully used to provide definitive measurements of these quantities.[14]

Subsequently, the development of modern surgical techniques and instrumentation for the preparation and maintenance of chronically catheterized pregnant animals made it possible to measure placental blood flow using radioactive microspheres and/or electromagnetic flow probes. These developments were of great importance, because the effects of anesthesia and surgical stress appear to linger for several days and to have effects upon physiological responses of the fetus and placenta.[15,16]

Oakes et al.[17] have implanted electromagnetic flowmeters on the common umbilical vein, thereby providing a direct and continuous measurement of umbilical blood flow in a chronic preparation. Berman et al.[18] have described a similar technique, whereby the probe is placed on the common umbilical artery in the fetus.

Most of these above-mentioned studies are performed on animals (mainly on fetal lambs). In relating animal data to the human fetus, numerous problems exist, including differences between species, the effects of anesthesia and surgical procedures, and the difficulty of maintaining a suitable controlled environment.[19,20]

The work of Haselhorst and Stromberger in 1932 was the first attempt at calculating umbilical blood flow in the human.[21] Since that first communication, besides the above-mentioned studies, various remarkable papers have been published by Assali and co-workers,[22,23] Stembera et al.,[24] McCallum et al.,[25] and others.[21] However, although those experimental studies have given fundamental information about the fetal physiology, they could not be used for studies and clinical purposes in human fetus due to their invasive nature, low reproducibility, and potential hazards for the mother and fetus.

ULTRASONIC MEASUREMENT OF BLOOD FLOW

The measurement of blood flow velocity, using ultrasound, is based on the effect which is named after Christian Johan Doppler (1803 to 1853), professor of elementary mathematics and practical geometry at the University of Vienna. In 1842, he published in Prague his famous paper entitled "Uber das farbige Licht der Doppelsterne under einiger anderer Gestirne des Himmels".[26] He described the shifts in red light from binary stars and explained that the color perceived by the eye varies with the frequency. The phenomenon, that when a wave source is moving in relation to an observer, the perceived wave frequency is different from the emitted one, was predicted on theoretical grounds.

Then, 3 years later, Buys Ballot (1817 to 1890) applied the Doppler effect to sound.[27] Two trumpet players with the sense of absolute pitch and a locomotive were needed for the verification of the Doppler theory and its applicability to the sound. One trumpet player was put on the locomotive and the other along the track. A horn was blown on the train once while approaching the observer, and then after passing him. It appeared that the difference in the two sounds was almost a complete note. The perceived tone was a half tone higher from the original sound when the locomotive was approaching, and a half tone lower after it has passed.[28]

However, more than a century had passed before it was realized that the red blood cells can also reflect sound waves producing the Doppler effect.[29] Briefly, if the erythrocytes move toward the wave source (ultrasound transducer), the frequency of the emitted signal will increase. If they move away from the wave source, the frequency of the emitted signal will decrease. During the measurements of the blood flow, the ultrasound wave is sent toward a blood vessel in which moving erythrocytes act as reflectors, causing a change of the reflected sound frequency. This change of frequency is called the Doppler shift and is directly proportional to the velocity of the blood stream.

The simplest Doppler instrument is a relatively cheap and highly portable continuous-wave Doppler unit. In such instruments, the transmitting and receiving of ultrasound and its frequency changes are done continuously. Consequently, it has no depth resolution and there are no limitations regarding high-velocity measurement *(vide infra)*. Continuous-wave Doppler systems have been widely used in the examination of superficial structures such as the carotid and superficial vessels of the limb. It is capable of detecting weak signals and, therefore, is preferred when the examination of ophthalmic, supraorbital, female breast vessels, etc. is needed. Unfortunately, when there are too many vessels present, as for example, in the upper abdomen and gravid uterus, the superimposition of several Doppler signals occurs.

The vast majority of Doppler ultrasound units for obstetrical purposes used pulsed-wave Doppler ultrasound. It is depth selective, which is its main advantage in comparison with continuous-wave Doppler. The same transducer is used for transmitting and receiving, and the last emitted short pulse of ultrasound has to travel to the vessel and back before the next one is emitted. Signals from a certain depth can be sampled and analyzed separately. It is achieved simply by changing the length of time that the system waits to open the sound gate; that allows it to receive the emitted pulse. Of course, the system is far more sophisticated and more expensive than a continuous-wave Doppler.

The advantage of range selectiveness is practically useless unless there is a possibility to guide the sample volume in the region of interest. The combination of real-time imaging for this purpose and a pulsed Doppler system (most commonly) is called a "duplex system". It can be a combination of Doppler with sector scanner (mechanical or phased array) or a phased array linear scanner. Another combination, especially convenient for the Doppler measurement in obstetrics, is the combination of linear array with offset Doppler transducer (Figure 1). An important advantage of the system is that it allows the possibility to measure all parameters necessary for volume flow calculation *(vide infra)*.

Regardless of the equipment used, the methods of transcutaneous blood flow measurement can be divided into two groups. There are those in which the sensitivity of the instrument is approximately uniform over the vessel cross-section and which give a mean Doppler shift proportional to the mean blood flow. If the angle of approach between the ultrasound and the vessel and the vessel diameter can be measured, the calculation of flow in milliliters per minute is performed automatically. This type is usually called volume flow measurement. The other type is a semiquantitative method of flow calculations, usually called flow velocity waveform (FVW) analysis.

VOLUME FLOW MEASUREMENT

The changes of the Doppler shift are proportional to the velocity of the blood stream. They are also proportional to the angle between blood vessel and emitted ultrasound wave. The Doppler shift can be calculated from the following equation:

$$F_d = \frac{F \times v \times 2 \cos O}{c} \tag{1}$$

where Fd is the Doppler shift, F is the frequency of the emitted ultrasound, v is the velocity of the blood stream, 0 is the angle between the sound wave and the direction of the blood stream, and c is the velocity of ultrasound in tissue (1540 cm/s).

The values of c and F are known and constant. Therefore, once the Doppler shift and the angle of Doppler beam to the vessel are measured, the average blood flow velocity can be easily calculated from the standard form of the Doppler equation:

$$V = \frac{F_d \times c}{F \times 2 \cos O} \tag{2}$$

By multiplying the cross-sectional area of the blood vessel with the spatial average blood velocity over the cross-section, the rate of blood flow can be calculated:

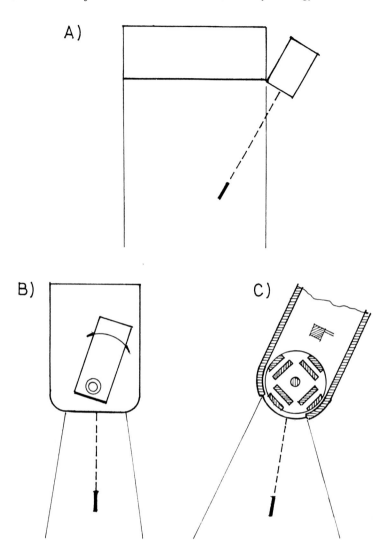

FIGURE 1. The schematic drawing of three types of Doppler duplex transducers. (A) Linear transducer with Doppler probe attached to it with the fixed angle; (B) mechanical sector probe with the built-in Doppler system; (C) phased array sector probe with built-in Doppler system.

$$\text{FLOW} = v \times [(\tfrac{D}{2})^2 \times 3.14] \qquad (3)$$

where v is the average velocity, and D is the vessel diameter.

Equations 2 and 3 show that for quantitative information of the total rate of blood flow *in utero*, three parameters should be known:

1. The Doppler shift
2. The angle between the Doppler ultrasound beam and the blood vessel
3. The vessel diameter

In 1979, Gill and Kossoff[30] described a method which made possible such noninvasive quantification of blood flow in the umbilical vein. The method involves a combination of

B mode ultrasound imaging (UI Octoson) and pulsed, 2-MHz Doppler ultrasound. The intra-abdominal part of the umbilical vein was located by the real-time scanner. Calipers were placed on the inner edges of the vessel to determine both the lumen diameter and the spatial orientation of the vessel. The pulsed Doppler units was then activated with known information of the angle between the beam and the vessel, and the Doppler shift was electronically measured. Due to its limitation of the range of velocity, the system did not allow recording of the high velocities, such as in arteries.

A more sophisticated system was described by Eik-Nes et al.[31] which could quantify blood flow in fetal veins as well as arteries. The duplex scanner, which can be handled easily on the abdomen of a pregnant woman, consists of a real-time B mode transducer and a pulsed Doppler transducer firmly attached to each other at an angle of 45°.

Current machines offer a choice of a fixed-angle Doppler transducer or a Doppler transducer attached to the B mode by a jointed arm.[32] The direction of the Doppler beam with the position of the time gate is displayed on the screen. In order to avoid artifacts, the obtained Doppler shift frequencies are analyzed before displaying by means of a real-time, on-line spectrum analyzer.

The distribution and intensities (represented by the gray scaling) of the Doppler shifts are displayed against the time (the Doppler sonogram).

The analyzer also has the ability to separate forward and reverse flow into opposite channels. The sonogram is displayed by means of a television monitor, its audio signal is fed to a loudspeaker, and it can be stored by means of a tape recorder for an off-line spectral analysis.

TECHNICAL CONSIDERATIONS AND POTENTIAL SOURCES OF PITFALLS

For the volume flow measurements in obstetrics, the duplex system with the pulsed Doppler is almost exclusively used. From the frozen picture of such a unit, the vessel diameter, the angle between the investigated vessel and Doppler beam, and the Doppler shift can be measured, thus allowing the calculation of blood flow velocity in milliliters per minute from Equations 2 and 3 (Figure 2).

Vessel Diameter

The error in vessel diameter measurement seems to be the most significant, since the error will be squared when calculating volume blood flow (Equation 3). For example, the error of 0.4 mm will cause a 10% error if the vessel diameter is between 6 to 8 mm, and up to 25% if the vessel diameter is below 5 mm.[33,34]

Another problem during vessel measurement is the pulsatility of the arterial vessel wall. The calculated errors, if measurement is carried out from one frozen real-time image, vary between +9 and −19%, and if the M mode recordings are used, the error can be decreased to 5%.[4]

In order to increase the reproducibility of the measurement, the vessel diameter should be measured in a zoomed real-time image, from inner to inner outline of the vessel wall. Although the measurement from outer to inner wall is theoretically more accurate, the previous method seems to be more feasible because the flow inside the vessel should be calculated.

Angle Measurement

The correct angle measurement is also important for the flow velocity calculation. Fortunately, for measurements around 50°, the velocity calculation with ±4° angle error would still be within a ±5% accuracy range.[34] If the angle between the investigated vessel and the Doppler beam exceeds 60°, the error becomes unacceptably high.[4,34] This is the major reason why the sector scanners with the same crystal or aperture for imaging and Doppler do not allow reliable volume flow measurement.[34,35]

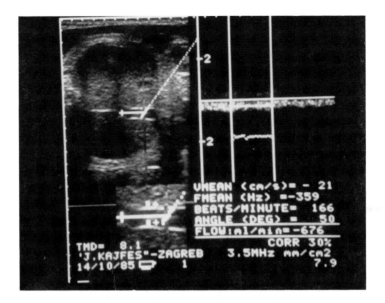

FIGURE 2.   Volume flow measurement in the umbilical vein. Cross-section of the
fetal abdomen with the umbilical vein is displayed on the left side of the image.
Vessel diameter is measured in the zoomed part of the image. The Doppler signal
is displayed on the right side of the image. Once the image is frozen and the angle
between the estimated flow direction and the Doppler beam and the vessel diameter
are measured, flow is calculated automatically.

Doppler Shift

The quality of the Doppler signal depends on the type and quality of the equipment,
and clinicians usually can do very little to improve its quality. Generally speaking, the quality
of the obtained signal is better if the real-time image is frozen while the Doppler signal is
acquired. Modern electronic equipment is capable of switching between imaging and Doppler
modes to permit real-time duplex imaging. However, it is at the expense of signal-to-noise
performance, thus decreasing the quality of the Doppler signal.[36]

A potential problem could be the depth limitation of the pulsed Doppler system determined by pulse repetition frequency (PRF). If the vessel of interest lies deep in the gravid
uterus and has high velocities (fetal aorta), the highest Doppler frequency can be picked up
with ambiguity.

According to the Nyquist theorem, the aliasing occurs when the Doppler shift exceeds
half the volume of the PRF. With the insonation angle of 40 to 60°, the PRF should be at
least 5 kHz for accurate recording of peak maximum velocities in investigated vessels,
especially when the Doppler shifts from fetal aorta and uterine circulation are recorded.
Fortunately, aliasing can be easily detected during measurements. In the currently used
Doppler units, the peak velocities that exceed half the value of PRF are shifted on the other
side of the zero line (see chapter on basic physics of ultrasound).

Two other possible sources of errors, especially as far as volume flow measurement is
concerned, are incorrect positioning of sample gate and incorrect high-pass filters.

It should be borne in mind that the sample gate should cover the entire lumen of the
vessel in order to detect all moving structures inside the vessel. On the other side, the sample
volume should not be too large, since it might include signals from other moving structures
in the surrounding tissue.

Before spectral analysis, the Doppler audio signal must go through a high-pass filter in
order to remove low-frequency signals produced by surrounding slow-moving tissue. Filters
of 600 Hz used a few years ago caused underestimation of flow calculation;[32] 150 Hz, as

a cut-off frequency, is nowadays generally accepted in the recent studies, although it should be even lower, especially in the FVW analysis *(vide infra)*.

Estimation of Fetal Weight

The volume flow is expressed in milliliters per minute per kilogram. Such calculation provides an answer to the question of whether the flow is reduced only in proportion to the fetal size, or whether the reduction is more severe. However, the problems in the antenatal ultrasound estimation of fetal weight[37,38] can significantly contribute to the error in volume flow measurement.

CLINICAL APPLICATION OF VOLUME FLOW MEASUREMENT

Besides the various limitations of volume flow measurement, the possibility of noninvasive and relatively simple investigation of circulatory changes in pregnancy resulted in significant interest and wide clinical application of the method. It was used in the early 1980s in order to detect impaired circulation in various pathological states in pregnancy, such as intrauterine growth retardation (IUGR), preeclampsia, Rh incompatibility, etc.[39-45]

However, the first published experiences were human *in vivo* studies in which the rate of umbilical blood flow was calculated in normal pregnancies.[31,39,46-50] An almost constant flow of approximately 110 ml/min/kg was found, with a gradual decrease toward the end of pregnancy.[30,33,40,50,51]

Further investigations claimed that volume flow measurement may have diagnostic value, especially in cases of IUGR. The average umbilical flow was significantly lower when compared with the normal values. In our study, 155 measurements were carried out in 45 patients with ultrasonic and clinical signs of IUGR by means of Kranzbuehler 8130 Doppler duplex equipment. The average umbilical blood flow was 73.4 ml/min/kg, significantly lower when compared with a flow of 106 ml/min/kg in the control group.

In the study of the Australian group, the estimated sensitivity and specificity for prediction of IUGR was 69 and 90%, respectively.[52]

The volume flow was also measured in the fetal aorta.[31,51,53,54] The flow estimation in normal pregnancies ranged between 200 and 246 ml/min/kg.[33,45,51]

All above-mentioned data suggest that volume flow measurement is a valuable diagnostic tool. Reduced flow seems to be strongly associated with pathologic pregnancy, especially growth retardation. However, it must be emphasized that satisfactory high sensitivity, specificity, and positive and negative predictive value were obtained only in the group of experts from Australia who introduced the technique.[52]

To achieve published results, expensive equipment, time-consuming examination, and specially trained and skilled personnel are indispensable. Therefore, it is hard to believe that the technique will be widely accepted for clinical purposes, especially today when faster and simpler FVW analyses have been introduced.

FLOW VELOCITY WAVEFORM ANALYSIS

Clinical trials all over the world have proved that measurement errors of flow are unacceptably high in routine work. The attention has been turned once again to the FVWs and their quantification. Actually, the first Doppler signals obtained from human circulation studies were FVWs from the umbilical artery.[55]

The FVW represents maximum Doppler shift throughout the cardiac cycle, reflecting the pulsatile nature of blood flow in arterial vessels. Its graphic representation is usually called the Doppler sonogram.

The shape of the waveform depends on the cardiac contraction force, the density of the blood, peripheral resistance, and other characteristics of the cardiovascular tree.[56]

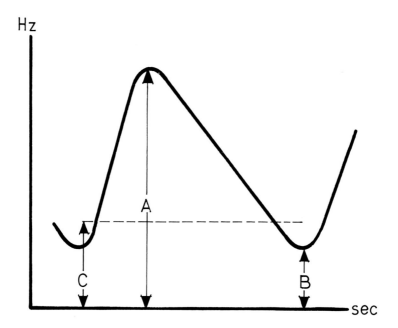

FIGURE 3.   Three parameters needed for FVW analysis: A = peak systole, B = end diastole, and C = mean velocity over one cardiac cycle.

Its major advantage in comparison with volume flow measurement is simple and angle-independent analysis. Furthermore, during analysis there is no need for simultaneous vessel visualization and diameter measurement.

More than ten various indices describing FVW have been used for assessment of vascular bed resistance in pregnancy.[32,57] Three of them, shown in Figure 3, which are predominantly used are

1.   A/B ratio[58] $= \dfrac{A}{B}$

2.   Resistance index (RI)[51] $= \dfrac{A - B}{A}$

3.   Pulsatility index (PI)[60] $= \dfrac{A - B}{C}$

The A/B ratio is sometimes also called the systolic/diastolic, or S/D, ratio. According to the recently published data, there are no arguments regarding preference of one index to the other.[61]

SOURCES OF ERRORS IN FVW ANALYSIS

Aliasing phenomenon as a potential source of error, i.e., underestimation of pulsatility, has already been described.

The presence of end diastolic flow is probably the most important information which can be obtained during the Doppler examination without measurement. Therefore, if the high-pass filter exceeds 50 Hz, data should be interpreted with extreme caution (Figures 4 and 5). Fortunately, with current machines, both potential sources of error could be easily overcome.

Fetal movements, breathing, and behavioral states alter the shape of the waveform

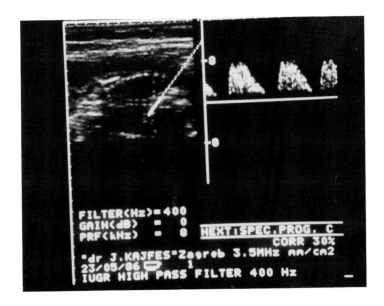

FIGURE 4. The Doppler sonogram of the fetal aorta with the high-pass filter set on 400 Hz. Complete absence of end diastolic flow indicating pathological peripheral resistance is present.

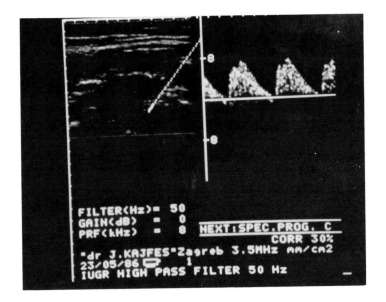

FIGURE 5. Same signal with high-pass filter set on 50 Hz. The lack of end diastolic flow is present only at the very end of diastole.

making the FVW analysis inaccurate.[62,63] There is a general agreement that recording and analysis of Doppler sonograms should be performed during fetal apnea and quiescence.

CLINICAL APPLICATION OF FVW ANALYSIS

UMBILICAL ARTERY

The FVWs can be obtained from at least three different points of the fetal circulation:

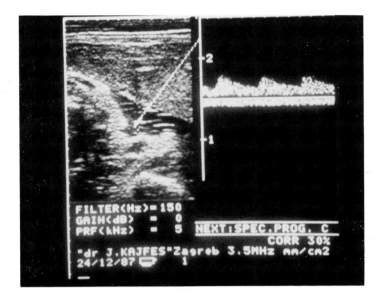

FIGURE 6.   Doppler sonogram of normal third-trimester umbilical artery flow.
The reverse flow of umbilical vein is displayed on the opposite side, below the zero
line.

fetal trunk, fetal brain, and umbilical cord. In the vast majority of reported studies, the
FVWs of the umbilical artery have been recorded and their value in the prediction of
pathologic pregnancy evaluated. The major reason for this is the fact that the signals from
the umbilical artery are very characteristic and easy to obtain (Figure 6). Even continuous-
wave equipment without simultaneous visualization of the umbilical cord on real-time image
can be used.[64,65]

We prefer combined real-time B mode imaging and pulsed Doppler system for clinical
purposes, in order to enable complete evaluation of uteroplacental and fetal circulation. The
real-time scanner is used to locate a loop of umbilical cord in the amniotic fluid, the sample
volume is placed in the luminal center of the artery, and the characteristic signal obtained.
The signal should be, if possible, analyzed when the FVWs from the umbilical artery and
low frequency signal of the umbilical vein are displayed simultaneously (Figure 6).

The pulsatility of the obtained signals decreases over the second half of pregnancy,
indicating a decrease in peripheral vascular resistance in the normal placenta (Figures 7 and
8).

Several groups of authors have found increased values of indices, mainly in IUGR
fetuses, suggesting increased peripheral placental resistance.[61,64-71] In severe cases, lack of
end diastolic flow or even reverse flow in the umbilical artery can be found, indicating an
extreme rise in peripheral resistance (Figures 9 to 11).

The estimated sensitivity of 78.3%,[65] or 58.3%[61] of the method, as a prospective diagnostic test for IUGR, is rather low. However, it should be borne in mind that our present
definition of IUGR (birth weight less than the tenth percentile) includes constitutionally
small fetuses.

Apart from IUGR, the umbilical artery waveforms have been also analyzed in diabetic
pregnancies,[72] placenta praevia,[73] twin gestation,[74] etc. As a general rule, the pathology was
always accompanied by increased pulsatility of the FVWs. Therefore, in the further evaluation of the method, the emphasis should be on its ability to predict fetal jeopardy regardless
of etiology.

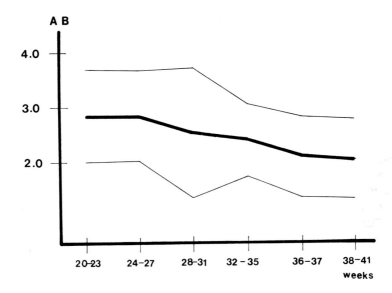

FIGURE 7.   A/B ratio in the umbilical artery during pregnancy. The data (n = 260) measured represent the means ± 2 SD.

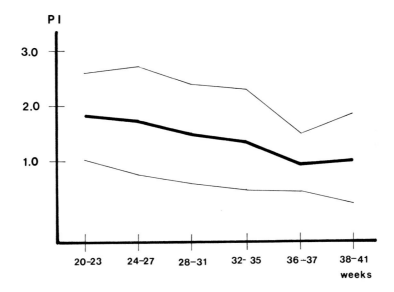

FIGURE 8.   Pulsality index values measured in umbilical artery (means ± 2 SD, n = 260).

FETAL AORTA

The fetal aorta is studied by orienting the transducer longitudinally along the fetus. Either the thoracic or abdominal part is visualized, and the sample volume of the Doppler beam placed over it.

If the pregnancy is normal, the FVW with the rather high pulsatility is obtained with the evident diastolic flow throughout the whole cardiac cycle (Figure 12).

The values of FVW indices of the fetal aorta have been measured in normal pregnancies[75,76] (Figures 13 and 14), as well as in pathologic ones.[75,77,79] The results suggest significantly elevated pulsatility expressed either by increased values of resistance index or pulsatility index.

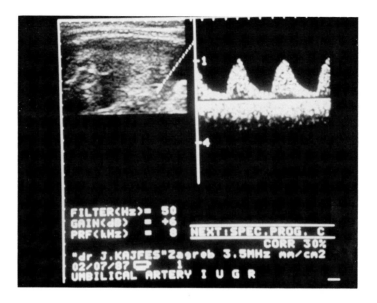

FIGURE 9.   Decreased end diastolic flow in the umbilical artery of a growth-retarded fetus.

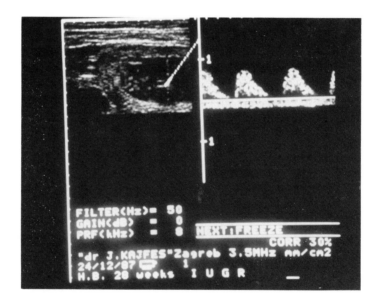

FIGURE 10.   Umbilical artery FVWs. Absent end diastolic flow in the severely growth-retarded fetus.

It seems that diminished flow through the descending aorta is a consequence of increased peripheral vascular resistance and selective redistribution of the cardiac output to the vital organs.

Especially important is the finding of absent end diastolic flow (Figure 15). Hackett et al.[80] compared 26 growth-retarded fetuses with absent end diastolic flow in the fetal aorta with 20 growth retarded fetuses with evident end diastolic flow. The former group were more likely to suffer perinatal death, necrotizing enterocolitis, and hemorrhage.

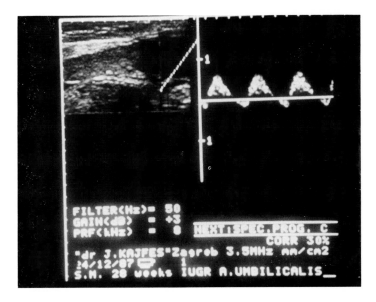

FIGURE 11.   Reverse flow in the umbilical artery. Ominous sign indicating extreme peripheral resistance.

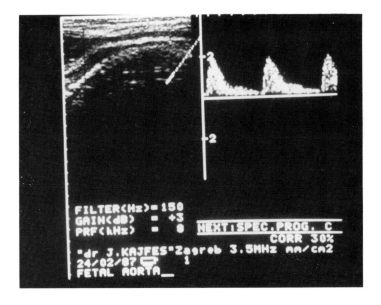

FIGURE 12.   Normal Doppler sonogram of fetal aorta.

   The presented data suggest that Doppler ultrasound visualization of circulatory changes (increased peripheral resistence) could provide a more sensitive sign of critical fetal compromise.

   If reproducible lack of end diastolic flow is observed, either in umbilical artery or fetal aorta, elective induction of labor or Cesarean section should be strongly considered.

INTRACRANIAL CIRCULATION

   The new generation of duplex system Doppler units enables the investigation of fetal

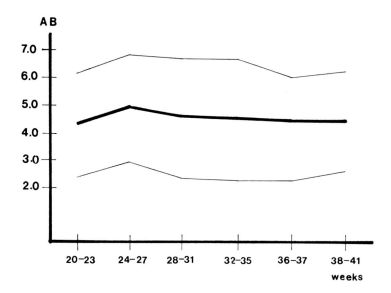

FIGURE 13.   A/B ratio measured in fetal aorta during pregnancy (means ± 2 SD, n = 260).

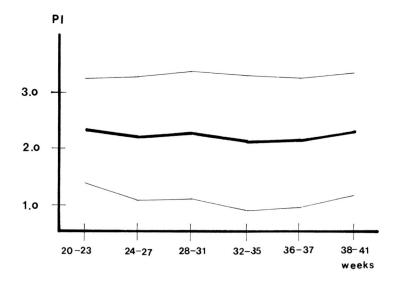

FIGURE 14.   Pulsality index values in fetal aorta (means ± 2 SD, n = 260).

intracranial circulation. Those investigations have been a logical extension of animal studies. It was shown that in animals, asphyxia *in utero* results in increased systemic vascular resistance, thus enabling the redistribution of oxygenated blood toward the brain and heart.[81,82]

Recent Doppler studies have suggested the presence of the same protective mechanism, the so-called "brain-sparing effect" in humans.[83,84]

The first reported studies of fetal cerebral circulation were reported in 1984 by Marsal et al.[83] They have recorded the FVWs of common carotid artery by visualizing its longitudinal axis in the fetal neck. It can be rather difficult to visualize the common carotid artery in frequently curved fetal neck and to obtain satisfactory FVWs. According to our opinion, the main disadvantage of the method is the fact that only one branch of the investigated vessel (internal carotid artery) actually represents cerebral blood flow.

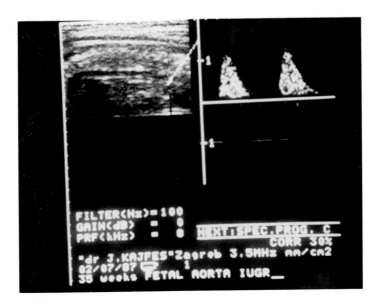

FIGURE 15. Doppler sonogram of fetal aorta in severe growth retardation. Note complete absence of end diastolic flow.

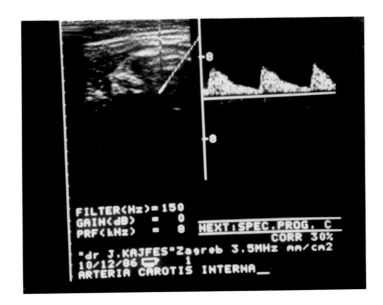

FIGURE 16. Normal Doppler sonogram of fetal internal carotid artery obtained in the third trimester.

The problem has been overcome by Wladimiroff et al.[84] They reported a technique for recording the FVWs from the intracranial part of internal carotid artery at the level of its bifurcation into the anterior and middle cerebral artery. To visualize the intracerebral portion of this vessel, it is necessary to direct the ultrasound transducer towards the base of the skull. Two pulsating structures in front of the heart-shaped brain stem representing the terminal parts of the internal carotid artery are visualized. The sample volume of the duplex system is placed on one of them (Figures 16 and 17).

Using the described technique, Wladimiroff et al.[84] have shown marked reduction of

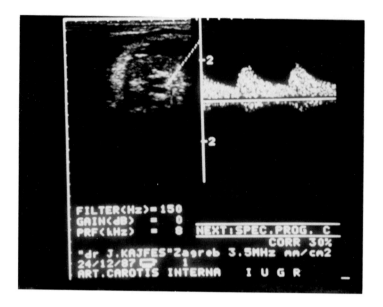

FIGURE 17.   Decreased pulsatility of Doppler sonogram of fetal carotid artery indicating "brain-sparing effect".

the pulsatility index (PI) in the internal carotid artery with its concomitant rise in fetal aorta and umbilical artery in nine antenatally detected and postnatally confirmed growth-retarded fetuses.

Two other arteries have been also used in order to detect changes in cerebral blood flow during fetal compromise. Kurjak et al.[85] have started to record FVWs from the fetal middle cerebral artery (MCA). A high level of reproducibility and the possibility of direct comparison with postnatal events was reported.

Arabeille et al.[86] suggested a technique to record FVWs at the level of anterior cerebral artery by performing a parasagittal view of the fetal face and directing the transducer towards the base of the skull.

Regardless of the investigated vessel, the isolated examination of cerebral blood flow in fetuses at risk seems to be of limited usefulness in the prediction of growth defects. Several reports have suggested that the value of prediction can be increased if the ratio between indices of umbilical and intracranial circulation are used.[86,89]

PELVIC CIRCULATION

Using the full-bladder technique, it is possible to analyze not only the anatomical structures of the female pelvis, but also the blood flow in pelvic vessels.[90,91] The FVWs of iliac vessels are characterized by high pulsatility that reflects high peripheral resistance. Ovarian arteries can be demonstrated on real-time images in 66% of cases. By placing the sample volume over the anterior and lateral part of the ovary, the signals that represent ovarian blood flow can be obtained in 55% of nonvisualized ovarian arteries.[91]

Taylor et al.[90] have performed invasive studies of pelvic circulation at open surgery and through the vaginal fornices directly by applying the Doppler transducer over the external and internal iliac and ovarian arteries. Characteristics of obtained signals correlated well with the previously performed transabdominal studies.

An important observation was the difference in FVWs from contralateral ovarian arteries. The FVWs from the artery that supplied the ovary with the dominant follicle had lower PI values, indicating low pulsatility and increased blood flow. The ovarian artery from the contralateral side showed absence of diastolic flow that implied high peripheral resistance.

The described differences can be observed early in the follicular phase of the menstrual cycle, well before the dominant follicle can be visualized on real-time ultrasound images.

We have not been able to find the significant differences in characteristics of the ovarian blood flow FVWs during the follicular, periovulatory, and early luteal phase of the cycle. Although it was suggested that midcycle luteinizing hormone (LH) surge could cause marked dilatation of ovarian artery and increased blood flow,[92] it was not supported in our investigation.

Signals from the uterine artery at the level of the cervix are regularly recorded. They are similar to the shape of internal iliac artery FVWs. On the contrary, terminal branches of the uterine artery are inconstantly recorded. When obtained, they are similar to the waveforms of the ovarian artery on the side of the nonfunctioning ovary.

At present, Doppler studies of pelvic circulation cannot be used for better prediction and more accurate diagnosis of ovulation. Their value in the assessment of adequacy of follicle development, diagnosis of luteal phase defects, and early diagnosis of ovarian neoplasms should be carefully evaluated in the future.

EARLY PREGNANCY

The Doppler studies of the pelvic circulation have been expanded to the first trimester of pregnancy.[90,93,94] Preliminary results failed to recognize a difference in blood flow pattern in threatened abortion.[94] However, further investigation, especially with transvaginal sonography, may be of clinical interest.[93]

ARCUATE ARTERIES

During the first trimester of pregnancy, more than 100 uteroplacental arteries convert into low-resistance vessels.[95,96] The process is known as "trophoblast invasion" and has two stages. The wave of trophoblast migration from the decidua invades the decidual segments of the spiral arteries in the first trimester, and the myometrial segments in the second trimester.[97,98]

Further pathohistologic investigations have shown that in preeclampsia and in a proportion of pregnancies with IUGR infants, the physiological vascular changes are restricted to the decidual segments of uteroplacental arteries.[97,99,100] It has been speculated that absence of "trophoblast invasion" could reduce perfusion of intervillous space because the myometrial arteries retain their musculo-elastic coat. Indeed, Campbell et al.[101] demonstrated that in pregnancy complicated by hypertension and IUGR, decreased end diastolic flow in uterine circulation could be found.

The FVWs of arcuate artery can be obtained either abdominally[101] or vaginally.[102] We prefer the abdominal approach in which the transducer should be directed to the lateral pelvic wall to identify FVWs of external or internal iliac artery. When the transducer is tilted closer to the amniotic cavity, the typical signal of arcuate artery showing a pattern of low pulsatility with high velocities in diastole is obtained (Figures 18 to 20).

A highly pulsatile waveform in that region would imply a pathological finding (Figures 21 and 22). Therefore, *"quid pro quo"* with the internal iliac artery or uterine artery should be avoided. If the arcuate artery FVWs are recorded in the opposite channel of that in which iliac artery signals are obtained, the possibility of error will be decreased to the minimum.

Campbell has studied 126 singleton pregnancies at 18 weeks of gestation in order to assess the predictive value of a pathological finding in the arcuate artery for pregnancy-induced hypertension, IUGR, and fetal asphyxia.[103] The satisfactory results were reported (66% of IUGR was predicted correctly), and the method was proposed as an early second-trimester screening test to indicate high-risk pregnancies.

Undoubtedly, there are cases of growth retardation in which changes in uterine perfusion are the primary event. On the other hand, there is also much speculation whether the fetus determines its placenta and uteroplacental blood flow.[16] Unfortunately, the proportions of

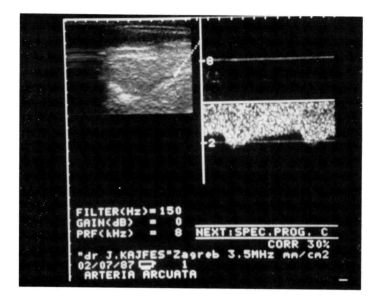

FIGURE 18. Doppler sonogram of the normal second-trimester arcuate artery.

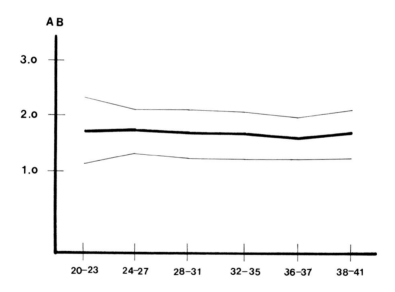

FIGURE 19. A/B ratio in arcuate artery (means ± 2 SD, n = 260).

both events are not known, neither in a low- nor in a high-risk population. Therefore, the belief that screening for only one possible factor of impaired fetal growth can be cost effective seems to be too enthusiastic for the time being.

Until the cost effectiveness of such a screening program is fully evaluated, the FVW analysis of the arcuate artery should remain an important part of comprehensive Doppler blood studies in a high-risk pregnant population.

CONCLUSION

From all that was said, it is obvious that with Doppler ultrasound, perinatologists finally

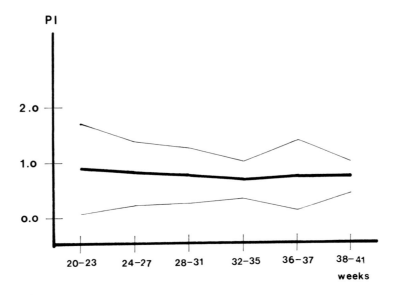

FIGURE 20.   PI values measured in arcuate artery (means ± 2 SD, n = 260).

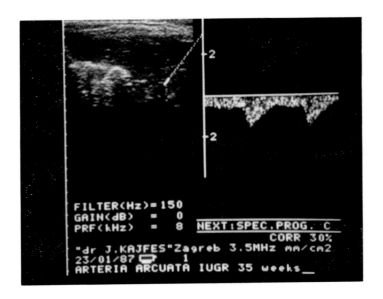

FIGURE 21.   Increased pulsatility in the arcuate artery. Reproducible finding would indicate increased peripheral resistance in uterine circulation.

have the opportunity to perform noninvasive studies of circulatory changes in human pregnancy under physiological circumstances. In the last few years, the method has proven valid in the detection of altered blood flow in already recognized pathologic pregnancies. However, the two most important questions of perinatology still have to be answered.

1.   Is the fetus really jeopardized regardless of the mother's status?
2.   Has the time to deliver the baby come?

We are still waiting to see whether Doppler ultrasound is capable of giving the answers to these two crucial questions of perinatology.

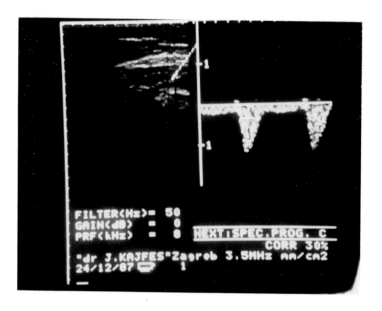

FIGURE 22.   Extreme pulsatility in Doppler sonogram of arcuate artery in a case of severe EPH gestosis.

REFERENCES

1. **Assali, N. S.,** Ontogenic developments of neurohumoral control of fetal and neonatal cardiovascular functions, in *Ultrasuoni in Obstetrica,* Destro, F., Ed., Monduzzi, Bologna, 1981, 121.
2. **Kuenzel, W.,** Umbilical circulation — physiology and pathology, *J. Perinat. Med.,* 9, 68, 1981.
3. **Salvadori, B. A.,** History of the measurement of fetal blood flow, in *Measurement of Fetal Blood Flow,* Kurjak, A., Ed., CIC, Rome, 1984, 1.
4. **Tonge, H. M.,** A Doppler Ultrasound Study of Human Fetal Vascular Dynamics, thesis, Drukkerij, J. H. and Pasmans, B. V., Grevenhage, 1987, 11.
5. **Cohnstein, J. and Zuntz, N.,** Untersuchungen uber das Blut, den Kreislauf, und die Athmung beim Saugethier Foetus, *Pfluger's Arch. Gesamte. Physiol. Menschen Tiere,* 39, 1056, 1975.
6. **Barcroft, J.,** Foetal circulation and respiration, *Physiol. Rev.,* 16, 103, 1936.
7. **Barcroft, J.,** *Researches on Pre-Natal Life,* Charles C Thomas, Springfield, IL, 1947, 1.
8. **Cooper, K. E. and Greenfield, A. D. M.,** A method for measuring blood flow in the umbilical vessels, *J. Physiol.,* 233, H465, 1949.
9. **Greenfield, A. D. M., Shepherd, J. F., and Whelan, R. F.,** The rate of blood flow in the umbilical cord, *Lancet,* ii, 422, 1951.
10. **Edelstone, D. I., Rudolph, A. M., and Heymann, M. A.,** Liver and ductus venosus blood flows in fetal lambs in utero, *Circ. Res.,* 42, 426, 1978.
11. **Dawes, G. S. and Mott, J. C.,** Changes in O_2 distribution and consumption in foetal lambs with variations in umbilical blood flow, *J. Physiol.,* 170, 524, 1964.
12. **Kirschbaum, T. H., Lucas, W. E., Dehaven, J. C., and Assali, N. S.,** The dynamics of placental oxygen transfer, *Am. J. Obstet. Gynecol.,* 98, 429, 1967.
13. **Meschia, G., Cotter, J. R., Breathnach, S., and Barron, D. H.,** The diffusibility of oxygen across the sheep placenta, *Q. J. Exp. Physiol.,* 50, 446, 1965.
14. **Meschia, G., Cotter, J. R., Makowski, E. L., and Barron, D. H.,** Simultaneous measurement of uterine and umbilical blood flows and oxygen uptakes, *Q. J. Exp. Physiol.,* 52, 1, 1966.
15. **Makowski, E. L., Meschia, G., Droegenmueller, W., and Battaglia, F. C.,** Distribution of uterine blood flow in the pregnant sheep, *Am. J. Obstet. Gynecol.,* 101, 409, 1968.
16. **Rankin, P. G. H. and McLaughlin, M. K.,** The regulation of the placental blood flows, *J. Dev. Physiol.,* 1, 3, 1979.

17. **Oakes, G. K., Walker, A. M., Ehrenkranz, R. A., and Chez, R. A.,** Effect of propranolol infusion on the umbilical artery and uterine circulations of pregnant sheep, *Am. J. Obstet. Gynecol.*, 41, 197, 1976.
18. **Berman, W., Goodlin, R. C., Heymann, M. A., and Rudolph, A. M.,** Measurement of umbilical blood flow in fetal lambs in utero, *J. Appl. Physiol.*, 39, 1056, 1975.
19. **Longo, L. D. and Reneu, D. D., Eds.,** *Fetal and Newborn Cardiovascular Physiology,* Garland STPM Press, New York, 1978, 1.
20. **Longo, L. D., Wyatt, J. F., Hewitt, C. W., and Gilbert, R. D.,** A comparison of circulatory responses to hypoxic hypoxia and monooxide hypoxia in fetal blood flow and oxygenation, in *Fetal and Newborn Cardiovascular Physiology,* Longo, L. D. and Reneu, D. D., Eds., Garland STPM Press, New York, 1978, 256.
21. **Stembera, Z. K., Hodr, J., and Janda, J.,** Umbilical blood flow in newborn infants who suffer intrauterine hypoxia, *Am. J. Obstet. Gynecol.*, 91, 568, 1965.
22. **Assali, N. N., Douglass, R. A., Baird, W. W., Jr., Nicholson, D. B., and Suyemoto, R.,** Measurement of uterine blood flow and uterine metabolism. IV. Results in normal pregnancy, *Am. J. Obstet. Gynecol.*, 66, 248, 1953.
23. **Assali, N. S., Rauramo, L., and Peltonen, T.,** Measurement of uterine blood flow and uterine metabolism. VIII. Uterine and fetal blood flow and oxygen consumption in early pregnancy, *Am. J. Obstet. Gynecol.*, 79, 86, 1960.
24. **Stembera, Z. K., Hodr, J., Ganz, V., and Fronek, A.,** Measurement of umbilical cord blood by thermodilution, *Am. J. Obstet. Gynecol.*, 90, 780, 1964.
25. **McCallum, W. D.,** Thermodilution measurement of human umbilical blood flow at delivery, *Am. J. Obstet. Gynecol.*, 127, 491, 1977.
26. **Doppler, J. C.,** Uber das farbige Licht der Dopplersterne und einiger anderer Gestirne des Himmels, *Abh. Konig. Bohem. Ges. Wiss.*, 11, 465, 1842.
27. **Buys Ballot, C. H. D.,** Akustische Versuche auf der Niederlandishen Eisenbahn, nebst gelegentlichen Bemerkungen zur Theorie des Hrn. Prof. Doppler, *Pogg. Ann. Bd. LXVI*, 11, 321, 1845.
28. **Jonkman, E. J.,** An historical note. Doppler research in the nineteenth century, *Ultrasound Med. Biol.*, 6, 1, 1980.
29. **Satomura, S.,** A study on examining the heart with ultrasonics. I. Principles. II. Instrument, *Jpn. Circ. J.*, 20, 227, 1956.
30. **Gill, R. W. and Kossoff, G.,** Pulsed Doppler combined with B-mode scanning for blood flow measurement, *Contrib. Gynecol. Obstet.*, 6, 139, 1979.
31. **Eik-Nes, S. H., Marsal, K., Brubbakk, A. O., Kristoffersen, K., and Ulstein, M.,** Ultrasound measurement of human fetal blood flow, *J. Biomed. Eng.*, 4, 28, 1982.
32. **Cohen-Overbeek, T., Pearce, J. M., and Campbell, S.,** The antenatal assessment of utero-placental and fetoplacental blood flow using Doppler ultrasound, *Ultrasound Med. Biol.*, 11, 329, 1985.
33. **Eik-Nes, S. H., Marsal, K., and Krisoffersen, K.,** Noninvasive measurement of human fetal blood flow, in *Measurements of Fetal Blood Flow,* Kurjak, A., Ed., CIC, Rome, 1984, 73.
34. **Warnking, K.,** Errors in quantitative Doppler measurements, in *Doppler Techniques in Obstetrics,* Jung, H. and Fendel, H., Eds., Georg Thieme Verlag, Stuttgart, 1986, 2.
35. **Griffin, D., Cohen-Overbeek, T., and Campbell, S.,** Fetal and utero-placental blood flow, *Clin. Obstet. Gynecol.*, 10, 565, 1983.
36. **Burns, P. N.,** The physical principles of Doppler and spectral analysis, *J. Clin. Ultrasound*, 15, 567, 1987.
37. **Kurjak, A. and Breyer, B.,** Estimation of fetal weight by ultrasonic abdominometry, *Am. J. Obstet. Gynecol.*, 125, 962, 1976.
38. **Hill, L. M., Breckie, R., Wolfgram, K. R., and O'Brien, P. C.,** Evaluation of three methods for estimating fetal weight, *J. Clin. Ultrasound*, 14, 171, 1986.
39. **Kurjak, A. and Rajhavjn, B.,** Ultrasonic measurements of umbilical blood flow in normal and complicated pregnancies, *J. Perinat. Med.*, 10, 3, 1982.
40. **Kurjak, A., Ed.,** *Measurements of Fetal Blood Flow,* CIC, Rome, 1984, 103.
41. **Kirkinen, P., Jouppila, P., and Eik-Nes, S. H.,** Umbilical vein blood flow in rhesus isoimmunization, *Br. J. Obstet. Gynaecol.*, 90, 7, 1983.
42. **Tonge, H. M., Struijk, P. C., and Wladimiroff, J. W.,** Blood flow measurements in the fetal descending aorta: technique and clinics, *Clin. Cardiol.*, 7, 323, 1984.
43. **Gill, R. W., Warren, P. S., Garrett, W. J., and Kossoff, G.,** Measurement of umbilical blood flow, a potential diagnostic test?, in *Measurements of Fetal Blood Flow,* Kurjak, A., Ed., CIC, Rome, 1984, 91.
44. **Gill, R. W., Kossoff, G., Warren, P. S., and Garrett, W. J.,** Umbilical venous flow in normal and complicated pregnancies, *Ultrasound Med. Biol.*, 10, 349, 1984.
45. **Jouppila, P. and Kirkinen, P.,** The role of fetal blood flow in obstetrics, in *Measurements of Fetal Blood Flow,* Kurjak, A., Ed., CIC, Rome, 1984, 127.

46. **Gill, R. W.,** Pulsed Doppler with B-mode imaging for quantitative blood flow measurement, *Ultrasound Med. Biol.,* 5, 223, 1979.

47. **Gill, R. W., Trudinger, B. J., Garrett, W. J., Kossoff, G., and Warren, P. S.,** Fetal umbilical venous flow measured in utero by pulsed Doppler and B-mode ultrasound. I. Normal pregnancies, *Am. J. Obstet. Gynecol.,* 139, 720, 1981.

48. **Eik-Nes, S. H., Brubbakk, A. O., and Ulstein, M. K.,** Measurement of human fetal blood flow, *Br. Med. J.,* 280, 283, 1980.

49. **Wladimiroff, J. W. and McGie, J.,** Ultrasonic assessment of cardiovascular geometry and function in the human fetus, *Br. J. Obstet. Gynaecol.,* 88, 870, 1981.

50. **Jouppila, P., Kirkinen, P., Eik-Nes, S. H., and Koivula, A.,** Fetal and intervillous blood flow measurements in late pregnancy, in *Recent Advances in Ultrasound Diagnosis,* Kurjak, A. and Kratochwill, A., Eds., Excerpta Medica, Amsterdam, 1981, 226.

51. **Griffin, D., Teague, M. J., Tallet, P., Willson, K., Bilardo, K., Massini, L., and Campbell, S.,** A combined ultrasonic linear array scanner and pulsed Doppler velocimeter for the estimation of blood flow in the foetus and adult abdomen. II. Clinical evaluation, *Ultrasound Med. Biol.,* 11, 37, 1985.

52. **Gill, R. W., Kossoff, G., Warren, P. S., Stewart, A., and Garrett, W. J.,** Umbilical artery velocity waveform and umbilical vein volume flow in the assessment of high risk pregnancies in the third trimester, in *Recent Advances in Ultrasound Diagnosis,* Vol. 6, Kurjak, A. and Kossoff, G., Eds., Anali Opce bolnice "Dr. Josip Kajfes", Zagreb, 1987, 41.

53. **Laurin, J., Marsal, K., Persson, P., and Lingman, G.,** Ultrasound measurement of fetal blood flow in predicting fetal outcome, *Br. J. Obstet. Gynaecol.,* 94, 940, 1987.

54. **Marsal, K., Lindblad, A., Lingman, G., and Eik-Nes, S. H.,** Blood flow in the fetal descending aorta; intrinsic factors affecting fetal blood flow, i.e., fetal breathing movements and cardiac arrhythmia, *Ultrasound Med. Biol.,* 10, 339, 1984.

55. **FitzGerald, D. E. and Drumm, J. E.,** Non-invasive measurement of the fetal circulation using ultrasound: a new method, *Br. J. Obstet. Gynaecol.,* 2, 1450, 1977.

56. **McDonald, D. A.,** *Blood Flow in Arteries,* 2nd ed., Edward Arnold, London, 1974, 1.

57. **Thompson, R. S., Trudinger, B. J., and Cook, C. M.,** A comparison of Doppler ultrasound waveform indices in the umbilical artery. I. Indices derived from the maximum velocity waveform, *Ultrasound Med. Biol.,* 12, 835, 1986.

58. **Stuart, B., Drumm, J., FitzGerald, D. E., and Duignan, N. M.,** Fetal blood velocity waveforms in normal pregnancy, *Br. J. Obstet. Gynaecol.,* 87, 780, 1980.

59. **Pourcelot, L.,** Applications cliniques de l'examen Doppler transcutane, in *Velocimetrie Ultrasonore Doppler,* Vol. 34, Peronneau, P., Ed., Seminaire INSERM, Paris, 1974, 213.

60. **Gosling, R. G. and King, D. H.,** Ultrasound angiology, in *Arteries and Veins,* Marcus, A. W. and Adamson, L., Eds., Churchill Livingstone, Edinburgh, 1975, 61.

61. **Mulders, L. G. M., Wijn, P. F. F., Jongsma, H. W., and Hein, P. R.,** A comparative study of three indices of umbilical blood flow in relation to prediction of growth retardation, *J. Perinat. Med.,* 15, 3, 1987.

62. **Mires, G., Dempster, J., Patel, N. B., Crawford, J. W.,** The effect of fetal heart rate on umbilical artery flow velocity waveforms, *Br. J. Obstet. Gynaecol.,* 94, 665, 1987.

63. **Van Eyck, J., Wladimiroff, J. W., Van den Wijngaard, J. A. G., Noordam, M. J., and Prechtl, H. F. R.,** The blood flow velocity waveform in the fetal internal carotid and umbilical artery; its relation to fetal behavioural states in normal pregnancy at 37—38 weeks, *Br. J. Obstet. Gynaecol.,* 94, 736, 1987.

64. **Trudinger, B. J., Giles, W. B., Cook, C. M., Bombardieri, J., and Collins, L.,** Fetal umbilical artery flow velocity waveforms and placental resistance: clinical significance, *Br. J. Obstet. Gynaecol.,* 92, 23, 1985.

65. **Fleisher, A., Shulman, H., Farmakides, G., Bracero, L., Blattner, P., and Randolph, G.,** Umbilical artery velocity waveforms and intrauterine growth retardation, *Am. J. Obstet. Gynecol.,* 151, 502, 1985.

66. **Reuwer, P. J. H. M., Bruinse, H. W., Stoutenbeek, P., and Haspels, A. A.,** Doppler assessment of the fetoplacental circulation in normal and growth-retarded fetuses, *Eur. J. Obstet. Gynecol. Reprod. Biol.,* 18, 199, 1984.

67. **Oakes, G. K., Walker, A. M., Ehrenkranz, R. A., and Chez, R. A.,** Effect of propranolol infusion on the umbilical artery and uterine circulations of pregnant sheep, *Am. J. Obstet. Gynecol.,* 41, 197, 1976.

68. **Trudinger, B. J., Cook, C. M., Jones, L., and Giles, W. B.,** A comparison of fetal heart rate monitoring and umbilical artery waveforms in the recognition of fetal compromise, *Br. J. Obstet. Gynaecol.,* 93, 171, 1986.

69. **Rochelson, B. L., Schulman, H., Flesiher, A., Farmakides, G., Bracero, L., Ducey, J., Winter, D., and Penny, B.,** The clinical significance of Doppler umbilical artery velocimetry in the small for gestational age fetus, *Am. J. Obstet. Gynecol.,* 156, 1223, 1987.

70. **Rochelson, B., Schulman, H., Farmakides, G., Bracero, L., Ducey, J., Fleisher, A., Penny, B., and Winter, D.,** The significance of absent end-diastolic velocity in umbilical artery velocity waveforms, *Am. J. Obstet. Gynecol.,* 156, 1213, 1987.

71. **McCowan, L. M., Erskine, L. A., and Ritchie, K.,** Umbilical artery Doppler blood flow studies in the preterm, small for gestational age fetus, *Am. J. Obstet. Gynecol.,* 156, 655, 1987.

72. **Bracero, L., Schulman, H., Fleisher, A., Farmakides, G., and Rochelson, B.,** Umbilical artery velocimetry in diabetes and pregnancy, *Obstet. Gynecol.,* 68, 654, 1986.

73. **DeVore, G. R., Brar, H. S., and Platt, L. D.,** Doppler ultrasound in the fetus: a review of current applications, *J. Clin. Ultrasound,* 15, 687, 1987.

74. **Giles, W. B., Trudinger, B. J., and Cook, C. M.,** Fetal umbilical artery flow velocity-time waveforms in twin pregnancies, *Br. J. Obstet. Gynecol.,* 92, 490, 1985.

75. **Griffin, D., Bilardo, K., Masini, L., Diaz-Recasens, J., Pearce, J. M., Wilson, K., and Campbell, S.,** Doppler blood flow waveforms in the descending thoracic aorta of the human fetus, *Br. J. Obstet. Gynaecol.,* 91, 997, 1984.

76. **Lingman, G. and Marsal, K.,** Fetal central blood circulation in the third trimester of normal pregnancy — a longitudinal study. II. Aortic blood velocity waveform, *Early Hum. Dev.,* 13, 151, 1986.

77. **Jouppila, P. and Kirkinen, P.,** Increased vascular resistance in the descending aorta of the human fetus in hypoxia, *Br. J. Obstet. Gynaecol.,* 91, 853, 1984.

78. **Jouppila, P and Kirkinen, P.,** Blood velocity waveforms of the fetal aorta in normal and hypertensive pregnancies, *Obstet. Gynecol.,* 67, 856, 1986.

79. **Tonge, H. M., Wladimiroff, J. W., Noordam, M. J., and Van Kooten, C.,** Blood flow velocity waveforms in the descending fetal aorta: comparison between normal and growth-retarded pregnancies, *Obstet. Gynecol.,* 67, 851, 1986.

80. **Hackett, G. A., Campbell, S., Gamsu, H., Cohen-Overbeek, T., and Pearce, J. M. F.,** Doppler studies in growth retarded fetus and prediction of neonatal necrotising enterocolitis, haemorrhage, and neonatal morbidity, *Br. Med. J.,* 294, 13, 1987.

81. **Kjellmer, I., Karlsonn, K., Olsson, T., and Rosen, K. G.,** Cerebral reactions during intrauterine asphyxia in the sheep. I. Circulation and oxygen consumption in the fetal brain, *Pediatr. Res.,* 8, 50, 1974.

82. **Johnson, G. N., Palahnuik, R. J., Tweed, W. A., Jones, M. V., and Wade, J. G.,** Regional cerebral blood flow changes during severe fetal asphyxia produced by slow partial umbilical cord compression, *Am. J. Obstet. Gynecol.,* 135, 48, 1979.

83. **Marsal, K., Lingman, G., and Giles, W.,** Evaluation of the carotid, aortic and umbilical blood flow velocity, in Proc. Soc. for the Study of Fetal Physiology, XI Annu. Conf., Oxford, 1984, C33.

84. **Wladimiroff, J. W., Tonge, H. M., and Stewart, P. A.,** Doppler ultrasound assessment of cerebral blood flow in the human fetus, *Br. J. Obstet. Gynaecol.,* 93, 471, 1986.

85. **Kurjak, A., Alfirevic, Z., Rizzo, G., and Arduini, D.,** Utero-placental and fetal circulation in intrauterine growth retardation, in *Intrauterine Growth Retardation — Diagnosis and Treatment,* Kurjak, A. and Beazley, J., Eds., CRC Press, Boca Raton, FL, 1988, in press.

86. **Arbeille, P., Roncin, A., Berson, M., Patat, F., and Pourcelot, L.,** Exploration of the fetal cerebral blood flow by Duplex Doppler — linear array system in normal and pathological pregnancies, *Ultrasound Med. Biol.,* 13, 329, 1987.

87. **Wladimiroff, J. W., Van Wijngaard, J. A. G. W., Degani, S., Noordam, M. J., Van Eyck, J., and Tonge, H. M.,** Cerebral and umbilical arterial blood flow velocity waveforms in normal and growth-retarded pregnancies, *Obstet. Gynecol.,* 69, 705, 1987.

88. **Wladimiroff, J. W., Noordam, M. J., Van Wijngaard, J. A. G. W., and Deagani, S.,** Pulsatility index in fetal and umbilical vessels during normal pregnancy and intrauterine growth retardation, in *Recent Advances in Ultrasound Diagnosis,* Vol. 6, Kurjak, A. and Kossoff, G., Eds., Anali Opce Bolnice "Dr. Josip Kajfes", Zagreb, 1987, 59.

89. **Rizzo, G., Arduini, D., Romanini, C., and Mancuso, S.,** The value of blood flow assessment in predicting growth retardation, in *Recent Advances in Ultrasound Diagnosis,* Vol. 6, Kurjak, A. and Kossoff, G., Eds., Anali Opce Bolnice "Dr. Josip Kajfes", Zagreb, 1987, 23.

90. **Taylor, K. J. W., Burns, P. N., Wells, P. N. T., Conway, D. I., and Hull, M. G. R.,** Ultrasound Doppler flow studies for the ovarian and uterine arteries, *Br. J. Obstet. Gynaecol.,* 92, 240, 1985.

91. **Kurjak, A. and Jurkovic, D.,** Ultrasound Doppler studies of blood flow in the pelvic vessels, in *Ultrasound and Infertility,* Kurjak, A., Ed., CRC Press, Boca Raton, FL, 1988, in press.

92. **Trimor-Tritsch, I. E. and Rottem, S.,** The appearance of the early abnormal pregnancy by a 6.5 MHz transvaginal probe, in *Euroson '87,* Proc. 6th Congr. of the European Federation of Societies for Ultrasound in Medicine and Biology, Bondstam, A., Alanen, A., and Jouppila, P., Eds., Finnish Society for Ultrasound in Medicine and Biology, Helsinki, 1987, 208.

93. **McSweeney, M. B., Warren, P. S., Baber, R. J., Kossoff, G., and Gill, R. W.,** Transvaginal Doppler assessment of pelvic vascularity in early pregnancy: a collaborative study, in Book of Abstracts, Australian Society for Ultrasound in Medicine, 17th Annual Scientific Meeting, Canberra, ACT, 1987, 38.

94. **Stabile, I., Bilardo, K., Campbell, S., and Grudzinskas, J. G.,** Doppler assessed uterine blood flow in the first trimester of pregnancy, in *Euroson '87,* Proc. 6th Congr. of the European Federation of Societies for Ultrasound in Medicine and Biology, Bondestam, S., Alanen, A., and Jouppila, P., Eds., Finnish Society for Ultrasound in Medicine and Biology, Helsinki, 1987, 184.

95. **Brosens, I. and Dixon, H. G.,** Anatomy of the maternal side of the placenta, *J. Obstet. Gynecol. Br. Commonw.,* 73, 357, 1966.

96. **Brosens, I., Robertson, W. B., and Dixon, H. G.,** The physiological response to the vessels of the placental bed to normal pregnancy, *J. Pathol. Bacteriol.,* 93, 569, 1967.

97. **Robertson, W. B., Brosens, I., and Dixon, H. G.,** Uteroplacental vascular pathology, *Eur. J. Obstet. Gynecol. Reprod. Biol.,* 5, 47, 1975.

98. **Pijnenborg, R., Bland, J. M., Robertson, W. B., and Brosens,** I. Uteroplacental arterial changes related to interstitial trophoplast migration in early human pregnancy, *Placenta,* 2, 303, 1983.

99. **Sheppard, B. L. and Bonnar, J.,** An ultrastructural study of uteroplacental spiral arteries in hypertensive and normotensive pregnancy and fetal growth retardation, *Br. J. Obstet. Gynaecol.,* 88, 695, 1981.

100. **McFadyen, I. R., Price, A. B., and Geirsson, R. T.,** The relation of birthweight to histological appearances in vessels of the placental bed, *Br. J. Obstet. Gynaecol.,* 93, 476, 1986.

101. **Campbell, S., Diaz-Recasens, J., Griffin, D. R., Cohen-Overbeek, T., Pearce, J. M., Willson, K., and Teague, M. J.,** New Doppler technique for assessing uteroplacental blood flow, *Lancet,* i, 675, 1983.

102. **Fleisher, A., Schulman, H., Farmakides, G., Bracero, L., Grunfeld, L., Rochelson, B., and Koenigsberg, M.,** Uterine artery Doppler velocimetry in pregnant women with hypertension, *Am. J. Obstet. Gynecol.,* 154, 806, 1986.

103. **Campbell, S., Pearce, J. M. F., Hackett, G., Cohen-Overbeek, T., and Hernandez, C.,** Qualitative assessment of uteroplacental blood flow: early screening test for high-risk pregnancies, *Obstet. Gynecol.,* 68, 649, 1986.

Chapter 5

BLOOD FLOW AND BEHAVIORAL STATES IN THE HUMAN FETUS

J. van Eyck and J. W. Wladimiroff

INTRODUCTION

Since Fitzgerald and Drumm[1] first reported on the measurement of blood flow velocity in the umbilical cord by means of continuous wave Doppler ultrasound, our knowledge of the human fetal cardiovascular system has rapidly expanded. Measurements on volume blood flow in umbilical vein and fetal descending aorta using pulsed wave Doppler ultrasound were first described by Gill and Kossoff[2] and Eik-Nes et al.[3] However, errors that arise from single measurement of vessel diameter and fetal weight estimations by ultrasound have resulted in attention turning to two alternative methods of assessing fetal blood flow. First, combined analysis of the blood flow velocity and pulsatile vessel diameter waveforms has been used for more accurate calculation of volume flow in the lower part of the fetal descending aorta.[4] It was demonstrated that the marked rise in aortic stroke volume (= pulsatile flow integrated over one cardiac cycle) during normal late pregnancy is entirely correlated with the pronounced increase in aortic diameter. Moreover, it was calculated that the percentage of total cardiac stroke volume directed to the descending aorta varies between 65 and 80%. Second, calculation of angle-independent parameters such as the A/B ratio, resistance index, and pulsatility index (PI) is a method used in the lower thoracic part of the fetal descending aorta,[5-7] umbilical artery,[8-10] and fetal common carotid[11,12] and internal carotid artery.[13] For a correct interpretation of recorded data, it is of importance to establish the effect of internal variables, e.g., fetal breathing movements, fetal heart rate (FHR) and rhythm, and fetal behavioral states. Blood flow velocity waveforms in the fetal descending aorta, umbilical artery,[14] and internal carotid artery[15] are clearly modulated by fetal breathing movements. In a study of fetal cardiac arrhythmias (atrioventricular blocks and supraventricular tachycardias), Tonge et al.[16,17] were able to confirm an earlier report by Marsál et al.[14] that despite alterations in rhythm, blood flow in the fetal descending aorta is maintained within the normal range. In the human fetus, behavioral states were studied from FHR recordings alone[18,19] and in conjuction with body movements,[20,21] resulting in the description of quiet and activity phases. The observations did not provide conclusive proof of the presence of true behavioral states in the human fetus, since both FHR and FHR variability are affected by fetal motility.[22]

Nijhuis et al.[23] stated that the presence of behavioral states can only be established following fulfillment of a number of criteria: (1) particular conditions of several variables must recur in specific, fixed combinations; (2) these combinations must be temporarily stable; and (3) there should be clear state transitions. It was therefore necessary to study several independent variables with respect to the consistency and stability of their association and the simultaneity of their transition from one condition to another. Nijhuis et al.[23] clearly identified four distinct fetal behavioral states on the basis of eye and body movements and FHR patterns in low-risk multigravidae as from 36 to 38 weeks of gestation.

State 1F — Quiescence, which can be regularly interrupted by brief gross body movements, mostly startles. Eye movements absent. Heart rate stable, with a small oscillation band width (less than ten beats per minute [bpm]); isolated accelerations occur. These are strictly related to movements. This heart rate pattern is called FHRP-A.

State 2F — Frequent and periodic gross body movements — mainly stretches and retroflexions — and movements of the extremities. Eye movements continually present (REMs and SEMs). Heart rate (called FHRP-B) with a wider oscillation band width (>10 bpm) than FHRP-A, and frequent accelerations during movements.

State 3F — Gross body movements absent. Eye movements continually present. Heart rate (called FHRP-C) stable, but with a wider oscillation band width than FHRP-A and no accelerations.

State 4F — Vigorous, continual activity including many trunk rotations. Eye movements continually present (when observable). Heart rate (called FHRP-D) unstable, with large and long-lasting accelerations, frequently fused into a sustained tachycardia.

At 38 weeks of gestation, the distribution of percentages of stage 1F to 4F is respectively 32, 42, 1, and 7%.[23]

Based on the marked changes in FHR pattern and incidence of fetal body movements between different behavioral states, it is not unlikely that these changes are associated with alterations in fetal cardiovascular performance. Doppler flow measurements are increasingly performed during the early first trimester of pregnancy for the early detection and evaluation of intrauterine growth retardation (IUGR). At 27 to 28 weeks of gestation, there already is a clear periodicity of state variables. Still, there is no proper synchronization in their cyclic appearance, thus allowing elucidation of the relation between separate state variable and the blood flow velocity waveform in the fetal descending aorta.

The purpose of this chapter is to review the latest reports on the relationship between the blood flow velocity waveform in the lower thoracic part of the fetal descending aorta, fetal internal carotid, and umbilical artery and fetal behavioral states, in particular, stage 1F and 2F according to the classification of Nijhuis et al.[23] in the normal growing and growth-retarded human fetus at term. Second, the relationship will be discussed between separate state variables and the blood flow velocity waveform in the lower thoracic part of the fetal descending aorta in the human fetus at 27 to 28 weeks of gestation.

NORMAL GROWING FETUS AT 37 to 38 WEEKS OF GESTATION

FETAL DESCENDING AORTA (n = 13)

Using a combined real-time scanner and pulsed Doppler system as described by Eik-Nes et al.,[3] the mean blood flow velocity at the lower thoracic level of the fetal descending aorta was recorded. Mean flow velocity waveforms were recorded during fetal behavioral states 1F and 2F according to Nijhuis et al.[23] These two behavioral states were studied because of the high incidence of 1F (32%) and 2F (42%) at 38 weeks and the marked differences in FHR pattern, fetal eye movements, and fetal body movements between these two behavioral states.[23]

In order to establish fetal behavioural states, the following parameters were simultaneously recorded:

1. The FHR, which was obtained from a Doppler ultrasound Cardiotocograph (Hewlett Packard 8040A, carrier frequency 1 MHz).
2. Fetal eye movements which were studied from a transverse view of the fetal face using the Diasonics CV 400 (carrier frequency 3.5 MHz).
3. Fetal body movements from a two-dimensional real-time linear array scanner (Toshiba Sal 20A, carrier frequency 3.5 MHz) for a sagittal view of the fetal trunk.

The three transducers were placed in such a way, that there was minimal interference between the three ultrasound modes (Figure 1). Flow velocity recordings were only performed when a clear fetal behavioral state was identified and when this state had been present over

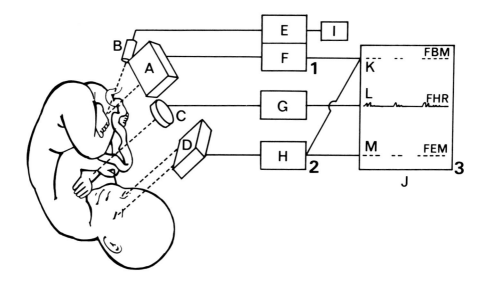

FIGURE 1. Schematic design of the way a recording is performed. (A) Real-time linear array scanner (fetal body movements); (B) pulsed Doppler system fixed to A under an angle of 45°; (C) FHR transducer; (D) real-time linear array scanner (fetal eye and head movements); (E) Organon Teknika Cadiovisor 03; (F) Pedoff (pulsed Doppler); (G) Hewlett Packard 8040A cardiotocograph; (H) Toshiba SaL 20 A; (I) Apple® III microcomputer for analysis of the flow velocity data; (J) three-channel writer; (K) input fetal body movements (head, trunk, extremities); (L) input FHR pattern; (M) input fetal eye movement; (1) person 1 who registers fetal body movements and performs flow velocity measurements; (2) person 2 who registrates fetal eye and head movements; (3) person 3 who identifies fetal behavioral states and gives the signal to start flow velocity measurements.

a period of at least 3 min. All recordings were performed during fetal apnea, with the subject in the semirecumbent position. All studies were carried out 2 h following a meal and had to last at least 1 h. The maximum amount of time for the completion of a flow velocity recording following a state determination was 3 min. The blood flow velocity waveform at the lower thoracic part of the fetal descending aorta was recorded over a 5-s period which included, on average, ten consecutive cardiac cycles. In each flow velocity recording, at least seven optimal cardiac cycles were selected, and the mean value for the peak velocity (PV, (centimeters per second), end diastolic velocity (EDV, (centimeters per second), averaged velocity (AV, centimeters per second), and instantaneous FHR was calculated (Figure 2).

The degree of pulsatility of the waveform was quantified by calculating the PI according to Gosling and King[24] using a microcomputer (Apple® III). The PI changes predominantly reflect changes in peripheral vascular resistance. Since at normal fetal heart rates, changes in cardiac output are mainly regulated through changes in FHR,[25,26] it was decided to standardize cardiac output by dividing the PI values in each subject and for each fetal behavioral state into groups, each of which representing an FHR range of 5 bpm. This standardization will also rule out the effect of cardiac cycle length dependency of the PI when comparing PI values between behavioral states 1F and 2F. The mean number of cardiac cycles studied for all 13 patients was 55 (minimum 26; maximum 95) in state 2F, a total of 1480 cycles. FHR in state 1F ranged between 103 and 171 bpm and in state 2F between 94 and 185 bpm. Paired analysis of the PI data in state 1F and 2F was feasible in the FHR range between 121 to 150 bpm in a total number of 1320 cardiac cycles.

Table 1 shows the statistical significance of the paired differences in PI, EDV, PV, and AV between states 1F and 2F per FHR range. A lower PI and higher EDV was observed in state 2F as compared with state 1F. PV and AV demonstrated no statistical significant

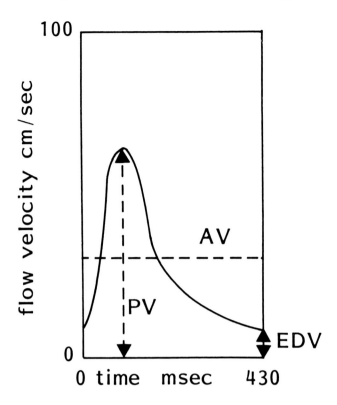

FIGURE 2.   Flow velocity profile at the lower thoracic level of the fetal descending aorta at 37 to 38 weeks of gestation. PV = peak velocity (cm/sec); EDV = end diastolic velocity (cm/sec); AV = averaged velocity (cm/sec).

difference between states 1F and 2F per FHR ranges studied. A significant reduction (p <0.001) in PI with increasing FHR was established, which was mainly determined by a significant rise (p <0.02) in EDV. Figure 3 depicts for each FHR the mean PI in state 1F and 2F for all 1480 cardiac cycles studied (93 to 185 bpm).

The elevated EDV in the fetal descending aorta suggesting reduced fetal peripheral vascular resistance in behavioral state 2F may be explained by the need for an increased perfusion of the fetal skeletal musculature (trunk and lower extremities) to meet the energy demands during raised muscular activity in this particular behavioral state.[27]

FETAL INTERNAL CAROTID AND UMBILICAL ARTERY (n = 15)

A combined mechanical sector scanner and pulsed Doppler system (Diasonics CV 400) was used for recording the maximum flow velocity waveform in the fetal internal carotid artery at the level of the bifurcation into the middle and anterior cerebral artery (Figure 4)[13] and for recording the maximum flow velocity waveform in the umbilical artery. Only recordings depicting simultaneous arterial venous flow velocity patterns were accepted as originating from the umbilical cord. Venous blood flow had to be constant to ensure fetal apnea. In the fetal internal carotid and umbilical artery, the blood flow velocity waveforms were recorded on videotape over a 15-s period which included an average of 30 consecutive cardiac cycles. In each subject, a minimum of three flow velocity waveform recordings in each vessel in each behavioral state (1F and 2F) was obtained. From hard copies of each flow velocity recording, an average 20 cardiac cycles of optimal quality were selected.

In three subjects, the blood flow velocity recordings in the fetal internal carotid artery in either behavioral state 1F or 2F had to be rejected due to poor quality or was not obtained

TABLE 1
Statistical Significance of the Paired Differences in Pulsatility Index (ΔPI), End Diastolic Velocity (ΔEDV), Peak Velocity (ΔPV), and Averaged (ΔAV) per FHR range

FHR range (bpm)	n	Δ 1F-2F	PI (SD)	p	Δ 2F-1F	EDV (SD)	p	Δ 1F-2F	PV (SD)	p	Δ 2F-1F	AV (SD)	p
121—125	8	0.43	0.21	<0.001	2.70	2.78	<0.05	7.36	4.75	<0.01	1.06	1.82	<0.20*
126—130	9	0.36	0.17	<0.001	2.66	1.53	<0.001	3.41	6.09	<0.20*	1.99	1.76	<0.01
131—135	10	0.35	0.18	<0.001	2.98	2.40	<0.01	4.80	8.07	<0.20*	1.26	2.78	<0.20*
136—140	9	0.33	0.21	<0.002	4.48	3.05	<0.01	2.47	2.32	<0.02	2.04	2.66	<0.10*
141—145	10	0.38	0.24	<0.001	5.01	2.21	<0.001	2.00	6.22	>0.20*	2.57	3.07	<0.05
146—150	6	0.26	0.19	<0.05	3.05	2.49	<0.05	3.44	7.92	>0.20*	1.05	2.89	>0.20*

Note: Statistical significance as determined by paired student t test; n = number of paired observations per FHR range; asterisk denotes statistically insignificant values.

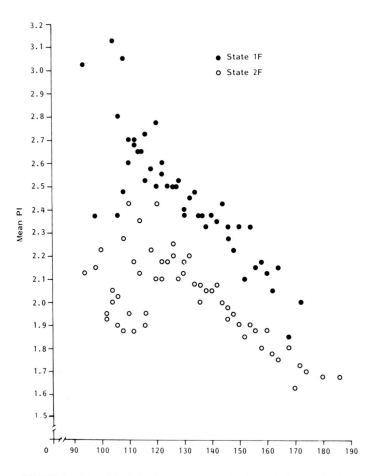

FIGURE 3. Mean PI of the flow velocity profile for each FHR at the lower thoracic level of the fetal descending aorta relative to FHR in all cardiac cycles studied.

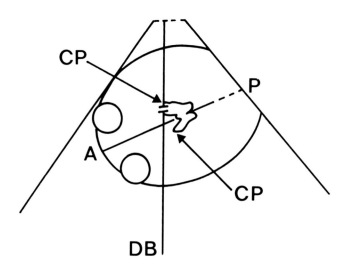

FIGURE 4. Schematic representation of the fetal head at the level of the bifurcation of the fetal internal carotid artery into the middle and anterior cerebral artery. A — anterior; P — posterior; DB — Doppler beam; CP — cerebral peduncle.

TABLE 2

**Mean Paired PI Difference (Δ PI ± 1 SD) between Fetal Behavioral
States 1F and 2F in the FHR Range between 121 and 145 bpm in the
Fetal Internal Carotid Artery for Normal Pregnancy**

FHR range (bpm)	Number of paired observations	Mean PI		ΔPI	SD	Significance
		State 1F	State 2F			
121—125	8	1.58	1.20	0.38	0.13	$p < 0.001$
126—130	10	1.59	1.23	0.36	0.16	$p < 0.001$
131—135	9	1.49	1.18	0.31	0.16	$p < 0.001$
136—140	10	1.60	1.24	0.36	0.21	$p < 0.001$
141—145	8	1.54	1.19	0.35	0.18	$p < 0.001$

at all as a result of hiccups, breathing, or excessive body movements or deep engagement of the fetal head. The mean number of cardiac cycles studied in the fetal internal carotid artery for all 12 subjects was 56 (minimum 47; maximum 68) in state 1F and 59 (minimum 26; maximum 76) in state 2F, a total of 1381 cycles.

FHR in state 1F ranges between 109 and 164 bpm, and in state 2F between 109 and 185 bpm. Paired analysis of the PI data in state 1F and 2F was feasible in the FHR range between 121 and 145 bpm in a total number of 1021 cardiac cycles. There is a statistically significant difference in mean PI between states 1F and 2F for all of the FHR ranges studied (Table 2). Figure 5 demonstrates the regression lines for the correlation between PI and FHR in states 1F (continuous lines) and 2F (dotted lines) for all 12 subjects. A significant reduction in PI with increasing FHR was established in states 1F ($p < 0.005$) and 2F ($p < 0.001$). The decrease in PI in the internal carotid artery during behavioral state 2F, as demonstrated in our study, suggests a reduction in peripheral vascular resistance in the fetal brain. The mean number of cardiac cycles studied in the umbilical artery for all 15 subjects was 59 (minimum 38; maximum 82) in state 1F and 58 (minimum 33; maximum 76) in state 2F, a total of 1752 cycles. FHR ranged in state 1F between 105 and 185 bpm. Paired analysis of the flow velocity data in states 1F and 2F was statistically feasible in the FHR range between 121 and 150 bpm in a total of 1449 cycles. The 95% confidence interval of the paired differences in mean PI between states 1F and 2F displayed a narrow distribution around zero, reflecting a virtual overlap of PI values originating from states 1F and 2F (Table 3). Figure 6 demonstrates for each FHR the mean PI in states 1F and 2F for all 15 subjects studied (102 to 188 bpm). An inverse relationship between PI and FHR both in behavioral states 1F ($p < 0.05$) and 2F ($p < 0.001$) was established. Whereas in normal pregnancies and under standardized FHR conditions the PI in the lower thoracic part of the fetal descending aorta[27] and fetal internal carotid artery[28] depicts significant changes with respect to the fetal behavioral state, this is not so for the umbilical artery.[28] This fetal behavioral state independency suggests a fetal regulatory mechanism for the state-dependent changes in the fetal descending aorta and internal carotid artery. The decrease in PI with rising FHR observed in all three vessels studied is mainly determined by the definition presented by Gosling and King[24] for PI calculations, i.e., at a lower FHR, a more gradual end diastolic slow-down of the blood flow velocity takes place.

GROWTH-RETARDED FETUS (<10%) AT 37 TO 38 WEEKS OF GESTATION

FETAL DESCENDING AORTA (n = 12)

The mean number of cardiac cycles studied for all 12 patients was 81 (minimum 32; maximum 127) in state 1F and 86 (minimum 52; maximum 153) in state 2F, a total of 2004

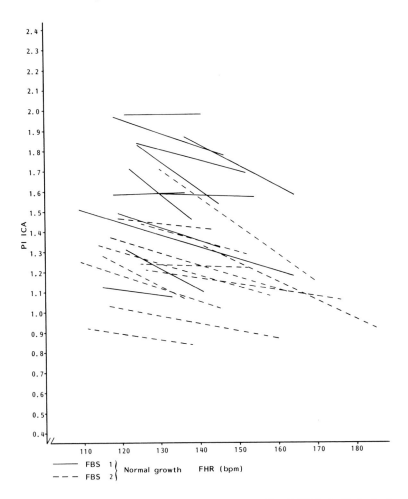

FIGURE 5. Regression lines for the correlation between PI and FHR in fetal behavioral states 1F (continuous lines) and 2F (dotted lines) in the fetal internal carotid artery for all 12 normal pregnancies.

TABLE 3
Mean Paired PI Difference (ΔPI $\pm$ 1 SD) between Fetal Behavioral States 1F and 2F in the FHR Range between 121 and 150 bpm in the Umbilical Artery for Normal Pregnancy

FHR range (bpm)	Number of paired observations	Mean PI		ΔPI	SD	Significance	95% confidence interval
		State 1F	State 2F				
121—125	9	0.83	0.83	0.00	0.05	$p >0.20$ (NS)[a]	−0.04,0.04
126—130	12	0.84	0.80	0.04	0.08	$p >0.10$ (NS)	−0.01,0.09
131—135	14	0.84	0.82	0.02	0.11	$p >0.20$ (NS)	−0.04,0.08
136—140	11	0.80	0.79	0.01	0.09	$p >0.20$ (NS)	−0.05,0.07
141—145	11	0.79	0.76	0.03	0.10	$p >0.20$ (NS)	−0.04,0.10
146—150	7	0.83	0.77	0.06	0.09	$p >0.10$ (NS)	−0.02,0.14

[a] NS = not significant.

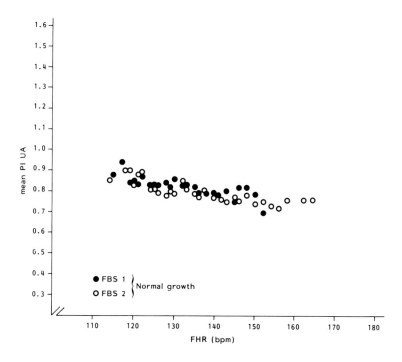

FIGURE 6.   Mean PI in the umbilical artery in fetal behavioral states 1F (FBS 1) and
2F (FBS 2) relative to FHR for all 15 normal pregnancies.

TABLE 4
The 95% Confidence Interval of the Paired Difference in Mean PI, EDV, AV, and PV between States 1F and 2F for Each of the FHR Ranges Studied

FHR range	Mean PI 1F minus mean PI 2F	95% confidence interval			
		PI	EDV (cm/s)	AV (cm/s)	PV (cm/s)
121—125	0.02	−0.14, +0.18	−1.99, +0.81	−0.88, +1.68	−3.60, +3.60
126—130	0.01	−0.12, +0.14	−1.20, +1.54	−2.14, +2.06	−6.50, +5.14
131—135	0.09	−0.02, +0.22	−1.51, +2.07	−1.49, +1.23	−4.95, +3.05
136—140	0.02	−0.11, +0.03	−1.41, +0.77	−2.42, +1.12	−5.68, +3.96
141—145	−0.05	−0.01, +0.11	−0.40, +1.22	−1.97, +0.39	−6.54, +0.68
146—150	0.00	−0.08, +0.10	−1.17, +1.15	−1.85, +1.21	−6.66, +3.62
151—155	0.04	−0.06, +0.12	−1.01, +0.83	−2.28, +1.02	−6.77, +0.43
156—160	−0.04	−0.15, +0.09	−2.28, +1.70	−3.53, +3.67	−8.62, +7.42
161—165	0.01	−0.01, +0.03	−8.86, +5.90	−2.77, +2.21	−20.33, +15.11

cycles. FHR in state 1F ranged between 111 and 169 bpm, and in state 2F between 115 and 176 bpm. Paired analysis of the flow velocity data in states 1F and 2F was statistically feasible in the FHR range between 121 and 165 bpm, resulting in 9 groups, e.g., 121 to 125, 126 to 130, ... 161 to 165 bpm, a total of 1888 cardiac cycles. The 95% confidence interval of the paired difference in mean PI between states 1F and 2F displayed for each FHR range a narrow distribution around zero, reflecting a virtual overlap of PI values originating from states 1F and 2F (Table 4). Using Student t test, a significant reduction ($p < 0.001$) in PI with increasing FHR was established in both states 1F and 2F (Figure 7). In Figure 8, all PI values from the growth-retarded (Figure 7) and normal growing population (Figure 3) are plotted together. Note the markedly elevated PI levels in IUGR, particularly at lower heart rates, and their virtual overlap when relating these values to states 1F and 2F.[29]

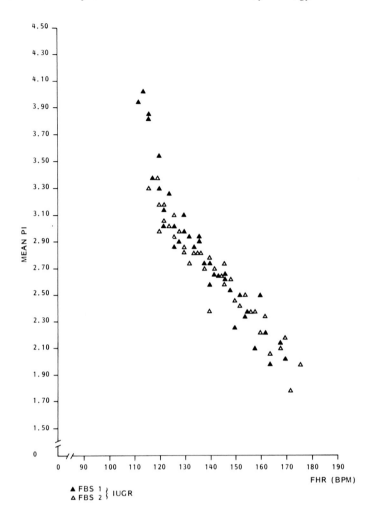

FIGURE 7.   Mean PI in states 1F (FBS 1) and 2F (FBS 2) relative to FHR in IUGR.

In IUGR, the PI in the descending aorta demonstrated a marked increase compared to normal pregnancy. Whereas in the normal fetus increased peripheral perfusion documented by a reduction in PI and rise in EDV was established in state 2F, this change did not occur in IUGR. This may be explained by the fact that chronic hypoxia present in IUGR stimulates the peripheral arterial chemoreceptors[30,31] and subsequent release of vasoconstrictive agents, such as vasopressin and catecholamines.[32-34] This peripheral vasoconstriction seems to overrule state-dependent PI fluctuations. Consequently, the increased energy demand needed for raised muscular activity during state 2F may not be adequately met.

FETAL INTERNAL CAROTID AND UMBILICAL ARTERY (n = 8)

The mean number of cardiac cycles studied in the fetal internal carotid artery for all 8 subjects was 50 (minimum 31; maximum 72) in state 1F and 48 (minimum 29; maximum 63) in state 2F, a total of 782 cycles. FHR in state 1F ranged between 98 and 158 bpm, and in state 2F between 115 and 167 bpm. When calculating the mean PI independent of FHR behavioral state, all eight values were situated below -1 SD and in two patients below -2 SD of the nomogram according to Wladimiroff et al.[35] The mean number of cardiac cycles studied in the umbilical artery was 47 (minimum 15; maximum 66) in state 1F and

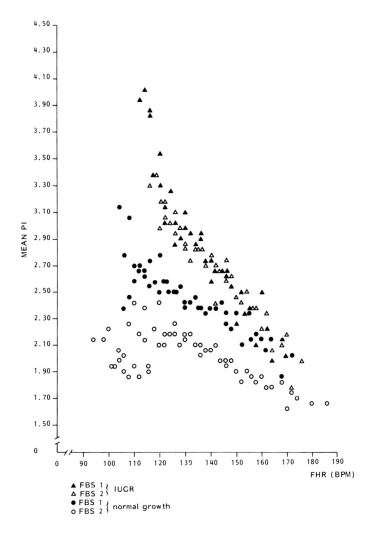

FIGURE 8. Mean PI in states 1F and 2F in IUGR and in normal growth (see Figure 3) relative to FHR.

41 (minimum 18; maximum 62) in state 2F, a total of 699 cycles. FHR in state 1F ranged between 99 and 171 bpm, and in state 2F between 107 and 162 bpm. The mean PI, irrespective of FHR and behavioral state, was situated above $+1$ SD in all eight patients and above $+2$ SD in five patients according to the nomogram by Wladimiroff et al.[36] Paired analysis of the PI data in states 1F and 2F was feasible for the fetal internal carotid artery in the FHR range between 126 and 145 bpm (561 cardiac cycles) and for the umbilical artery, also in the FHR range between 126 and 145 bpm (529 cardiac cycles). There was no statistically significant difference in mean PI between states 1F and 2F for all FHR ranges studied in the fetal internal carotid artery[37] (Table 5) and umbilical artery[37] (Table 6). Moreover, the 95% confidence interval of the paired differences in mean PI between states 1F and 2F displayed for each FHR range a narrow distribution around zero, reflecting a virtual overlap of PI values originating from states 1F and 2F. A significant inverse relationship between PI and FHR was established for both behavioral states 1F ($p < 0.001$) and 2F ($p < 0.01$) in the umbilical artery and for behavioral state 1F ($p < 0.001$) in the fetal internal carotid artery. Whereas flow velocity waveforms in the internal carotid artery of normal pregnancies demonstrated reduced PI values during state 2F, reflecting a decrease in cerebral vascular resistance during this behavioral state, this state dependency seems to be absent during IUGR.

TABLE 5
Mean Paired PI Difference (Δ PI ± 1 SD) and 95% Confidence Interval between Fetal Behavioral States 1F and 2F in the FHR Range between 126 to 145 bpm in the Fetal Internal Carotid Artery in IUGR

FHR range (bpm)	Number of paired observations	Mean PI		ΔPI	SD	Significance	95% confidence interval
		State 1F	State 2F				
126—130	7	1.09	1.14	−0.05	0.28	$p >0.20$ (NS)[a]	−0.31,0.21
131—135	7	1.05	1.14	−0.09	0.22	$p >0.20$ (NS)	−0.29,0.11
136—140	8	1.01	1.07	−0.06	0.18	$p >0.20$ (NS)	−0.21,0.09
141—145	7	0.97	1.10	−0.13	0.21	$p >0.10$ (NS)	−0.33,0.07

NS = not significant.

TABLE 6
Mean Paired PI Difference (Δ PI ± SD) and 95% Confidence Interval between Fetal Behavioral States 1F and 2F in the FHR Range between 126 to 145 bpm in the Umbilical Artery in IUGR

FHR range (bpm)	Number of paired observations	Mean PI		ΔPI	SD	Significance	95% confidence interval
		State 1F	State 2F				
126—130	5	1.13	1.17	−0.04	0.15	$p >0.20$ (NS)[a]	−0.23,0.15
131—135	6	1.26	1.27	−0.01	0.10	$p >0.20$ (NS)	−0.11,0.09
136—140	7	1.24	1.23	0.01	0.13	$p >0.20$ (NS)	−0.11,0.13
141—145	6	1.20	1.19	−0.01	0.13	$p >0.20$ (NS)	−0.15,0.13

[a] NS = not significant.

In contrast to the marked PI increase in the fetal descending aorta, state independency in the fetal internal carotid artery was associated with only moderate reduction in PI, suggesting the onset of circulatory redistribution with the aim of favoring cerebral blood flow (brain-sparing effect). The degree of PI reduction at this stage seems, however, to be sufficient to overrule behavioral state dependency. The inverse relationship between PI and FHR for both states 1F and 2F and the fetal descending aorta and umbilical artery and for state 1F if the fetal internal carotid artery is mainly determined by the cycle length dependency of the formula from which the PI is calculated.

NORMAL GROWING FETUS AT 27 TO 28 WEEKS OF GESTATION

FETAL DESCENDING AORTA (n = 13)

At 27 to 28 weeks of gestation, there are episodes of low (<10 bpm) heart rate variability (FHRP-A) and high (>10 bpm) heart rate variability (FHRP-B), with and without fetal eye movements (FEM) and fetal body movements (FBM). There is no proper synchronization in the cyclic appearance of these variables. Periods of coincidence occur often by change and will result in the occurrence of eight combinations of state parameters.

The data analysis was carried out in two steps.[38] First, all PI values obtained from epochs with combined presence (code 111) or absence (code 000) of FHRP-B, FEM, and FBM were compared. Analysis of the mean PI differences per FHR range of 5 bpm was performed using the paired Student t test. Second, the relationship between individual state

TABLE 7
Code and Mean Duration for Each State
Parameter Combination as Percentage of Time

State variable combinations			Code	Time %	SD
FHRP-A	FEM −	FBM −	000	15.4	6.1
FHRP-A	FEM −	FBM +	001	7.6	5.7
FHRP-A	FEM +	FBM −	010	1.9	3.2
FHRP-A	FEM +	FBM +	011	3.9	6.8
FHRP-B	FEM −	FBM −	100	8.6	7.2
FHRP-B	FEM −	FBM +	101	33.4	10.0
FHRP-B	FEM +	FBM −	110	1.3	2.1
FHRP-B	FEM +	FBM +	111	27.9	10.0

variables and PI was studied. Analysis of the relationship with FHRP consisted of comparison of the following four pairs of coincidences of state parameters: 000-100, 001-101, 010-110, and 011-111. In this way, flow velocity waveforms were obtained from epochs, in which FHRP was the only variable in combination with the same FEM and FBM distribution. Analysis of the relationship with FEM consisted of comparison of 000-010, 001-011, 100-110, and 101-111; analysis of the relationship with FBM led to the comparison of 000-001, 010-011, 100-101, and 110-111. Again, the PI data were standardized for FHR and divided into groups of 5 bpm each. Analysis of the mean PI differences per FHR range of 5 bpm was performed using the paired student t test when at least five or more paired observations per FHR range were obtained. The mean duration of a recording was 69.5 ± 9.5 min, which may be considered sufficient for completion of a quiet-active cycle.[39] Table 7 shows that episodes of low FHR variation (FHRP-A) were observed in 28.8%, and episodes of high FHR variation were observed in 71.2% of the total recording time. The mean number of cardiac cycles studied in the fetal descending aorta for each subject during epochs with the state variable combination FHRP-A, FEM (−), FBM (−) was 27 (minimum 7; maximum 57) and with the state variable combination FHRP-B, FEM (+), FBM (+) was 28 (minimum 8; maximum 64), a total of 722 cardiac cycles.

Paired analysis of the PI data for both combinations was feasible in the FHR range between 136 to 160 bpm, resulting in 5 groups, i.e., 136 to 140, 141 to 145, ... 156 to 160 bpm, a total of 458 cardiac cycles.

There is a statistically significant reduction in mean PI in the presence of state parameter combination FHRP-B, FEM (+), FBM (+) (Table 8). A statistically significant inverse relationship between PI and FHR was established in both combinations ($p < 0.05$).

The mean PI differences (PI ± 1 SD) per FHR range between state variable combinations in which FHRP-A or FHRP-B is present, is depicted in Table 9. Paired analysis was feasible between the combinations 011-111 and 001-101 in a total of 255 cardiac cycles. A statistically significant reduction in mean PI is demonstrated in the presence of FHRP-B as compared with FHRP-A. In the combinations 010-110 and 000-100, the number of paired observations was too small to allow statistical analysis. In Table 10, the mean PI difference (PI ± 1 SD) per FHR range between state variable combinations in which FEM are absent or present is shown. Paired analysis was feasible between the combinations 101-111 and 000-010 in a total of 528 cardiac cycles. There is no statistically significant change in mean PI relative to the absence or presence of FEM. In the combinations 100-110 and 001-011, statistical analysis was not feasible. There is no absence or presence of FBM, as can be seen in Table 11. Paired analysis was feasible in the combinations 000-001 and 100-101 in a total of 233 cardiac cycles. In the combinations 110-111 and 010-011, the number of paired observations was not sufficient to allow statistical analysis. The presented data at 27 to 28 weeks of

TABLE 8

Mean Paired PI Difference (Δ PI $\pm$ 1 SD) per FHR Range between Combined Absence (Code 000) and Presence (Code 111) of FHRP-B, FEM, and FBM in the Fetal Descending Aorta

FHR range (bpm)	Number of paired observations	Mean PI for code 000	Mean PI for code 111	ΔPI	SD	Statistical significance
136—140	8	2.47	1.99	0.48	0.22	$p <0.001$ (S)[a]
141—145	9	2.39	1.96	0.43	0.44	$p <0.02$ (S)
146—150	7	2.32	1.84	0.48	0.18	$p <0.001$ (S)
151—155	7	2.33	1.95	0.38	0.31	$p <0.02$ (S)
156—160	6	2.35	2.03	0.32	0.18	$p <0.01$ (S)

[a]   S = significant.

TABLE 9

Mean Paired PI Difference (Δ PI $\pm$ 1 SD) per FHR Range between State Parameter Combinations in which FHRP-A or FHRP-B is Present

FHR range (bpm)	Number of paired observations	Mean PI for code 011	Mean PI for code 111	ΔPI	SD	Statistical significance
146—150	5	2.36	1.91	0.45	0.29	$p <0.02$ (S)[a]
151—155	5	2.49	1.97	0.52	0.33	$p <0.02$ (S)
156—160	5	2.39	1.95	0.44	0.29	$p <0.02$ (S)
146—150	5	2.43[b]	2.05[c]	0.38	0.16	$p <0.01$ (S)

[a]   S = significant.
[b]   Mean PI for code 001.
[c]   Mean PI for code 101.

TABLE 10

Mean Paired PI Difference (Δ PI $\pm$ 1 SD) per FHR Range between State Parameter Combinations in which FEM are Absent or Present

FHR range (bpm)	Number of paired observations	Mean PI for code 101	Mean PI for code 111	ΔPI	SD	Statistical significance
131—135	5	2.33	2.29	0.04	0.37	$p >0.2$ (NS)[a]
136—140	10	2.11	1.97	0.14	0.33	$p >0.2$ (NS)
141—145	8	2.12	1.91	0.21	0.25	$p <0.1$ (NS)
146—150	7	2.11	2.01	0.10	0.28	$p >0.2$ (NS)
151—155	6	2.11	2.00	0.11	0.37	$p >0.2$ (NS)
156—160	5	2.02	2.13	-0.11	0.40	$p >0.2$ (NS)
146—150	5	2.61[b]	2.40[c]	0.21	0.22	$p <0.1$ (NS)

[a]   NS = not significant.
[b]   Mean PI for code 000.
[c]   Mean PI for code 010.

TABLE 11
Mean Paired PI Difference (Δ PI $\pm$ 1 SD) per FHR Range between State Parameter Combinations in which FBM are Absent or Present

FHR range (bpm)	Number of paired observations	Mean PI for code 000	Mean PI for code 001	ΔPI	SD	Statistical significance
141—145	6	2.42	2.32	0.10	0.35	$p > 0.2$ (NS)[a]
146—150	6	2.51	2.39	0.12	0.17	$p < 0.2$ (NS)
151—155	5	2.33	2.20	0.13	0.45	$p > 0.2$ (NS)
136—140	5	1.92[b]	2.02[c]	−0.10	0.15	$p > 0.2$ (NS)

[a]   NS = not significant.
[b]   Mean PI for code 100.
[c]   Mean PI for code 101.

gestation are in agreement with the existence of fetal rest-activity cycles[39] and their relationship with low and high heart rate variation as early as 27 to 28 weeks of gestation.[35,40]

The distribution of FHRP-A and FHRP-B demonstrates a predominance of the latter pattern, i.e., 71.2% of the total recording time, which is close to that (80.4%) observed by Arduini et al.[41] Fetal body movements are clearly present during episodes with FHRP-B at this time of pregnancy (61.3%), as has also been pointed out in previous studies.[21,40,42] Following the introduction of FEM studies using real-time ultrasound[43] and the recognition of various types of eye movements with their characteristic sequence of development,[44] it was Nijhuis et al.[23] who investigated the biological implications of these movements relative to fetal behavioral states. Both from the present study and that by Inoue et al.,[45] the percentage of incidence of eye movements at 27 to 28 weeks of gestation seems to vary between 35 and 45%.

In the present study, only a change in PI relative to the FHR pattern was established. In chronically instrumented fetal lambs it was demonstrated that arterial baroreceptors are important in regulating variability of the arterial pressure and heart rate in fetal life, and they also may play a significant role in maintaining the normal peripheral vascular resistance.[46,47] Differences in sensitivity of the baroflex during different behavioral states were demonstrated in fetal lambs[48] and in cats.[49] In fetal sheep, an increased baroreceptor sensitivity was observed during high-voltage electrocortical activity.[48] As the FHR pattern is one of the state variables, it could well be that this state is related to baroreceptor sensitivity. The assumption that the human fetus exhibits increased baroreceptor sensitivity during episodes of high FHR variability would explain the observation that PI changes in the fetal descending aorta are related to FHR variability, i.e., reduced PI in the presence of high FHR variability. In earlier studies, a relationship between PI and fetal behavioral states was demonstrated in the human fetus at term.[27,28] It might well be that at term, PI is also related to only one state variable, i.e., FHRP, and not to the others. Similar to term pregnancy,[27,28] an inverse relationship between FHR and FHR variability should therefore be taken into account when studying velocity waveform in the fetal descending aorta at 27 to 28 weeks of gestation.

CONCLUSIONS

In this chapter, the relationship was studied between blood flow velocity waveforms in various fetal vessels and fetal behavioral states, in particular, states 1F and 2F, according to the classification of Nijhuis et al.[23] In the normal growing human fetus at term, blood flow velocity waveforms obtained from the lower thoracic part of the fetal descending aorta show fetal behavioral state dependency. In state 2F, PI values are statistically significant reduced as compared with state 1F. This reduction in PI is mainly determined by a rise in EDV. The reduced PI and elevated EDV reflects a reduced peripheral vascular resistance, suggesting an increased perfusion of skeletal musculature. The reduced PI in the fetal internal carotid artery in fetal behavioral state 2F in the normal growing human fetus at term suggests increased cerebral perfusion. Due to the increased muscular and electrocortical activity in behavioral state 2F, there is a raised energy demand. During the last 4 weeks of pregnancy, there is a fall in PI in the fetal internal carotid artery with maintenance of behavioral state dependency. Fetal behavioral state dependency should be taken into account when blood flow velocity waveforms in the lower thoracic part of the fetal descending aorta and fetal internal carotid artery are studied in the normal growing fetus at term. At 27 to 28 weeks of gestation, the PI in the lower thoracic part of the fetal descending aorta displays a statistically significant reduction during periods with high FHR variability as compared with periods with low FHR variability, irrespective of FEM or FBM. It is suggested that baroreceptor sensitivity is related to PI fluctuations in different fetal behavioral states in general and FHR variability in particular. The fetal origin of the behavioral state-dependent PI fluctuations in the normal growing fetus at term is suggested by the absence of behavioral state-dependent PI fluctuations in the umbilical artery. This state independency in the umbilical artery is of practical importance, since in contrast to the above-mentioned fetal vessels, blood flow velocity waveform studies in the umbilical artery during the latter weeks of gestation may be carried out without taking the fetal behavioral state into account.

In IUGR, the PI in the lower thoracic part of the fetal descending aorta and in the fetal internal carotid artery show no fetal behavioral state dependency. This may be considered a vascular adaptation, which is instrumental in the redistribution of fetal circulation during IUGR. The rise in PI in the lower thoracic part of the fetal descending aorta and the reduction in PI in the fetal internal carotid artery, which reflect this redistribution, seem to overrule behavioral state-dependent PI fluctuations.

In all studies, there is a significant inverse relationship between PI and FHR. With increasing FHR, PI drops. FHR should, therefore, be taken into account when evaluating blood flow velocity waveforms.

REFERENCES

1. **Fitzgerald, D. E. and Drumm, J. E.,** Non-invasive measurement of human fetal circulation using Ultrasound: a new method, *Br. Med. J.,* 2, 1450, 1977.
2. **Gill, R. W. and Kossoff, G.,** Pulsed Doppler combined with B-mode imaging for blood flow measurement, *Contrib. Gynaecol. Obstet.,* 6, 139, 1979.
3. **Eik-Nes, S. H., Brubakk, A. O., and Ulstein, M. K.,** Measurement of human fetal blood flow, *Br. Med. J.,* 1, 283, 1980.
4. **Tonge, M. H., Struyk, P. C., Custers, P., and Wladimiroff, J. W.,** Vascular dynamics in the descending aorta of the human fetus in normal late pregnancy, *Early Hum. Dev.,* 9, 21, 1983.
5. **Griffin, D., Bilardo, K., Masini, L., Diaz-Recasens, J., Pearce, J. M., Willson, K., and Campbell, S.,** Doppler blood flow waveforms in the descending thoracic aorta of the human fetus, *Br. J. Obstet. Gynaecol.,* 91, 997, 1984.
6. **Jouppila, P. and Kirkinen, P.,** Increased vascular resistance in the descending aorta of the human fetus in hypoxia, *Br. J. Obstet. Gynaecol.,* 91, 853, 1984.
7. **Tonge, H. M., Wladimiroff, J. W., Noordam, M. J., and Van Kooten, C.,** Blood flow velocity waveforms in the descending aorta of the human fetus in the third trimester of pregnancy: comparison between normal and growth-retarded fetuses, *Obstet. Gynecol.,* 67, 851, 1986.
8. **Stuart, B., Drumm, J., Fitzgerald, D. E., and Duignan, N. M.,** Fetal blood velocity waveforms in normal pregnancy, *Br. J. Obstet. Gynaecol.,* 87, 780, 1980.

9. **Reuwer, P. J. H. M., Bruinse, H. W., Stoutenbeek, P., Haspels, A. A.,** Doppler assessment of the fetoplacental circulation in normal and growth-retarded fetuses, *Eur. J. Obstet. Gynecol. Reprod. Biol.,* 18, 199, 1984.
10. **Trudinger, B. J., Giles, W. B., and Cook, C. M.,** Uteroplacental blood flow velocity-time waveforms in normal and complicated pregnancy, *Br. J. Obstet. Gynaecol.,* 92, 39, 1985.
11. **Marsál, K., Lingman, G., and Giles, W.,** Evaluation of the carotid, aortic and umbilical blood velocity, in *Proc. Soc. for the Study of Fetal Physiololgy. XI Annu. Conf.,* Oxford, University Press, London, 1984, C33.
12. **Arabin, B., Bergman, P., and Saling, E.,** Simultaneous assessment of blood flow velocity waveforms in uteroplacental vessels, the umbilical artery, the fetal aorta and the common carotid artery, *Fetal Ther.,* 1987, in press.
13. **Wladimiroff, J. W., Tonge, H. M., and Stewart, P. A.,** Doppler ultrasound assessment of cerebral blood flow in the human fetus, *Br. J. Obstet. Gynaecol.,* 93, 471, 1986.
14. **Marsál, K., Lindblad, A., Lingman, G., and Eik-Nes, S. H.,** Blood flow in the fetal descending aorta; intrinsic factors affecting fetal blood flow, i.e., fetal breathing movements and cardiac arrhythmia, *Ultrasound Med. Biol.,* 10, 339, 1984.
15. **Wladimiroff, J. W. and Van Bel, F.,** Fetal and neonatal cerebral blood flow, *Seminars in Perinatology,* Creasy and Warshaw, Eds., 1987, 16, 335, 1987.
16. **Tonge, H. M., Stewart, P. A., and Wladimiroff, J. W.,** Fetal blood flow measurements during fetal cardiac arrhythmia, *Early Hum. Dev.,* 10, 23, 1984.
17. **Tonge, H. M., Wladimiroff, J. W., Noordam, M. J., and Stewart, P. A.,** Fetal cardiac arrhythmia and its effect on volume blood flow in the descending aorta of the human fetus, *J. Clin. Ultrasound,* 14, 607, 1986.
18. **de Haan, R., Patrick, J., Chess, J. F., and Jaco, M. T.,** Definition of sleep state in the newborn infant by heart rate analysis, *Am. J. Obstet. Gynecol.,* 127, 753, 1977.
19. **van Geyn, H. P., Jongsma, H. W., de Haan, J., Eskes, T. K. A. B., and Prechtl, H. F. R.,** Heart rate as an indicator of the behavioural state; studies in the newborn infant and prospects for fetal heart rate monitoring, *Am. J. Obstet. Gynecol.,* 136, 1061, 1980.
20. **Timor-Tritsch, I. E., Dierker, L. J., Zador, I., Hertz, R. H., and Rosen, M. G.,** Fetal movements associated with fetal heart rate accelerations and decelerations, *Am. J. Obstet. Gynecol.,* 131, 276, 1978.
21. **Natale, R., Nasello-Paterson, C., and Turliuk, R.,** Longitudinal measurement of fetal breathing, body movements, heart rate, and heart rate accelerations and decelerations at 24 to 32 weeks of gestation, *Am. J. Obstet. Gynecol.,* 151, 256, 1985.
22. **Wheeler, T. and Guerard, P.,** Fetal heart rate during late pregnancy, *J. Obstet. Gynaecol. Br. Commonw.,* 64, 348, 1974.
23. **Nijhuis, J. G., Prechtl, H. F. R., Martin, C. J., Jr., and Bots, R. S. G. M.,** Are there behavioural states in the human fetus?, *Early Hum. Dev.,* 6, 177, 1982.
24. **Gosling, R. G. and King, D. H.,** Ultrasound angiology, in *Arteries and Veins,* Marcus and Adamson, Eds., Churchill Livingstone, Edinburgh, 1975, 61.
25. **Kirkpatrick, S. E., Pitlick, P. T., Naliboff, J., and Friedman, W. F.,** Frank-Starling relationship as an important determination of fetal cardiac output, *Am. J. Physiol.,* 231 (2), 495, 1976.
26. **Tonge, H. M., Struyk, P. C., and Wladimiroff, J. W.,** Blood flow measurements in the fetal descending aorta: techniques and Clinics, *Clin. Cardiol.,* 7, 323, 1984.
27. **van Eyck, J., Wladimiroff, J. W., Noordam, M. J., Tonge, H. M., and Prechtl, H. F. R.,** The blood flow velocity waveform in the fetal descending aorta; its relationship to fetal behavioural states in normal pregnancy at 37—38 weeks, *Early Hum. Dev.,* 12, 137, 1985.
28. **van Eyck, J., Wladimiroff, J. W., van den Wijngaard, J. A. G. W., Noordam, M. J., and Prechtl, H. F. R.,** The blood flow velocity waveform in the fetal internal carotid and umbilical artery; its relationship to fetal behavioural states in normal pregnancy at 37—38 weeks of gestation, *Br. J. Obstet. Gynaecol.,* 94, 736, 1987.
29. **van Eyck, J., Wladimiroff, J. W., Noordam, M. J., Tonge, H. M., and Prechtl, H. F. R.,** The blood flow velocity waveform in the fetal descending aorta; its relationship to behavioural states in the growth-retarded fetus at 37—38 weeks of gestation, *Early Hum. Dev.,* 14, 99, 1986.
30. **Dawes, G. S., Lewis, B. V., Milligan, I. E., Roach, M. R., and Talner, N. S.,** Vasomotor responses in the hind limbs of foetal and new-born lambs to asphyxia and aortic chemoreceptor stimulation, *J. Physiol.,* 195, 55, 1968.
31. **Itskovitz, J., Goetzman, B. W., and Rudolph, A. M.,** The mechanism of late deceleration of heart rate and its relationship to oxygenation in normoxemic and chronically hypoxemic fetal lambs, *Am. J. Obstet. Gynecol.,* 142, 66, 1982.
32. **Iwamoto, H. S., Rudolph, A. M., Keil, L. C., and Heymann, M. A.,** Hemodynamic responses of the sheep to vasopressin infusion, *Clin. Res.,* 44, 430, 1979.
33. **Oosterbaan, H. P.,** Amniotic Oxytocin and Vasopressin in the Human and the Rat, *Ph.D. thesis, University of Amsterdam,* The Netherlands, 1985.

34. **Mott, J. C.,** Humoral control of the fetal circulation, in *The Physiological Development of the Fetus and Newborn,* Jones and Nathanielsz, Eds., Academic Press, New York, 1985, 133.

35. **Visser, G. H. A., Dawes, G. S., and Redman, C. W. G.,** Numerical analysis of the normal antenatal fetal heart-rate, *Br. J. Obstet. Gynaecol.,* 88, 792, 1981.

36. **Wladimiroff, J. W., van den Wijngaard, J. A. G. W., Degani, S., Noordam, M. J., van Eyck, J., and Tonge, H. M.,** Cerebral and umbilical arterial blood flow velocity waveforms in normal and growth-retarded pregnancies; a comparative study, *Obstet. Gynecol.,* 69, 705, 1987.

37. **van Eyck, J., Wladimiroff, J. W., Noordam, M. J., van den Wijngaard, J. A. G. W., and Prechtl, H. F. R.,** The blood flow velocity waveform in the fetal internal carotid and umbilical artery; its relationship to fetal behavioural states in the growth-retarded fetus at 37—38 weeks of gestation, *Br. J. Obstet. Gynaecol.,* 1988, in press.

38. **van Eyck, J., Wladimiroff, J. W., Noordam, M. J., Cheung, K. L., van den Wijngaard, J. A. G. W., and Prechtl, H. F. R.,** The blood flow velocity waveform in the fetal descending aorta; its relationship to fetal heart rate pattern, eye and body movements in normal pregnancy at 27—28 weeks of gestation, *Early Hum. Dev.,* 1988, in press.

39. **Sterman, M. B. and Hoppenbrouwers, T.,** The development of sleep-waking and rest-activity patterns from fetus to adult in men, in *Brain Development and Behaviour,* Sterman, McGinty and Adinolfi, Eds., Academic Press, New York, 1971, 203.

40. **Dawes, G. S., Houghton, C. R. S., and Redman, C. W. G.,** Baseline in human fetal heart rate records, *Br. J. Obstet. Gynaecol.,* 89, 270, 1982.

41. **Arduini, D., Rizzo, G., Giorlandino, C., Valensise, H., Dell-Acqua, S., and Romanini, C.,** The development of fetal behavioural states: a longitudinal study, *Perinat. Diagn.,* 6, 117, 1986.

42. **Sorokin, Y., Dierker, L. J., Pillay, S. K., Zador, I. E., Schreiner, M. L., and Rosen, M. G.,** The association between fetal heart rate patterns and fetal movements in pregnancies between 20 and 30 weeks' gestation, *Am. J. Obstet. Gynecol.,* 143, 243, 1982.

43. **Bots, R. S. G. M., Nijhuis, J. G., Martin, C. B., Jr., and Prechtl, H. F. R.,** Human fetal eye movements: detection in utero by ultrasonography, *Early Hum. Dev.,* 5, 87, 1981.

44. **Birnholtz, J. C.,** The development of human fetal eye movement patterns, *Science,* 213, 679, 1981.

45. **Inoue, M., Koyanagi, T., Nakahara, H., Hara, K., Hori, E., and Nakano, N.,** Functional development of human eye movement in utero assessed quantitatively with real-time ultrasound, *Am. J. Obstet. Gynecol.,* 155, 170, 1986.

46. **Itskovitz, J., La Gamma, E. F., and Rudolph, A. M.,** Baroreflex control of the circulation in chronically instrumented fetal lambs, *Circ. Res.,* 52, 589, 1983.

47. **Shinebourne, E. A., Vapaavuori, E. K., Williams, R. L., Heymann, M. A., and Rudolph, A. M.,** Development of baroreflex activity in unanesthetized fetal and neonatal lambs, *Circ. Res.,* 31, 710, 1972.

48. **Zhu, Y. and Szeto, H. H.,** Cyclic variation in fetal heart rate and sympathetic activity, *Am. J. Obstet. Gynecol.,* 156, 1001, 1987.

49. **Baccelli, G., Albertini, R., Mancia, G., and Zanchetti, A.,** Interactions between sino-aortic reflexes and the cardiovascular effects of sleep and emotional behaviour in the cat, *Circ. Res.,* 38, 30, 1976.

Chapter 6

TRANSVAGINAL ULTRASONOGRAPHIC DIAGNOSIS IN GYNECOLOGY AND INFERTILITY

Shraga Rottem,* Ilan E. Timor-Tritsch, and Joseph Itskovitz

INTRODUCTION

Ultrasound has continued to make rapid technological and diagnostic advances during the last 10 years. Its clinical usefulness in obstetrical practice has continuously expanded, not only as a diagnostic tool, but additionally as a guide for fetal therapy. However, because optimal ultrasound imaging of female pelvic organs is difficult to obtain, the impact of this imaging modality on gynecological practice did not keep up with its use in obstetrics.[1]

There are two reasons for the difficulty in identifying and differentiating anatomical and pathological details within the female pelvis using the conventional 3.5- to 5-MHz abdominal probes.

The first of these is the similar acoustic impedance of most pelvic organs, which makes it difficult to visualize tissue interfaces. A good example is the normal Fallopian tube. The second is the relatively large distance between the abdominal probe and the pelvic organs in question, which makes it necessary to use a low-frequency (3.5 to 5.0 MHz) transducer. The resolution of those transducers does not permit accurate characterization of the pathology involved. The use of higher frequency transducers with a better resolution cannot improve images of pelvic organs if used through the conventional abdominal route due to unacceptable attentuation.

Image quality is partially improved by performing transabdominal scans while the bladder is full, but many fine details will still be missed, even by expert sonographers. The practical solution to the problem is based on the combination of two important components.

First, by placing the ultrasound probe within the vaginal vault, pelvic organs come closer to the transducer, which decreases the attenuation to a great extent. Second, the close physical contact permits the use of higher frequency transducers (e.g., 6.5 to 7 MHz), with a considerable improvement of lateral and axial resolution (Figure 1).

The combination of ''near finding scanning'' and high-frequency transducer solves many of the problems presented by the abdominal scanning and makes it possible to obtain high-quality images of pelvic structures.[2]

A basic and brief knowledge of the pertinent physics is necessary to understand the ultrasound principles that are related to the abdominal and the vaginal sonographic examination and the differences between them.

This relatively new examination is easy to perform and improves diagnostic accuracy if simple principles concerning patient preparation and scanning techniques are adhered to.[3,4]

In this chapter, an overview of the transvaginal sonographic technique based on the authors' experience in performing 13,700 examinations of 11,500 women with gynecological and early pregnancy problems is described.

PATIENT PREPARATION AND SCANNING TECHNIQUE

A brief explanation is sufficient to ensure acceptance of the new scanning technique and full cooperation by all patients. By comparing the insertion of the probe with the insertion of a tampon, speculum examination, or pelvic bimanual examination, patient's fears are quickly dispelled.

* Supported by a grant from Chester & Taube Hurwitz Foundation Fellowship, U.S.A.

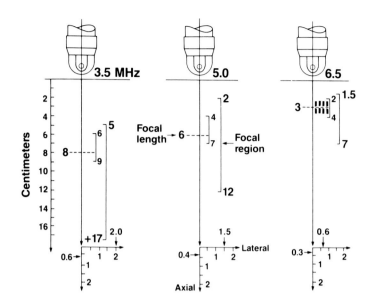

FIGURE 1.   Comparative figure demonstrating the focal region, focal length, and lateral and axial resolution of the 3.5-, 5.0-, and 6.5-MHz transducers. Note the combination of near focal length and high resolution of the 6.5-MHz transducer — the ''core'' of transvaginal sonography.

1.   Scanning is performed with an empty bladder; therefore, both patient and technician will not have to wait for the slowly filling bladder in order to receive pelvic images. This may be important in cases of emergency such as ectopic pregnancies, acute pelvic inflammatory disease, and other pathologies where the patient is potentially a subject for surgery and, therefore, may not drink to fill the bladder.

2.   A regular gynecological examination table with heel support is adequate for vaginal scanning, but a flat examination table can also be used if an 8- to 10-inch firm foam cushion is inserted below the pelvis. The patient lies in a lithotomy position with a slightly reversed Trendelenberg tilt, which allows the peritoneal fluid to pool into the pelvis. If present, this fluid creates tissue/fluid interfaces, which improves the outline of pelvic structures.

3.   The probe, covered with coupling gel, is introduced into one of the digits of a surgical rubber glove, and again lubricated with gel before insertion. Pelvic structures may be brought closer to the acoustical focal range by using the second hand on the patient's abdomen as in bimanual examination.

4.   The scanning is done systematically, starting with the uterus, next are the ovaries, then the Fallopian tubes, and finally the cul-de-sac. Various planes and depths are reached by the operator by tilting and angling the tip of the probe in the region of interest, or by rotation and push or pull motion of the probe, thus introducing various structures into the acoustical focal range (Figure 2).

PATIENT ACCEPTANCE

Initially, we thought that patients may reject the procedure because they would perceive it to be painful. However, after instruction, as mentioned earlier, patient acceptance has been almost universal.

In a sample study of 700 women, 91% of the examined women preferred transvaginal sonography (TVS) over transabdominal sonography (TAS), after they had tried both methods.

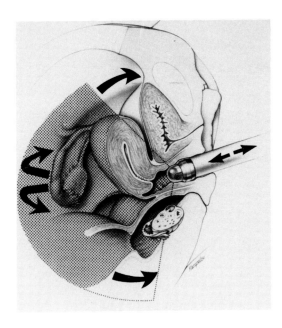

FIGURE 2. Schematic illutration of anatomic relationships
with tip of transvaginal probe and main manipulations starting
from the vertical (longitudinal) plane.

Of the women, 5% had no preference of one scanning route over the other, while 3% preferred the transabdominal route.

Of the patients, 88% reported no pain during the examination, and 10% reported some discomfort. Only 2% of all the tested women described TVS as being more painful than pelvic bimanual examination.

Women presenting with superficial dyspareunia (2.2% of the scanned patients) and with deep dyspareunia (0.7%) underwent TVS successfully. The relative discomfort did not reach the level of having to interrupt the procedure before its completion.

SCANNING THE UTERUS

Scanning in the longitudinal and transverse planes reveals the size of the uterus, its position, the myometrium, and the endometrial lining (Figure 3).

By virtue of being within the acoustical range of the high-frequency transducer, a retroverted uterus is easily scanned, and the transducer will first reveal the fundus of the uterus. In the case of an anteverted uterus, the first structure to appear on the screen is the cervix.

Systematic scanning of the uterus should start with the corpus uteri, then the endometrial cavity, and finally the cervix.[5] As the long axis of the body of the uterus is bent forward or backward at the level of the internal os (forming an angle which may vary from patient to patient), the probe should follow the direction of the endometrial cavity longitudinally, then, for the examination of the cervix, the probe will be inclinated at a suitable angle for each patient.

THE ENDOMETRIUM

The cyclic changes presented by the endometrium during the menstrual cycle can be depicted by the high-resolution TVS probe and, as described below, may be helpful in the management of the infertile women.

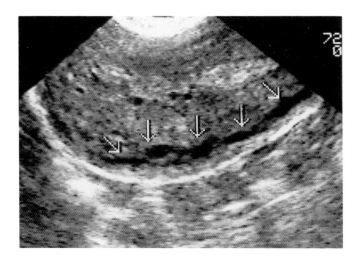

FIGURE 3.   Longitudinal scan of the uterus in midcycle. The arrows are pointing to the arcuate arteries.

Endometrial hyperplasia, especially if accompanied by an excess of estrogenic hormone production in postmenopausal women, should direct the attention of the sonographer to a rigorous scanning of the ovaries. An enlarged ovary with solid or semisolid components may represent a granulosa or theca cell tumor. However, TVS cannot differentiate between endometrial hyperplasia, endometrial polyps, and the early stages of endometrial carcinoma (Figure 4A and B).

The hydatiform mole can be detected by TVS starting from the 6th week of gestation, while later in pregnancy, a possible myometrial invasion can be reliably excluded by using the high-frequency transducer probe.

TVS also enables the investigation of problems related to intrauterine contraceptive devices (IUCD) such as uterine perforation (Figure 5), localization of the device in a case of missing string, and to demonstrate the relationship of the device with gestational structures in pregnant women.

CORPUS UTERI

The normal appearance of the corpus uteri and changes of the medium- to low-level homogeneous echoes of the myometrium are easily picked up by the 6.5-MHz TVS probe. Elderly patients present an atrophic uterus with occasional myometrial calcifications and retention of small amounts of clear fluid within the endometrial cavity (Figure 6), as described by Miller.[6] The high-resolution images enable the recognition of congenital anomalies, such as bicornuate uterus, this depending on uterine position.

TVS may detect uterine fibroid as small as 0.5 cm in diameter and define its location (e.g., intramural, subserous, submucous) and relationship to the endometrial cavity (Figure 7). TVS may also distinguish between uterine fibroid and other pelvic masses (e.g., pelvic inflammatory masses and solid ovarian tumors).

THE CERVIX

TVS displays fine details of the normal cervix (e.g., internal os, external os, cervical canal, and Nabothian cyst) and the changes that occur during the menstrual cycle (Figures 8 and 9). Minimal changes of the internal and external os and cervical canal can be accurately described by this method (Figure 10). Therefore, TVS may play an important role in the monitoring of cervical dynamics in pregnant women at risk for cervical incompetence.[7]

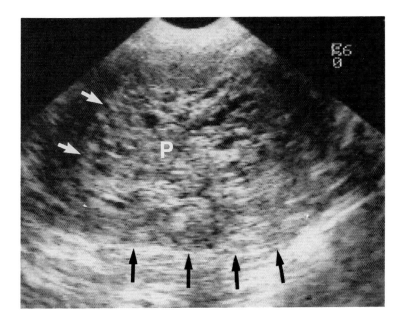

A

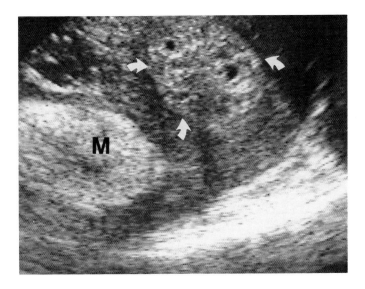

B

FIGURE 4. (A) Transverse scan of the uterus, demonstrating an endometrial polyp (P and white arrows). Black arrows demarcate the uterine border. (B) Transverse scan of the uterus with hyperplastic endometrium (white arrows), subsequently found to be a carcinoma. A calcified myoma is shown on the right (M).

Areas of increased echoes or hypoechoic areas with an irregular outline of the cervix may signify changes pertinent to a cervical carcinoma. The study of the extension of a mass beyond the cervix may be helpful in distinguishing stages of carcinoma of the cervix.

UTERINE VESSELS

The common, descending, and ascending uterine arteries are clearly displayed by TVS,

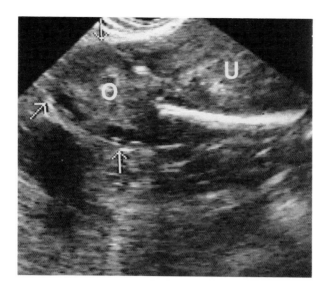

FIGURE 5.   Bulging of an intrauterine device into the adnexa.
U = uterus; O = ovary.

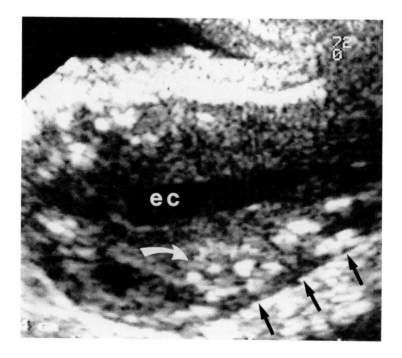

FIGURE 6.   A longitudinal scan of the uterus in a 72-year-old patient. Small calcifications are marked by a white arrow. The endometrial cavity (ec) is filled with fluid.

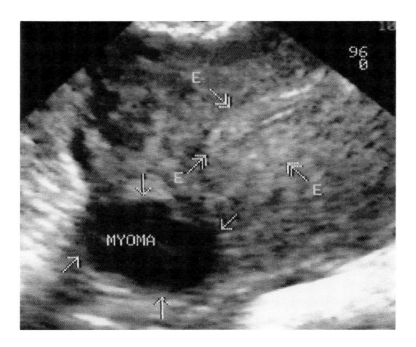

FIGURE 7.   A longitudinal scan of the corpus uteri showing a subserous degenerated myoma. E = endometrium.

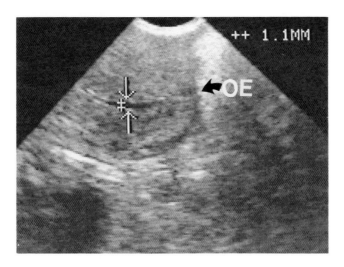

FIGURE 8.   Longitudinal scan of the cervix. Black arrow points to the cervical canal. White arrow shows a Nabothian cyst.

and the transvaginal probe is now used in blood flow studies employing the pulse Doppler method (Figure 11). The arcuate uterine vessels can also be seen by TVS. They are protruding during the midcycle and in case of an atonic, profusely bleeding uterus after curetage (Figure 12).

UTERINE LIGAMENTS

Both the round and the broad ligaments are displayed by TVS when a large amount of

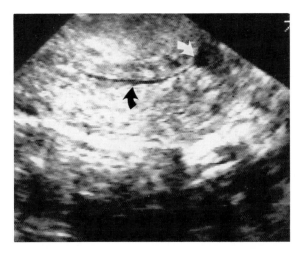

FIGURE 9.   A longitudinal scan of the cervix, demonstrating the cervical canal (1.1-mm width) on the 10th d of a normal cycle. OE = external os.

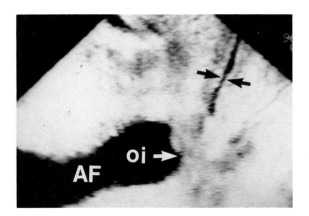

FIGURE 10.   A longitudinal scan of the cervix at 12 weeks gestation showing the cervical canal (black arrows), the internal os (oi), and the amniotic cavity (AF).

fluid is present in the pelvis. Pathological findings such as intraligamentary myomas are clearly shown by TVS (Figure 13), and the distinction between an intraligamentary myoma, a cornual pregnancy, or an ovarian cyst is readily made.

The ability to image normal uterine structures and to detect uterine pathology in the early stages of the disease is clearly improved by using a high-frequency transvaginal probe instead of the traditional 3.5- to 5-MHz transabdominal probes.

THE FALLOPIAN TUBES

One of the remarkable advantages of TVS is its capacity for studying the Fallopian tube.[8] Much more information can be derived about this organ by employing this new method than by scanning the patient via the transabdominal route. However, a normal Fallopian tube is not usually seen by TVS unless some fluid surrounds it. This pelvic fluid may originate from

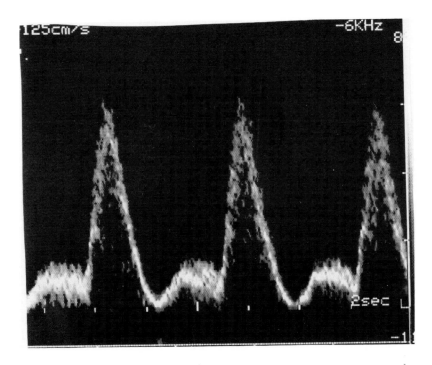

FIGURE 11.   A flow velocity waveform obtained from the ascending branch of the uterine artery in the follicular phase. This was obtained with a transvaginal pulsed Doppler duplex system.

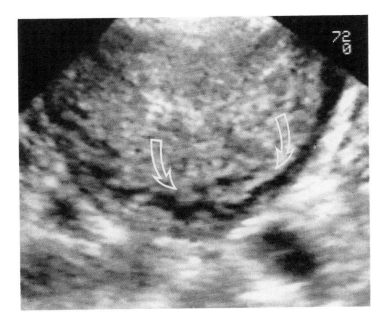

FIGURE 12.   An enlarged uterus 6 h following curettage due to inevitable abortion at 11 weeks gestation. The arcuate arteries are shown by arrows.

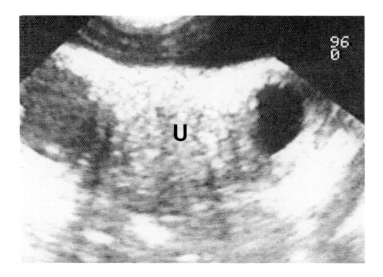

FIGURE 13.   A transverse scan of the uterus (U) at the level of the fundus, demonstrating two degenerated myomas on both sides.

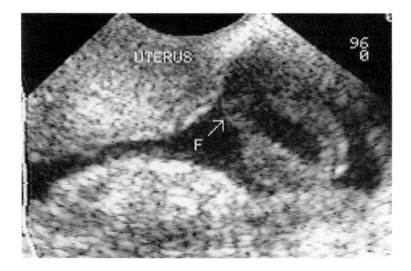

FIGURE 14.   A normal Fallopian tube lying in the cul-de-sac which is filled with a moderate amount of free fluid. F = fimbria.

1.   Normal peritoneal fluid present in the pelvis in healthy women.[9]
2.   Ovarian follicular fluid after ovulation.
3.   Blood (e.g., ruptured hemorrhagic corpus luteum).
4.   Ascitic fluid.
5.   Exudate associated with pelvic inflammatory disease.

When outlined, the normal Fallopian tube shows an undulating structure of 1 cm wide, while the lumen is not observed (Figure 14).

Inflammatory processes of the tube, such as hydrosalpinx, pyosalpinx, or involvement of the tube in a tubo-ovarian abscess, demonstrate typical patterns on TVS as described in Figure 15. Serial TVS examinations enable the evaluation of the efficacy of conservative antibiotic treatment.

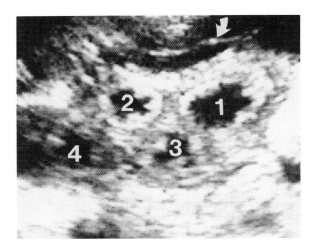

FIGURE 15. A tubo-ovarian abscess containing four loops of the Fallopian tube (1 to 4). A pelvic adhesion is shown by a white arrow.

TUBAL PREGNANCY

Ectopic pregnancy is frequently cited as a major cause of maternal mortality and morbidity. A marked global increase in its incidence in the last 2 decades has been demonstrated.[10,11] A three-week delay in making the correct diagnosis was reported in up to 14% of the cases using various diagnostic tests.[12] Part of the diagnostic delay is caused by the relatively low specificity and sensitivity rates associated with TAS. This method generally allows for the visualization of indirect findings (e.g., pelvic fluid and adnexal masses) which may not be present in many cases of ectopic pregnancy in its early stages, or, if present, may suggest other pathologies to be considered.

However, TVS, using a high-frequency transducer which provides high-resolution images, may be regarded as a better diagnostic tool than TAS in the work-up of patients suspected of having an ectopic pregnancy.[13-15] A systematic approach is presented.

SCANNING THE UTERUS

The uterus should be scanned first. An intrauterine gestational sac can be documented as early as 4 weeks and 3 days from the LMP, and in all patients at 4 weeks and 5 d from the LMP (Figure 16). The average level of serum β-hCG at this gestational age is 400 to 700 mIU/ml. A more detailed discussion of the improved sonographic recognition of early gestational structures using TVS is described elsewhere in this volume.

Various investigators using TAS described a gestational sac-like structure in patients with ectopic pregnancy which they termed "pseudogestational sac".[16,17] This pseudosac represents a highly echogenic thickened endometrium which has undergone degeneration and bleeding. In these cases, where "pseudogestational sac" was observed by TAS, TVS showed only a thick endometrium with a sonolucent area devoid of the decidual double ring of a normal gestation. When profuse uterine bleeding accompanied the ectopic gestation, TVS showed the cavity lined with blood and blood clots.

SCANNING THE FALLOPIAN TUBE

In a 2-year study of 725 patients scanned by TVS for suspected ectopic pregnancy, 84 of the 90 cases were correctly diagnosed by this tool.[18] TVS showed a sensitivity of 94.4% and a specificity of 99.8% in the diagnosis of tubal pregnancy. Fetal heart movements were observed in 21.4% of the cases. In most cases, a simple examination was sufficient to

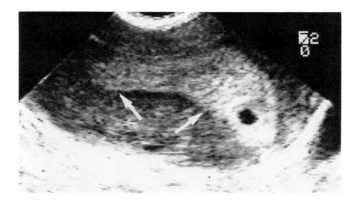

FIGURE 16.   Longitudinal scan of the uterus at 4 weeks and 4 d from LMP. A clear gestational sac of 5 mm is detected in the echogenic endometrium (white arrows).

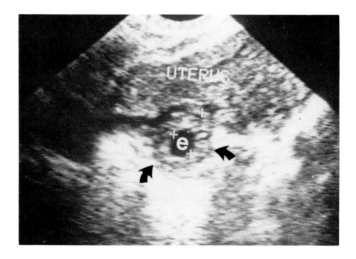

FIGURE 17.   Cross-section of the Fallopian tube at the level of the enlarged ampula (15 mm), outlined by arrows. The ectopic gestational sac (e) is only 8 mm in diameter.

establish the diagnosis. A few patients were reexamined up to four times until the diagnosis could be made. Three major distinct patterns of tubal pregnancy could be recognized:

1.   A Fallopian tube with clearly demonstrable gestational structures (direct diagnosis) consisted of a thickened Fallopian tube (the tubal ring) containing an ''empty'' gestational sac, a gestational sac with a yolk sac, or a gestational sac containing a yolk sac and an embryo (Figures 17 to 19). Almost 60% of the patients demonstrated this type of tubal pregnancy.
2.   A Fallopian tube containing blood clots (direct diagnosis) consisted of a dilated Fallopian tube containing an amorphous echogenic material, while a distinct tubal ring containing gestational products could not be visualized. In most cases, this pattern was accompanied by free fluid or blood clots in the cul-de-sac. Almost 30% of the cases were classified into this group. This pattern was compatible with a recent tubal abortion or rupture of the tube.

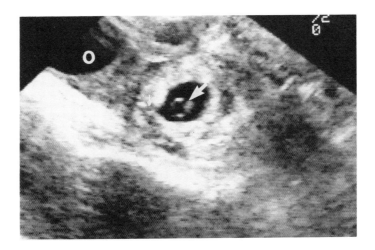

FIGURE 18.   Cross-section of the Fallopian tube containing gestational sac, yolk sac, and an embryonic pole of 2 mm (white arrow). Heart beats are evident on real-time scanning (6 weeks of gestation from LMP) A small white arrow points to the tubal wall. O = ovary.

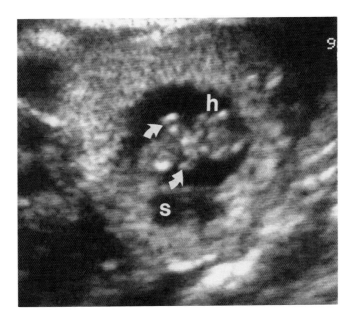

FIGURE 19.   Cross of the Fallopian tube containing a fetus of 1 cm (7 weeks 3 d from LMP). The fetal head (h) and limb buds (white arrows) are shown. Tubal wall is ''invaded'' by trophoplast. Lacunar structures (s) showing flow under real-time scaning can be observed.

3.   In the combined indirect pattern (indirect diagnosis), no distinct sonographic pattern of the Fallopian tube could be observed. The only finding was free blood or blood clots in the cul-de-sac and an empty uterus (Figure 20). Almost 10% of the cases showed this pattern, which was generally associated with either tubal abortion or cornual pregnancy. In the remaining cases, the tubal pregnancy was found at laparotomy to be adhered to the omentum above the uterine fundus, outside of the focal length of the ultrasound probe, and therefore could not be visualized.

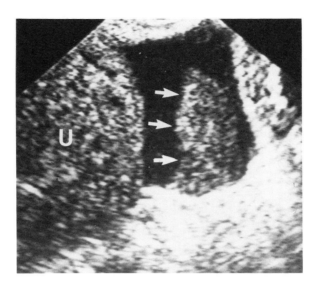

FIGURE 20.   A blood clot surrounded by free fluid (blood) is outlined
by arrows in the Douglas space. U = uterus.

It must be pointed out that the type 3 pattern (i.e., fluid or blood in the pelvic cavity) can represent other tubal or ovarian disorders, and, therefore, determination of serum β-hCG level or other diagnostic procedures are imperative. Serum β-hCG levels should also support the type 2 sonographic findings in making the diagnosis of tubal pregnancy.

Invasive diagnostic procedures such as culdocentesis, endometrial curettage, and laparoscopy were employed in less than 10% of the patients. We believe that the above-mentioned (sometimes superfluous) invasive diagnostic procedures should be uncommonly used and that the TVS with high-frequency transducer will become the main tool in the early diagnosis of ectopic pregnancy.

CUL-DE-SAC

The cul-de-sac can be demonstrated ultrasonigraphically only when it is filled by several milliliters of fluid. While the vaginal transducer is in place, the following information can be obtained:

1.   Free pelvic fluid with highly echogenic and homogeneous texture suggests the presence of blood in this space, while the blood clots are depicted as bizarre-shaped structures floating and moving when the position of the probe or patient changes.
2.   An empty cul-de-sac appears as a discrete echogenic line marked by the lining of the serosa on the posterior uterine wall (Figure 21). This usually excludes the possibility of active bleeding into the pelvis and permits a conservative work-up of the patient with suspected ectopic pregnancy, until the final diagnosis is made.

Using TAS, sonographers were commonly forced to issue vague reports stating, e.g., "...suspected adnexal mass of irregular echogenicity surrounded by some amount of fluid...ectopic pregnancy cannot be ruled out." These findings are not specific and may represent a multitude of pathological or physiological conditions. In a recent study, 22% of patients without ectopic pregnancy had adnexal masses observed on abdominal scans, while 20% of women with surgically confirmed ectopic pregnancy had normal adnexal findings.[19]

Using TVS, various "adnexal masses" can be readily distinguished as specific pathological entities in the Fallopian tube, ovary, or uterus.

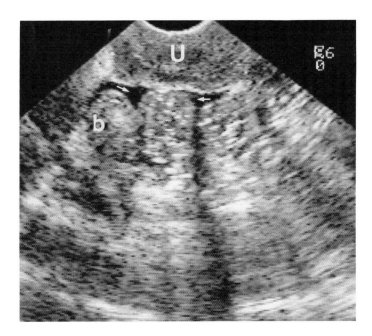

FIGURE 21.   Transverse scan of the uterus (U). A small amount of fluid is present in the cul-de-sac (small arrows) after ovulation has taken place. Three loops of bowels (b) are shown.

In conclusion, TVS, using a high-frequency transducer, which provides high-resolution images, may be regarded as a better diagnostic tool than TAS in the work-up of patients suspected of having an ectopic pregnancy. This is based on the ability to directly observe structural changes in the Fallopian tube and to obtain an early diagnosis without resorting to other diagnostic procedures, which are mostly invasive.

Therefore, TVS should become a "first-line" diagnostic tool in all patients who are suspected of having an ectopic pregnancy.

SCANNING THE OVARY

During the reproductive years, the ovaries are the most prominent landmarks of the adnexa, the Graafian follicles being the sonographic "markers" (Figure 22).

The diagnosis of ovarian masses using TAS is widely documented in the literature.[20-23] TVS is now reported as a powerful tool in the sonographic work-up of ovarian pathology.[24,25] The following ovarian pathologies can be diagnosed:

- Functional cysts are usually devoid of nodules or papillary structures and when followed serially, shrink either spontaneously or following a trial of oral contraceptives.
- Corpus luteum cysts are characteristic spherical masses extending across the ovarian surface. Blood clots and liquid content may appear as a scalloped, irregularly echogenic area or as a multilocular cyst (Figure 23). This is, of course, a normal phenomenon in the woman of child-bearing age and should not be mistaken with other disorders. As the natural progression and regression of the corpus luteum involves dramatic macroscopical changes (readily revealed by TVS), the sonographer may find the corpus luteum as the "great imitator" of many ovarian pathologies. The final diagnosis may incur the need for rescanning of the patient during the follicular phase of the following menstrual cycle, when the previous finding should have decreased in size, thus confirming the diagnosis.

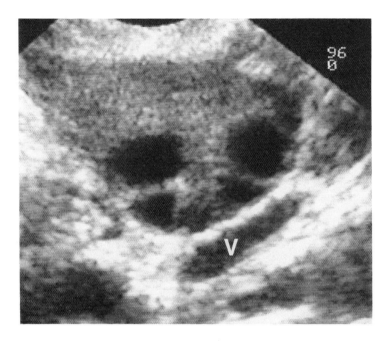

FIGURE 22.   Transvaginal sonographic image of the left normal ovary with four follicles of 4 to 7 mm. V = iliac vein.

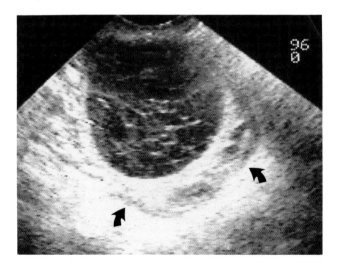

FIGURE 23.   A corpus luteum shows a multilocular content. Black arrows demarcate the ovarian border.

- Dermoid cysts may present a variety of typical sonographic patterns, depending on the presence or absence of sebaceous material, hair, teeth or bone (Figure 24).
- Multilocular cysts are easily detected by TVS. A proper TGC setting (equipment adjustment at 30 dB) enhances image brightness and enables the detection of tiny loculations. Occurring at any age, these lesions may represent variable histologic structures, such as cystadenomas, cystadenocarcinomas, endometrioidal carcinomas, dermoid cysts, or corpus luteum cysts.

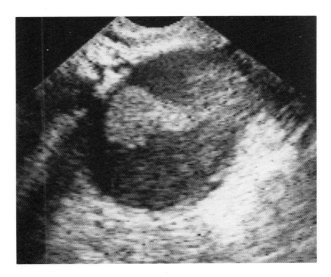

FIGURE 24. A 4.8 × 3-cm dermoid cyst with an inner tubercular protrusion surrounded by sebaceous fluid.

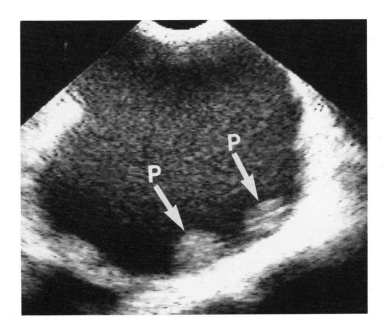

FIGURE 25.   Two of many papillary structures (P) on the inner surface of an ovarian adenocarcinoma.

- Papillary cysts should raise suspicion of malignancy even before detection of ascites (Figure 25). Papillary seedings of ovarian tumors can be detected on the pelvic walls if fluid is present (Figure 26).
- Solid ovarian cysts sometimes resemble the texture of a uterine fibroid (Figure 27) and should be distinguished from pedunculated or intraligamentous fibroids.
- Mixed tumors consist of more than one type of structural component (e.g., solid, semisolid, cystic) and must be distinguished from a hemorrhagic corpus luteum.

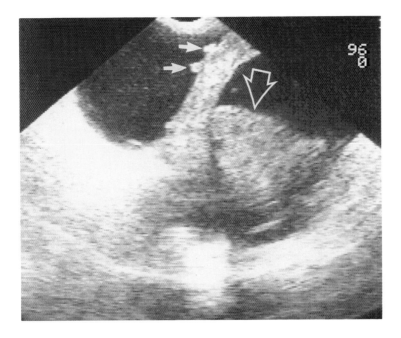

FIGURE 26. Two peritoneal seedlings (small arrows) highlighted by ascites and part of a stage-III ovarian carcinoma (arrow).

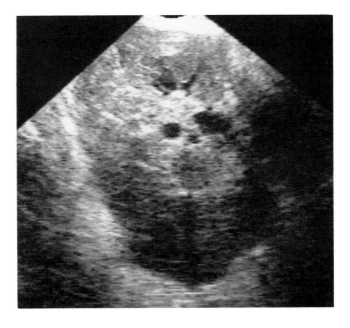

FIGURE 27. A solid ovarian tumor with inner loculations. Pathology revealed a granulosa all tumor.

TVS IN THE MANAGEMENT OF INFERTILITY

MONITORING OF FOLLICULAR DEVELOPMENT AND OVULATION INDUCTION

Monitoring of follicular size and the number of developing follicles are essential for the management of patients undergoing ovarian stimulation with gonadotropins.[26-29] Ovarian follicles can be easily visualized by TVS starting at a diameter of 2 to 3 mm. The normal developing follicle grows at a rate of 2 mm/d, reaching a diameter of 20 to 24 mm shortly before ovulation. In the natural menstrual cycle, most of the circulating estrogens originate from the growing dominant follicle, and there is a linear correlation between follicular diameter and serum estradiol level. In induced cycles when more than one follicle develops, the correlation between follicular diameter and estradiol level is lower than in the natural cycle, and total follicular volume seems to show the highest correlation with serum estradiol level. The value of ultrasonography is in making the decision to administer hCG at the appropriate time, when the sizes of the leading follicles have reached diameters of 16 to 18 mm, or to withhold its injection when estradiol levels are apparently ovulatory, but the developing follicles are too small.

For the measurement of ovarian follicles, the ovary is first located in the space between the posterolateral wall of the uterus and the iliac vein and artery, in which flow and pulsation can be easily recognized. Following pelvic surgery, the ovaries may be found at different sites, and in a few of these patients, the ovaries may only be located by TAS.

The anatomical structures that may assume the look of ovarian follicles and may impose some difficulty in distinguishing ovarian anatomy are ovarian cysts, hydrosalpinx, the cross-section of blood vessels, and the bowel. The latter is observed for some time and will show peristalsis. Blood vessels can be recognized by their pulsatility and by rotating the transducer scanning plane by 90° to provide a longitudinal section of the blood vessels. Ovarian functional (simple) cysts and hydrosalpinx do not grow in response to hormonal stimulation; therefore, several measurements will help to distinguish them from the growing follicles.

Ovulation can be detected by the demonstration of a previously nonexistent fluid in the pouch of Douglas, the disappearance of the dominant follicle(s), and the appearance of the corpus luteum. The corpus luteum is usually spheric, 2 to 3 cm in diameter (but may reach a greater diameter), and shows various degrees of wall thickness. As mentioned earlier, the recognition of the corpus luteum may be difficult because of the diversity of its appearance; it may appear as a sonolucent, trabecular, nodular, or multicolor structure.

OVARIAN PATHOLOGY

Other entities which are relevant to the management of the infertile woman and can be recognized by TVS include endometrioid cyst and the polycystic ovary.

The endometrioid cyst appears as a round, homogeneously echogenic structure that may resemble the sonographic appearance of the dermoid cyst. The polycystic ovary has a typical sonographic appearance characterized by a spherical enlarged ovary containing a large number of 3- to 6-mm-sized follicles crowded at its surface (Figure 28).

SCANNING THE UTERUS

Endometrial response to ovarian steroids can be detected and measured with greater precision by using the transvaginal approach (Figure 29). Four patterns (or grades) of endometrial response have been described and seem to correlate with the different phases of the menstrual cycle.[30]

Uterine malformations (e.g., bicornuate uterus) and small intramural or submucus fibroids can be more easily detected by transvaginal scanning. Intracavitary blood or fluid collection, endometrial polyp, or intrauterine adhesions (Asherman's syndrome) may also be demonstrated.

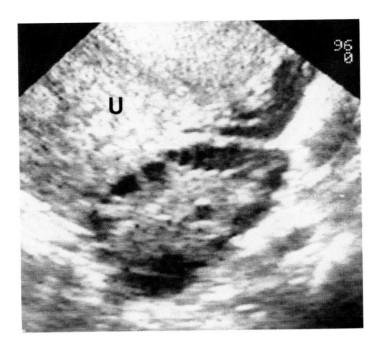

FIGURE 28.   A left polycystic ovary. Small follicles of 3 mm diameter are crowded at the surface of the ovary. U = uterus.

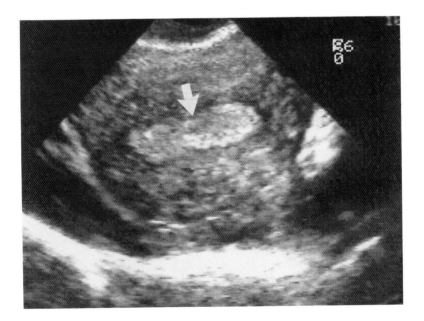

FIGURE 29.   Transverse scan of the uterus during the luteal phase. The white arrow points the highly reflective and thick endometrium. Menstruation occurred 3 d later.

TRANSVAGINAL FOLLICULAR ASPIRATION FOR *IN VITRO* FERTILIZATION

Ultrasound-directed follicular aspiration introduced by Dellenbach et al. in 1984,[31] has become the method of choice for egg retrieval in *in vitro* fertilization programs around the world. This method has replaced the laparoscopic follicular aspiration technique, obviating

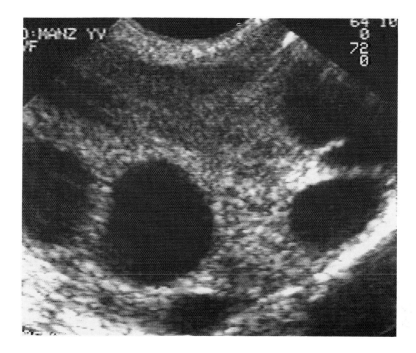

FIGURE 30.   Cross-section of the right ovary after hormonal induction of ovulation. Day of oocyte retrieval.

the need for general anesthesia. It also replaced another ultrasound-guided follicular aspiration technique which employs the transabdominal-transvesical approach. The advantages of the transvaginal over the transabdominal approach are related to the proximity of the vaginal transducer element to the pelvic organs, thus enhancing picture resolution of the ovary and the follicles.[32,33] The shorter puncture route and the more controlled and accurate puncture procedure, compared with the transabdominal approach, reduce the risk of puncturing blood vessels or bowel. The bladder is not entered, and the procedure is associated with less patient discomfort. Because the procedure can be done on an outpatient basis, the overall cost is significantly reduced.

Procedure

For vaginal disinfection, the patient is prepared with povidine-iodine vaginal suppositories the day before and the morning of the procedure. The patient is given intravenous pethidine (100 to 125 mg) and diazepam (10 mg) to induce sedation and analgesia. The vagina is thoroughly cleaned with povidone-iodine 10% solution and then with gauze soaked with saline. The transducer probe is covered with a sterile plastic bag that had sterile paraffin oil placed within it and was fitted with a needle guide.

The draped transducer tip is covered with a sterile paraffin oil and is introduced into the vaginal vault. The ovaries are then imaged (Figure 30), and the biopsy line is aligned with the target follicles. The follicles are punctured with a 35-cm-long, 1.6-mm outer diameter stainless steel needle serrated at the tip to facilitate its visualization (Figure 31). After all follicles have been aspirated, the pelvic organs are scanned to rule out active bleeding from the puncture sites. Occasional vaginal bleeding can be easily controlled by applying pressure to the vaginal vault.

Transvaginal ultrasound-directed follicular aspiration is the method of choice for egg retrieval in an *in vitro* fertilization program. In the uncommon situations where the ovaries cannot be approached vaginally, the transabdominal route can be employed. Laparoscopic

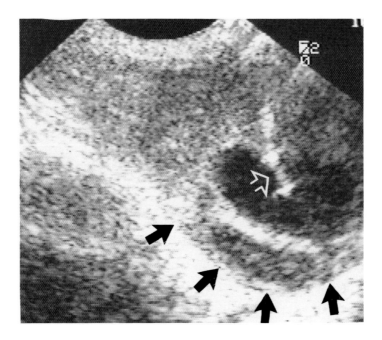

FIGURE 31.   Same ovary in Figure 30 during transvaginal follicular aspiration —
the needle is seen inside the follicle and shown by the white arrow. Black arrows
demonstrate ovarian border.

follicular aspiration is now reserved for patients in whom a simultaneous assessment of
pelvic anatomy is indicated.

TRANSVAGINAL SONOGRAPHIC SCANNING IN SPECIAL
CONDITIONS

The benefits of TVS can also be considered in special conditions, as follows:

VAGINAL BLEEDING

The use of the vaginal probe in all cases of gynecological bleeding from the reproductive
tract is not contraindicated. In the case of first- or second-trimester vaginal bleeding in
patients at risk for cervical incompetence, the use of the vaginal probe may be preceded by
speculum examination in order to rule out frank cervical dilation and to localize cervix
position. Cervical imaging is possible when the cervix is still 3 cm away from the tip of
the probe. Damage will not occur if a gentle scanning is performed, minimizing maneuvers
employed with the probe.

ACUTE ABDOMEN OR SEVERE PELVIC PAIN

TVS may add invaluable information where the pelvic bimanual examination is difficult
to perform. The examination should be carried out using minimal maneuvers. If pathology
is present in the small pelvis, the probe may be used as a direct diagnostic tool to detect
the point of maximal tenderness by touching the affected area itself.

VAGINISMUS AND ATROPHIC VAGINA
Vaginismus

The involuntary spasm reflex of the perineal and levator ani muscles surrounding the

outer third of the vagina in response to attempts at vaginal examination results in painful sensation for the patient, and also physician frustration. By instructing the patient regarding the TVS examination and employing a liberally lubricated probe (preferably introduced by the patient herself), women suffering from vaginismus cooperate during the transvaginal scanning better than during the pelvic bimanual examination with excellent results.

Atrophic Vagina

The vulnerability of the delicate vaginal introitus and wall in elderly patients should be taken into consideration during the examination. A bulky and thick or irregularly shaped vaginal probe may be awkward to insert and generally cause patient discomfort, reducing acceptance.

INTACT HYMEN

If TAS images do not provide reliable information in a case in which decisions involving possible laparoscopy or abdominal surgery have to be made, the sonographic examination via the vaginal route can be taken into consideration. However, in spite of the fact that we have successfully examined three such young girls without damage to the hymen, sonographic information should preferably be obtained by the transabdominal route, eventually completed by a transrectal sonographic examination before resorting to the vaginal route.

LIMITATIONS OF HIGH-FREQUENCY TRANSVAGINAL PROBES

Although the images of high-frequency transvaginal probes provide a better framework than TAS for recognizing gynecological pathology, limitations do exist. In our experience, at the end of a TVS scan, 2 to 5% of the patients with gynecological pathology would also require TAS. For example:

1. An enlarged myomatous uterus (e.g., 12 to 15 cm) may lie out of focus for the 6.5-MHz TVS probe and may not be visually encompassed on the screen.
2. Masses lying out of the true pelvis may not be observed at all using the 6.5-MHz probe.
3. A giant ovarian mass may present fine details on the near field area, but its boundaries may not be detected by this tool. Other pelvic organs may be displaced by this mass and pose the same problem.

In spite of the fact that many ovarian disorders exhibit textural changes that can be recognized using this tool, it is hard to display the normal ovary in elderly patients. The reasons for these limitations are the lack of follicles at this age, the ovarian atrophy, and the absence of peritoneal fluid in the pelvis of these patients, while a relatively atrophic vagina may not permit a reliable pelvic inspection using the vaginal probe.

Despite these drawbacks, in most patients the transvaginal approach can be applied and reward both the patient and the examiner with an optimal diagnostic scan, as previously described.

CLOSING REMARKS

TVS, especially when a high-frequency transducer is employed, presents unprecedented high-resolution pictures. The experience which was limited to the use of monitoring ovulation and transvaginal oocyte retrieval, unfolds with rapidity to the diagnosis of gynecological and early pregnancy problems. In most of the instances, TVS yields original information unavailable by the transabdominal route. The benefits of this new technology can be readily evaluated in every department of obstetrics and gynecology in a few minutes after starting to scan the first patient.

As good results of any type of technology depend on the skill and experience of the operator, the need for a rapid and high level of training is obvious. However, as TVS displays fine lesions at the stage when clinical signs are not yet present, and even before findings can be appreciated at the bimanual examination, this new technique will soon accompany the fingers of the gynecologists as one hundred eyes searching for lesions of less than 1 mm in size.

The ongoing investigations on the use of TVS have to validate and extend the initial good results already published or in press. This will lead to an ultimate improvement in patient care.

REFERENCES

1. **O'Brien, W. F., Buck, D. R., and Nash, T. D.,** Evaluation of sonography in the initial assessment of the gynecological patient, *Am. J. Obstet. Gynecol.,* 179, 598, 1984.
2. **Timor-Tritsch, I. E., Rottem, S., and Thaler, I.,** Review of transvaginal ultrasonography: a description with clinical application, *Ultrasound Q.,* 6(1), 1, 1988.
3. **Rottem, S., Thaler, I., et al.,** The transvaginal sonographic technique: targeted organ scanning without resorting to "planes", *J. Clin. Ultrasound,* May 1990 (in press).
4. **Timor-Tritsch, I. E., Bar-Yam, Y., Elgali, S., and Rottem, S.,** The technique of transvaginal sonography with the use of a 6.5 MHz probe, *Am. J. Obstet. Gynecol.,* 158(5), 1019, 1988.
5. **Lewit, N., Thaler, I., and Rottem, S.,** The uterus: a new look with transvaginal Sonography, *J. Clin. Ultrasound,* May 1990 (in press).
6. **Miller, E., Thomas, R. H., and Lines, P.,** The atrophic postmenopausal uterus, *J. Clin. Ultrasound,* 5, 261, 1976.
7. **Brown, J. E., Thieme, G. A., Shad, D. M., Fleischer, A. C., and Boehm, F. H.,** Transabdominal and transvaginal endosonography: evaluation of the cervix and lower uterine segment in pregnancy, *Am. J. Obstet. Gynecol.,* 155, 721, 1986.
8. **Timor-Tritsch, I. E. and Rottem, S.,** Transvaginal ultrasonographic study of the Fallopian tube, *Obstet. Gynecol.,* 70, 424, 1987.
9. **Davis, F. and Gosink, B. B.,** Fluid in the female pelvis, cyclic patterns, *J. Ultrasound Med.,* 5, 75, 1986.
10. **Westrom, L., Bengtsson, L., and Mardth, P. A.,** Incidence, trends and risk of ectopic pregnancy in a population of women, *Med. J.,* 282, 15, 1981.
11. **Rubin, G. L., Peterson, H. B., and Dorfman, S. F.,** Ectopic pregnancy in the United States, 1970 through 1978, *JAMA,* 249, 1725, 1983.
12. **Hazelkamp, J. T.,** Ectopic pregnancy: diagnostic dilema and delay, *Int. J. Gynecol. Obstet.,* 17, 598, 1980.
13. **Rottem, S., Timor-Tritsch, I. E., and Thaler, I.,** Assessment of pelvic pathology by high frequency transvaginal sonography, in *Textbook of Obstetric and Gynecologic Ultrasound,* Cherverak, F. A., Isaacson, G., and Campbell, S., Eds., Little, Brown, Boston, 1990.
14. **Rottem, S., Timor-Tritsch, I. E., and Brandes, J.,** Think ectopic — see ectopic, *Fertil. Steril. Suppl.,* October-November, 1986.
15. **Rottem, S. and Timor-Tritsch, I. E.,** Think ectopic, in *Transvaginal Sonography,* Timor-Tritsch, I. E. and Rottem, S., Eds., Elsevier, New York, 1987, chap. 8.
16. **Weiner, C.,** The pseudogestational sac in ectopic pregnancy, *Am. J. Obstet. Gynecol.,* 139, 959, 1981.
17. **Abramovici, H., Auslender, R., Lewin, A., et al.,** Gestational pseudogestational sac: a new ultrasonic criteria for differential diagnosis, *Am. J. Obstet. Gynecol.,* 145, 377, 1983.
18. **Rottem, S., Thaler, I., et al.,** Criteria for transvaginal ultrasonographic diagnosis of ectopic pregnancy,, *J. Clin. Ultrasound,* May 1990 (in press).
19. **Mahoney, B. S., Filly, R. A., Nyberg, D. A., and Callen, P. W.,** Sonographic evaluation of ectopic pregnancy, *J. Ultrasound Med.,* 4, 221, 1985.

20. **Campbell, S., Goessens, L., and Goswamy, R.,** Real time ultrasonography for determination of ovarian morphology and volume, *Lancet,* 1, 425, 1980.
21. **Reguard, K., Mettler, F., and Wicks, J.,** Preoperative sonography of malignant ovarian neoplasms, *Am. J. Radiol.,* 137, 79, 1981.
22. **Williams, A., Mettker, F., and Wicks, J.,** Cystic and solid ovarian neoplasms, *Semin. Ultrasound,* 4,(1), 166, 1983.
23. **Rifkin, M. D.,** Using ultrasound to diagnose gynecological malignancy, *Contemp. Obstet. Gynecol.,* 23, 200, 1984.
24. **Timor-Tritsch, I. E. and Rottem, S.,** High frequency transvaginal sonography: new diagnostic boon, *Contemp. Obstet. Gynecol.,* 31(4), 111, 1988.
25. **Mendelson, E. B., Bohm-Velez, M., Joseph, N., and Neiman, H. L.,** Gynecologic imaging: comparison of transabdominal and transvaginal sonography, *Radiology,* 166, 321, 1988.
26. **Funduk-Kurjak, B. and Kurjak, A.,** Ultrasound monitoring of follicular maturation and ovulation in normal menstrual cycle and in ovulation induction, *Acta Obstet. Gynecol. Scand.,* 61, 329, 1982.
27. **De Cresping, L., O'Herlhy, C., and Robinson, H. P.,** Ultrasonic observation of the mechanism of human ovulation, *Am. J. Obstet. Gynecol.,* 139, 616, 1981.
28. **De Cherney, A. H. and Laufer, N. D.,** The monitoring of ovulation induction using ultrasound and estrogen, *Clin. Obstet. Gynecol.,* 27 (4), 993, 1984.
29. **Siebel, M. M., McArdtle, C. R., and Thompson, I. E.,** The role of ultrasound in ovulation induction — a critical reappraisal, *Fertil. Steril.,* 36, 573, 1981.
30. **Smith, B., Porter, R., and Ahuja, K.,** Ultrasonic assessment of endometrial changes in stimulated cycles and in-vitro fertilization and embryo transfer program, *J. In Vitro Fertil. Embryo Transfer,* 1 (4), 233, 1984.
31. **Dellenbach, P., Nisand, I., and Moreau, L.,** Transvaginal Sonographically controlled ovarian follicle puncture for egretieval, *Lancet,* 1, 1467, 1984.
32. **Drugan, A., Blumenfeld, Z., Erlik, Y., Timor-Tritsch, I. E., and Brandes, J. M.,** The use of transvaginal sonography in infertility, in *Transvaginal Sonography,* Timor-Tritsch, I. E. and Rottem, S., Eds., Elsevier, New York, 1987, chap. 9.
33. **Timor-Tritsch, I. E. and Rottem, S.,** Transvaginal sonography in the management of infertility, in Kurjak, A., Ed., CRC Press, Boca Raton, FL, 1989.

Chapter 7

TISSUE CHARACTERIZATION IN OBSTETRICS AND GYNECOLOGY

K. Maeda and A. Akaiwa

INTRODUCTION

Quantitative measurements in obstetrics and gynecology are at present mainly geometrical and Doppler. Although these methods to a large extent make the quantitative assessment of pregnancy possible and are under further development, tissue characterization would open new horizons in this area of diagnostics. During the last 10 years, there have been many attempts to attach some kind of quantitative value to the tissue quality.

At present, two methods for such characterization yield promising results, i.e., the gray-level histogram and the radiofrequency attenuation analysis.

THE GRAY-LEVEL HISTOGRAM

The gray-scale B mode image consists of dots of different brightness, the brightness of which depends on the intensity of the ultrasound echo they represent. The abscissa of the histogram represents the brightness level, and the ordinate represents the number of pixels containing a specific brightness. The graph can be normalized at the most representative level.

The analysis is done within an area of interest in the two-dimensional image. The area of interest can, in a number of commercially available instruments, be chosen at will. In the experiments which illustrate the method in this chapter, Aloka scanners of the types SSD-258 and SSD-270 and UIP-100 computer system have been used. At the present state of development, this sort of analysis is applicable to tissues not containing severe structural changes like calcifications, teleangiectasia, and similar. Even so, there exist enough structures amenable to this analysis, like simple ovarian cysts, dermoid cysts, ovarian follicles, unruptured luteinized follicles, lutein cysts, fetal liver, fetal lungs, and placenta *in vitro* and *in vivo*. The following examples illustrate the method of the gray-level histogram.

Normal uterine muscle and fibromyoma tissue were compared with gray-level histograms (Figure 1). Fibromyoma showed larger width of the histogram than normal uterine muscle, probably due to the increase of connective tissue in the myoma and also from the difference of the structural complexity.

Simple ovarian and dermoid cysts were studied with gray-level histograms, and there was a clear difference between these two tissues. Ovarian follicle, unruptured luteinized follicle, and lutein cyst were compared by the histograms. Normal follicles and those of overstimulated ovary showed narrow and to the left-shifted histograms, whereas unruptured luteinized follicle and lutein cyst showed increased brightness, which was suspected to be from the high value of the average gray level and the histogram width, larger than the follicle (Figure 2).

Expelled placenta was immersed in water, and the linear scan transducer was placed at water level. B mode images and gray-level histograms were obtained at the same time. The placentas were divided into three visual grades from the B mode image, and the histograms were compared according to the grades (Figure 3). Average gray level was lowest in the grade I placenta, second highest in grade II, and the highest value was obtained in grade III. Histogram width showed the values increased along with the placental grade (Table 1).

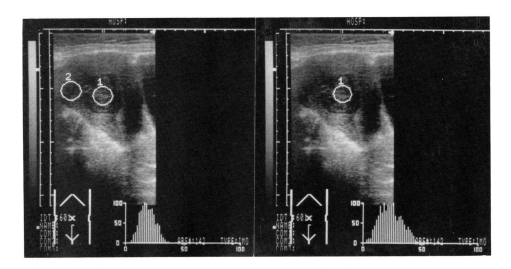

FIGURE 1.   Gray-level histograms obtained from normal uterine muscle (left) and fibromyomatous node (right). Wide histogram and a shift of the peak to higher gray level are observed in fibromyoma.

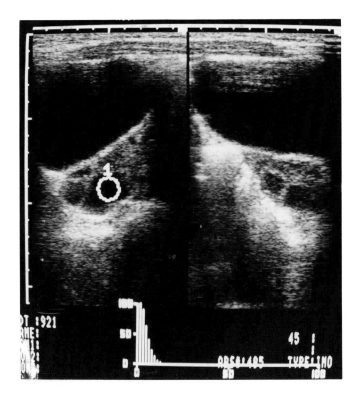

A

FIGURE 2.   Three gray-level histograms were obtained from periovulatory ovarian cysts. A is a preovulatory follicle which shows a narrow gray-level histogram at the lowest gray scale. B is a luteinized unruptured follicle (LUF), of which the histogram is wide and the peak is shifted to a higher gray scale than the follicle. C is an ovarian lutein cyst which shows a wide histogram and the peak located at a similar gray scale as LUF. (Courtesy of Drs. Y. Mio and T. Toda, Department of Obstetrics and Gynecology, Tottori University.)

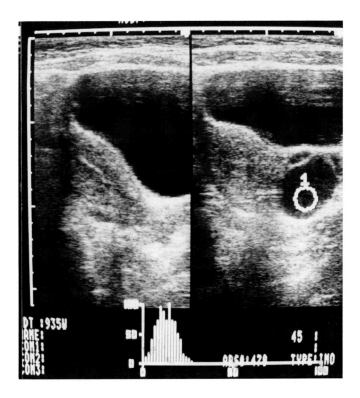

FIGURE 2B.

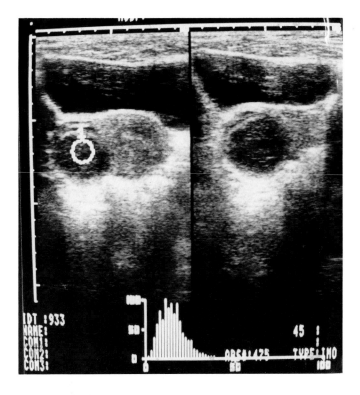

FIGURE 2C.

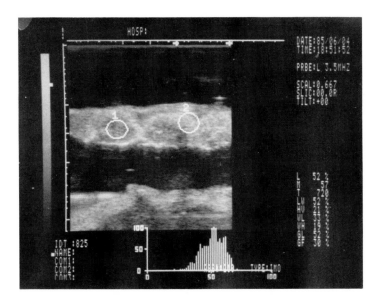

FIGURE 3.   A gray-level histogram obtained from expelled placenta which was examined in water. (Courtesy of Dr. P. E. Kihaile, Department of Obstetrics and Gynecology, Tottori University.)

TABLE 1
Ultrasonic Gray Level and Placental Grades[10]

Parameters	Placental grades		
	I	II	II
Number of cases	12	21	17
Gray level			
Mean	27.69	29.00	39.00
Deviation	18.20	30.20	34.05
Gray level histogram width (%)	40.58	49.95	51.00

In vivo placenta showed the same tendency as *in vitro* placenta. The width of a gray-level histogram was compared with the groups of several clinical abnormalities. The width value showed significant increases in the cases of intrauterine growth retardation (IUGR) and in those who exhibited fetal distress after histogram analysis, though the width value showed no correlation with the depth of the placenta in the detection of the region of interest (ROI) for the histogram analysis (Table 2). The most accurate test will be the comparison of the histograms obtained in the same case at the same time in consecutive multiple ROIs.

Akaiwa tried the comparison in the report of Maeda et al.[11] in five consecutive ROIs in the same *in vivo* placentas. Significantly clear coincidence of the histogram peaks were noted in grade I placenta, whereas grade III placenta showed widely distributed peaks of the histograms. This scanning method for ROI setting will show the characteristics of the placenta tissue more clearly than the simple histogram (Figure 4).

Akaiwa and Maeda[1] further reported the classification of the placental grades by multiple histograms and a discrimination function with statistical significance.

FETAL LUNG AND LIVER

The histograms and mean gray levels were determined in fetal lung and liver in several stages of gestation. At 24 to 26 weeks of pregnancy, most of the cases showed a higher

TABLE 2
Comparison of Gray Level Width in Several Abnormal Conditions to Normal Pregnancy[7]

Condition	No. of patients	No. of scans	Gray level width per 63 gray scales (mean and SD)	p[a]
Fetal distress	69	110	54.4 ± 5.39	<0.001
IUGR	28	56	50.1 ± 5.65	<0.001
EPH-gestosis	13	26	47.2 ± 8.47	N.S.
Elderly primi-gravid	23	35	47.5 ± 7.85	N.S.
Control	148	192	46.8 ± 7.30	

[a] p = comparison to the control value; N.S. = not significant.

From Kihaile, P. E., *Yonago Acta Med.,* 1988, in press. With permission.

gray level value in the liver than in the lung. However, in late stage of pregnancy after 32 weeks, the mean gray level was larger in fetal lung than the liver in most of the cases (Figure 5).

AN EXAMPLE OF RADIOFREQUENCY SIGNAL ANALYSIS

An UIP-100 computer system was used in radiofrequency (RF) signal processing. The computer system was composed of a PDP-11 minicomputer, the peripherals and softwares, and it was connected to a B mode scanner with an analog-to-digital converter. The combination of these devices prepared various functions for the analysis of ultrasonic signals, including several biometries, the estimation of gestational age, organ volume determination, velocity measurement in M mode, gray-level histogram, RF signal processing, and others. RF signal analysis will be more significant in tissue characterization, since there is reduced interference of artifacts in the RF signal processing. High sampling rates must be used. In our case, sampling frequency was 25.2 MHz, and AD conversion was done in eight bits. RF signal sampling points were 512 in each of 64 ultrasound beams which were included in an ROI. The data were stored on floppy disk, reproduced, and processed in the computer. The results were displayed on CRT. Amplitude histograms were obtained in the analysis. Fast Fourier transform (FFT) was done in the frequency analysis, and power spectrum was obtained. Two power spectrums were obtained from shallow and deep parts of the tissue, and the subtracted result of one spectrum from another was obtained in the form of frequency-dependent attenuation (FDA). Regression analysis was performed, and the attenuation coefficient was obtained from the FDA, peak frequency, and the distance between the two parts of the tissue. The RF signal processing was done in heparinized blood, hemorrhagic cyst of endometriosis, placenta, fetal liver, and fibromyoma.

RF ultrasound histogram was recorded and evaluated in some tissues, and the results showed the difficulty of interpretation and poor usefulness in clinical tissue characterization. Therefore, the main technique has been the investigations of the attenuation coefficient obtained from FDA. The technique was used on the tissues which scatter ultrasound homogeneously. The tissues which were suitable for analysis were studied in our department.

Two ROIs were selected in the tissue on the B mode image in shallow and deep parts of the tissue. Power spectrums were obtained from the two parts, FDA was displayed, and attenuation coefficient was obtained (Figure 6).

Attenuation coefficient showed low values in heparinzed blood and hemorrhagic cyst that contained rich blood. The highest value was obtained in uterine fibromyoma. The placenta showed a higher value than the blood. Fetal liver showed an intermediate value between the placenta and fibromioma (Figure 7).

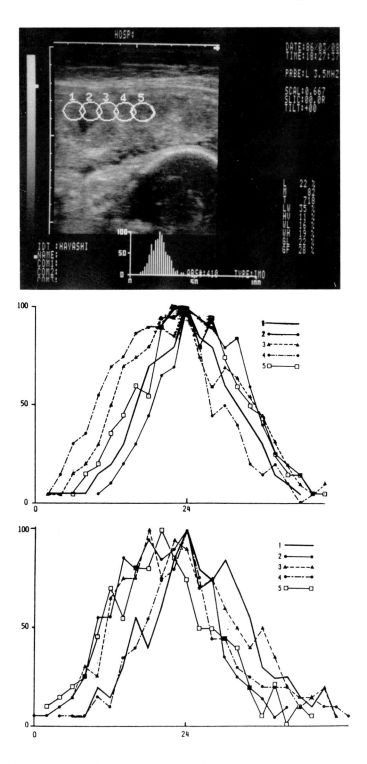

FIGURE 4. (Top) Scanning gray-level histograms obtained from *in vivo* placenta during pregnancy. (Middle) The envelopes of the histograms of homogeneous and low-grade placenta. The histograms are almost uniform in low-grade placenta. (Bottom) Scanning gray-level histograms of a high-grade placenta. The peaks are distributed in a wider range than low-grade placenta.

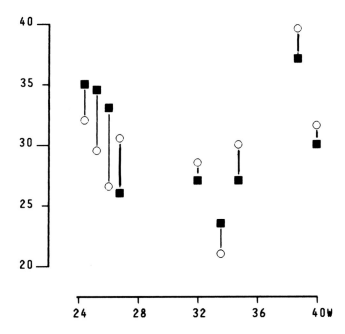

FIGURE 5.   Mean gray levels of fetal lung (open circle) and fetal liver (black square) are shown. Gray level of fetal lung is lower than the liver in the early stage of pregnancy, whereas the lung shows a higher gray level than the liver in late stage of gestation.

DISCUSSION

The body of knowledge is still in its initial growth stage, and the contributions, sometimes controversial, are yet to be matched. Kihaile et al.[7] reported the significant increase of grade III placenta in cases of IUGR[6] and those who exhibited fetal distress sign on CTG after the histogram examination. Gray-level histogram width showed the same results;[8] therefore, the quantified technique could be useful in clinical evaluation of the placenta states.

Garrett et al.[5] reported increased B mode brightness in fetal lung in late pregnancy. Morris[12] stated that fetal lung to liver ratio correlated with amniotic L/S ratio. There had been much criticism concerning the opinion that ultrasonic B mode was able to be used in the evaluation of fetal lung maturity.[2-4] We studied gray-level histogram and mean gray level in fetal lung and liver. There was a smaller value of mean gray level in the fetal lung than in fetal liver, and, on the contrary, the lung showed a higher mean gray level than the liver in the late stage of pregnancy. This result, which was obtained by quantified objective method, indicates increased brightness of the fetal lung image in late pregnancy, as reported by Garrett et al.,[5] and, therefore, there still remains the possibility of direct assessment of fetal lung maturity with the use of such a tissue characterization technique as gray-level histogram with its quantification.

Ultrasonic tissue characterization has been tried with the determination of sound velocity in the tissue, but it was difficult to determine ultrasonic propagation velocity in living tissue of pregnant cases, and clinical results have not been reported. The attenuation of ultrasound during insonation and reflection in living tissue will reflect the ultrasound absorption and scattering in the tissue, and the attenuation coefficient determination has been carried out in living tissue. FDA has been particularly expected to be the most useful in tissue characterization.[13] Namely, ultrasound shows its attenuation according to the increase in ultrasonic frequency. The attenuation in every frequency differs according to the tissue character and therefore reflects the nature of the tissue. Hence, it is suggested that the attenuation

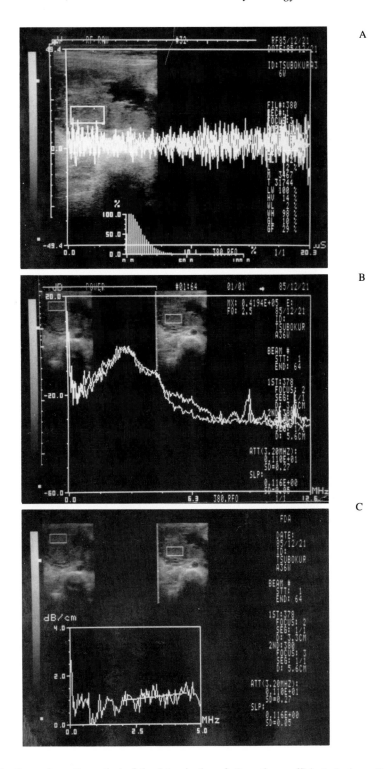

FIGURE 6. The figure shows the method of the determination of attenuation coefficient. A shows the ROI, reflected ultrasonic wave, and RF histogram. B is two frequency spectra which were obtained from shallow and deep parts of the tissue. C shows the result of subtraction of a power spectrum from another, and attenuation coefficient is calculated from the linear regression.

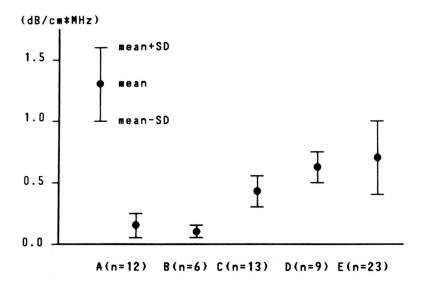

FIGURE 7. Attenuation coefficients are shown in heparinized blood (A), hemorrhagic cyst (B), *in vivo* placenta (C), fetal liver (D), and uterine fibromyoma (E).

coefficient obtained by FDA will show the clinical applicability of ultrasound tissue characterization. Studies have been done on the attenuation with several methods, and the most precise technique seems to be the spectral-difference method, which was reported by Kuc.[9] Several *in vivo* materials have been investigated in our department, and some useful results have been obtained.

CONCLUSION

Gray-level histogram of the ultrasonic A mode signal and the determination of the attenuation coefficient with the FDA method have showed their usefulness in the estimation of tissue character in obstetrics and gynecology. Particularly, the combined use of common real-time B mode with the tissue characterization technique will be very effective for further progress of the study in our field.

REFERENCES

1. **Akaiwa, A. and Maeda, K.,** Ultrasonic tissue characterization of fetus and placenta, Proceedings of the 2nd Autumn Congress of the JSMEBE, *Jpn. J. Med. Electron. Biol. Eng.,* Suppl., 46, 1987.
2. **Cayea, P. D., Grant, D. C., Doubilet, P. M., and Jones, T. B.,** Prediction of fetal lung maturity: inaccuracy of study using conventional ultrasound instruments, *Radiology,* 155, 473, 1985.
3. **Feingold, M., Scollins, J., Cetrulo, C. L., and Koza, D.,** Fetal lung to liver reflectivity ratio and lung maturity, *J. Clin. Ultrasound,* 15, 384, 1987.
4. **Fried, A. M., Loh, F. K., Umer, M. A., Dillon, K. P., and Kryscio, A. R.,** Echogenicity of fetal lung: relation to fetal age and maturity, *Am. J. Radiol.,* 145, 591, 1985.
5. **Garrett, W. J., Warren, P. S., Picker, R. H., and Kossoff, G.,** Fetal lung reflectivity, *Ultrasound Med. Biol.,* 8, 63, 1982.
6. **Grannum, P. A. T., Berkowitz, R. L., and Hobbins, J. C.,** The ultrasonic changes in maturing placenta and their relation to fetal pulmonic maturity, *Am. J. Obstet. Gynecol.,* 133, 915, 1979.
7. **Kihaile, P. E., Akaiwa, A., and Maeda, K.,** Relationship between grade III placenta maturation changes and fetal well-being, *Yonago Acta Med.,* 31, 75, 1988.
8. **Kihaile, P. E.,** Ultrasonic grey-level histogram of prenatal placenta and its relation to fetal well-being, *Yonago Acta Med.,* 1988, in press.

9. **Kuc, R.,** Clinical application of an ultrasound attenuation coefficient estimation technique for liver pathology characterization, *IEEE Trans. Biomed. Eng.,* BME-27, 312, 1980.
10. **Maeda, K., Sakao, A., Mio, Y., Kikukawa, A., Akaiwa, A., and Kihaile, P. A.,** The quantification of ultrasonic B-mode images with the trials of tissue characterization in obstetrics and gynecology, in *Recent Advances in Ultrasound Diagnosis,* Vol. 5, Kurjak, A. and Kossoff, G., Eds., Elsevier, Amsterdam, 1986, 215.
11. **Maeda, K., Akaiwa, A., Kihaile, P. E., Ishihara, H., and Takeuhi, Y.,** Ultrasonic tissue characterization in perinatal medicine, in *Recent Advances in Ultrasound Diagnosis,* Vol. 6, Kurjak, A. and Kossoff, G., Eds., Dr. Josip Kajfes, Zagreb, 1987, 17.
12. **Morris, S. E.,** Ultrasound: a predictor of fetal lung maturity, *Med. Ultrasound,* 8, 1, 1984.
13. **Ophir, J., Shawker, T. H., Maklad, N. F., Miller, J. G., Flax, S. W., Narayana, P. A., and Jones, J. P.,** Attenuation estimation in reflection: progress and prospect, *Ultrason. Imag.,* 6, 349, 1984.

Chapter 8

ENDOSONOGRAPHY FOR THE DIAGNOSIS OF UTERINE MALIGNOMAS

Gerhard Bernaschek and Josef Deutinger

INTRODUCTION

In cases of uterine malignomas, the use of abdominal sonography enabled one to only investigate suspected areas, if anamnesis and results of clinical investigations were available. The borders of tumor spread could only be detected if the tumor extended the boundary of the organs. Like other noninvasive methods, endosonography also does not allow to differentiate between benign and malignant diseases. However, in cases of known histologic diagnosis of cancer, localization and tumor extent can be imaged more precisely.[1] The numerous advantages of endosonography have led to an improved pretherapeutical staging. A better survey of the true pelvis is warranted and the intracorporal position of the scanner opens the possibility of using higher frequencies which improve resolution capacity. The scanner is positioned closely to the uterus. In each patient, the small distance between the probe and the investigated organs is nearly equal, and the investigation can be performed under standardized settings of the ultrasound equipment. Therefore, the obtained results can also be compared visually. Additionally, embarrassing layers located in the beam between the abdominal transducer and the investigated organs, like filled loops of intestine and bone structures, can be excluded by intracorporal placement of the scanner. Therefore, ''blind areas'' may be excluded. This is especially important in patients with severe adhesions after surgery or radiation therapy or in cases of inflammation or endometriosis. Transabdominal sonography might be hindered by obesity or in case of an empty bladder, whereas endosonography is not affected by these circumstances.

Vaginal sonography and hysterosonography are particularly useful for the staging in cases of endometrium cancer. Recto- and cystosonography bear advantages for the diagnosis of cervical cancer and especially for the diagnosis of recurrences after surgery and/or radiation treatment.

ENDOMETRIUM CANCER

Endosonography provides a better visualization of the endometrial echoes. Vaginal sonography is superior to hysterosonography in estimating the localization and the extension of endometrial cancer, mainly because of the simple investigation procedure. Vaginal sonography is performed with an empty bladder. Therefore, the well-known problems of the full-bladder technique (e.g., after radiation therapy) when performing transabdominal sonography do not occur. Therefore vaginal sonography can be performed immediately after bimanual palpation or, if necessary, simultaneously. The hand on the abdominal wall may also lead the uterus closer to the scanner.

Vaginal sonography may be performed by means of curved array probes that perform as well as the frontally radiating sector probes with the narrow sector. A curved array scanner provide a better view in the area close to the probe. The advantage of rotor scanners is their ability to provide a better survey of the small pelvis.

The clinical classification of endometrial cancer is performed, due to the length of the Hegar's dilator, when performing diagnostic dilatation and curretage. Vaginal sonography, however, allows the measurement of the extension of the length of the uterus and of the endometrial echoes. Differentiation and localization of myometrial infiltration are also pos-

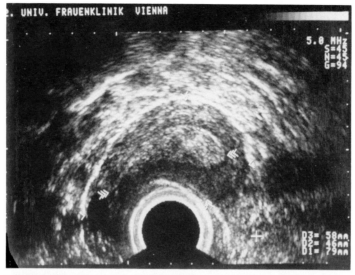

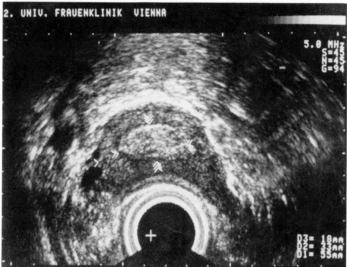

FIGURE 1.   Vaginal sonography in a patient with postmenopausal bleeding with histologically proven endometrium cancer, which is confined to the mucosa. (Above) Longitudinal section of the anteverted uterus. The endometrial echo is thickened; the myometrium appears to be inconspicuous. (Below) Cross-section of the corpus uteri in the same case.

sible. Pathologic proliferation of the endometrium may be visualized by vaginal sonography much before symptoms are apparent. In cases of endometrial cancer, the echoes of the endometrium are thickened and inhomogeneous, and no liquid is visible in this area as in the case of mucometra (Figure 1). Advanced carcinomas of the endometrium always show a pathologically thickened endometrium with typical "fuzzy", inhomogeneous margins toward the myometrium and a typical echo-poor area of invasion of the carcinoma into the myometrium (Figure 2). The boundary towards the myometrium is mostly not sharp. In contrast, myomas show a clearly recognizable delineation and are separated by a capsule. Since the corpus uteri and also the cervix can be imaged at the same time, an additional invasion of the cervical area can be ascertained. Therefore, the depth of an endometrial carcinoma, its longitudinal dimension, and the possible occupation of the cervical region

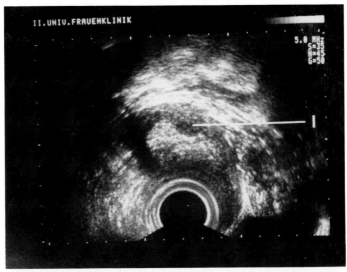

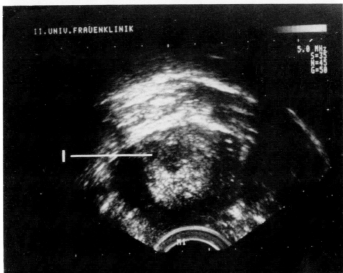

FIGURE 2.   Vaginal sonography in a patient with postmenopausal bleeding with histologically proven endometrium cancer. (Above) Longitudinal section of the retroverted uterus, the endometium appears to be thickened with irregular boundaries. Additionally, an area with low echogenity refers to an infiltration (I) of the myometrium. (Below) Cross-section of the corpus uteri in the same case.

can be evaluated, and stage II of the endometrium cancer may be diagnosed preoperatively. This allows for preoperative planning of the extent of intervention.

Hysterosonography is usually carried out by means of slim rotating scanners with a 360° transverse scanner (same scanners as for cystosonography). For protection of the endometrium, a cover had been used originally, however, this proved unnecessary. In order to also provide an evaluation of the fundus of the uterus, most of these scanners offer a switchable angle of frontal radiation of 90 and 135°.[2] The probes can be sterilized and the depth of the insertion into the cavum uteri can read off the shaft of the probes.

For performing hysterosonography, general anesthesia is required, because a cervical dilatation up to Hegar 8 or 10 is necessary. This disadvantage restricts the routine use of

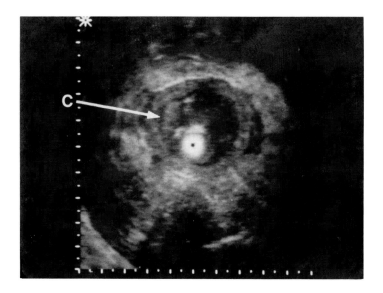

FIGURE 3. Hysterosonography in a case of histologically proven endometrium cancer. The cross-section of the corpus uteri shows an area with high echogenity; this local cancer area (C) is confined to the mucosa.

this method, and it is usually performed in combination with dilatation and diagnostic curettage. Since the scanner is introduced directly into the cavum uteri, it is possible to image the origin and the localization of carcinomas, which are located only in the endometrium (Figure 3). The optimum modality for radiation therapy can be determined in the course of therapy planning by means of a computer. Computer-aided processing of equally spaced hysterosonographic scan images is also a prerequisite for the determination of tumor volume.[2-4]

In cases of known histological and clinical findings of an endometrium carcinoma, the use of vaginal and hysterosonography may help to evaluate the localization, the boundaries, and the extent of myometrial invasion. Preoperatively, the extent of intervention or the best method for radiation therapy can be planned, and performance individualized therapy is possible.[5]

CERVICAL CANCER

Particularly, rectosonography is useful for objectifying the pretherapeutic staging of cervical cancer.[6,7] Cystosonography is used for the verification of infiltrations of the bladder wall. Rectosonography is superior to vaginal sonography because transverse sections can provide a better survey of the uterine cervix. It is advantageous if the structures that are to be examined are located higher in the small pelvis and the vaginal length is insufficient for performing vaginal sonography. Rectosonography is usually carried out with linear array scanners or with rotor scanners with a sector of 360°. The latter provide the diagnosis of dislocation of the uterus towards the infiltrated parametrium and allow to image lateral deviations of the parametria. The patient has to be prepared as for rectoscopy, and the bladder is filled with 400 ml of saline. The filled bladder tilts the normally anteverted uterus over and serves, together with the pelvic walls, as landmarks. After insertion of the scanner into the rectum, a condom-like cover, previously slipped over the transducer, is filled with approximately 50 ml of water in order to establish a short water delay. In the same way as for other endosonographical methods, dorsal lithotomy position of the patient is preferred.

This position improves the motility of the scanner. Systematic transversal scans up to a penetration depth of 17 cm, which also can be read off the shaft of the probes, enable one to carry out a precise exploration of the small pelvis.

Compared with vaginal sonography, rectosonography stresses the patient more. However, after a short explanation of the procedure, the invasivness of the investigation can be compared with rectal palpation. Like digital palpation, rectosonography is also restricted or even impossible in cases with painful hemorrhoids, highly obstructive tumors, and irritation of the rectal mucosa after previous radiation. In cases of cervical cancer, a precise staging is required for the decision of the kind of therapy and for comparison of the results of different treatments. Staging can only be performed before treatment. The guidelines, which were established by the FIGO, are primarily based on the continuous tumor spread and infiltration depth. Stage I A cannot be evaluated by means of endosonography. If a histological diagnosis is available, it is for the first time possible by means of rectosonography to pretherapeutically make a further differentiation within the stage I B classification in regard to the size and the depth of the infiltration of the tumor (Figure 4). In most cases, carcinomas are characterized by echo-poor areas (Figure 5), and in some cases, they have a higher echogenity than the surrounding cervical tissue. The use of standard settings of ultrasound equipment is possible because in each case, cervical tissue is adjacent to the rectal tissue. This is important in terms of computerized texture analyses of ultrasound images aimed at a future sonographical definition of subtle criteria of malignancy. The advantage of rectosonography is especially noticeable in patients with stage II B carcinoma not extending beyond the parametria. An irregular boundary of the parametrium with cervical dislocation toward the infiltrated side will cause suspicion of extrauterine tumor extension (Figure 6).

In comparison with rectal palpation, there is an essential advantage because not only the rectal, but also the vesical boundary can be assessed. In stage III B, the infiltrated parametrium, which is characterized by low echogenity and irregular boundaries, reaches the pelvic wall (Figure 7). Like rectal palpation, histologic diagnosis of malignancy must be known beforehand, because rectosonography does not provide a differentiation between inflamed and carcinomatously infiltrated tissues. In cases of carcinoma, mostly irregular boundaries and nodular alterations are found.

Stages II A and III A, defined by an infiltration of the vagina, may also be diagnosed by means of rectosonography, or even better by means of vaginal sonography. In stage IV, the continuous growth of the tumor leads to an invasion of bladder and/or rectum (Figure 8). In cases of infiltration of the rectum, this is imaged by an interruption of the typical contour of the rectal wall. Infiltration of the bladder wall is also displayed by inhomogeneity of the bladder contour. In this case, however, cystosonography should be performed subsequently.

Cystosonography is usually carried out by means of slim rotating scanners with a 360° transverse radiation.[8] Anesthetic catheter jelly is applied into the urethra under aseptic conditions, whereupon the scanner is inserted into the bladder via the urethra via a CH 24 resectoscope sheath. For imaging all areas of the bladder walls, most scanners allow the selection of the angle of radiation for an additional 45° forward and 45° backward viewing with regard to their long axis. Compared with cystoscopy, cystosonography also images the deeper layers of the bladder wall and provides images of the paravesical region, whereas by means of cystoscopy, only surface areas of the bladder wall can be investigated. The carcinomatous invasion of the bladder wall leads to an interruption of the typical contour (Figure 9). Edema of the bladder mucosa, where the mucosa is imaged irregularly and broadened, does not necessarily imply bladder invasion (Figure 10). Cystosonography is most helpful in those cases where cystoscopically a bullous edema is seen. Then, cystosonography allows to confirm or to reject the diagnosis of bladder infiltration. Additionally,

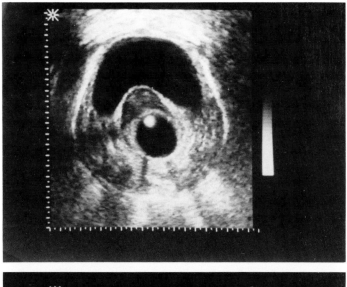

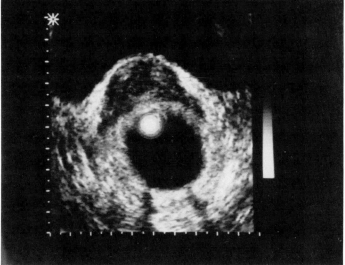

FIGURE 4.   Rectosonography in a case of histologically proven cervical cancer.
(Above) Cross-section of the uterine cervix. Bilaterally inconspicuous tapering off
and smoothly shaped features of the parametrium with uniform thickness. (Below)
Zoomed image.

it reveals ascertainment by mere endosonographic demonstration of deeper layers of the
bladder. In case of a bullous edema diagnosed by means of cystoscopy, the diagnosis of an
infiltration of the bladder wall cannot be made. However, if subsequently performed cystosonography shows an interruption of the typical bladder contour, it refers to cervical cancer
stage IV. An additional advantage of cystosonography is in the possibility of performing
biopsy under ultrasound guidance from deeper layers, whereas by means of cystoscopy, a
biopsy can be carried out only from a surface area.

RECURRENT CARCINOMA

A good survey is essential for the diagnosis of recurrences located in the small pelvis.
Therefore, those types of scanners are preferred which provide the image of a great sector.[9]

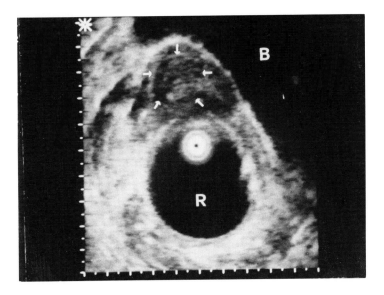

FIGURE 5.   Rectosonography in a case of histologically proven cervical cancer; cross-section of the uterine cervix. In the center, an area with low echogenity is imaged, which refers to malign alteration (arrows).

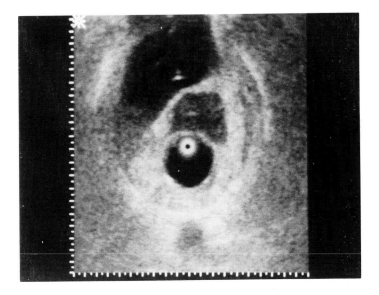

FIGURE 6.   Rectosonography in a case of histologically proven cervical cancer; cross-section of the uterine cervix. The uterus is displaced to the left, where the parametrium is infiltrated. The left parametrium appears to be thickened with irregular boundaries.

The diagnosis of recurrent malignomas is usually carried out by means of rectosonography. Applying vaginal sonography may be hindered by shortening or stenosis of the vagina after surgical or radiation treatment. By means of the above-mentioned method, local recurrences show as areas with low echogenity (Figure 11). Also their size, location, and state can be determined, as well as eventual infiltration of adjacent organs. Above all, however, rectosonography provides the assessment of recurrences located at the pelvic wall. Particularly,

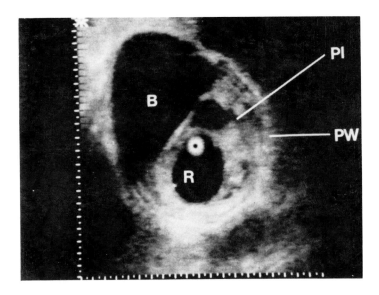

FIGURE 7. Rectosonography: cross-section through a cervix displaced to the left. The right parametrium appears to be inconspicuous, the left parametrium (Pl) is nodular and infiltrated to the pelvic wall (PW). Bladder, B; rectal balloon, R.

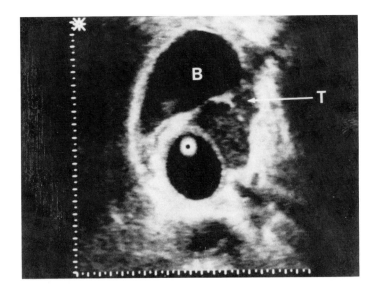

FIGURE 8. Rectosonography: cross-section through a cervix displaced to the left. The right parametrium appears to be inconspicuous; the left parametrium is thickened and infiltrated; the tumor (T) has broken through the anterior wall of the cervix and is infiltrating the bladder (B). The bladder contour is interrupted at this point.

if recurrences are located higher and impossible to reach by rectal palpation, the advantages of rectosonography are obvious (Figure 12). With recurrences located high in the lumbar region, where the rectal probe cannot be inserted in most cases, computer tomography is the method of choice compared to sonographical methods.

On the other hand, rectosonography allows the assessment of the lower pole of a tumor that can eventually extend cranially. In case of the lack of clinical signs, repeated endo-

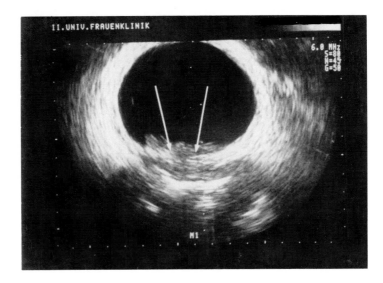

FIGURE 9. Cystosonography: irregular structures at the base of the bladder refer to a bullous edema of the mucosa. Additionally, a central interruption of the typical bladder contour and, therefore, infiltration of the bladder wall is imaged (arrows).

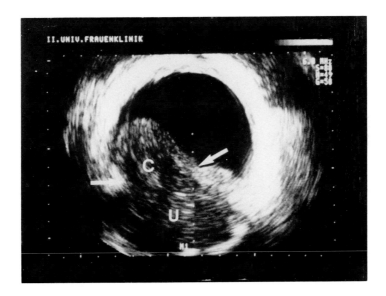

FIGURE 10. Cystosonography in a case of histologically proven cervical cancer (C). The tumor has broken through the anterior wall of the uterus (U), interrupting the bladder contour (arrows). Cystoscopy revealed only a bullous edema, which is imaged sonographically as a continuous area with higher echogenity above the cancer area (C).

sonographic investigation of suspected areas might be helpful. As with all noninvasive diagnostic methods, only a high degree of suspicion of a recurrent malignancy can be stated by means of rectosonography. The definitive diagnosis is finally possible by histologic evaluation. Up to now, the puncture of tumors has been restricted to those that were reachable by palpation. Now, rectosonography and vaginosonography provide the chance to puncture

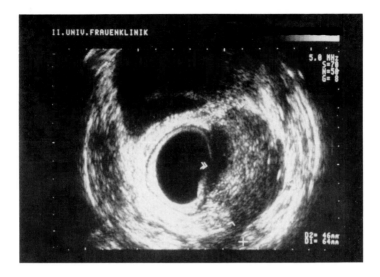

FIGURE 11. Rectosonography: cross-section of the small pelvis 1 year after Wertheim surgery performed in another hospital with subsequent radiation therapy. Recurrent cancer area at the pelvic wall on the left side.

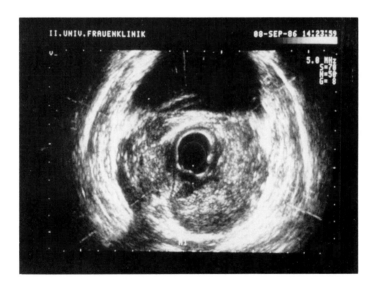

FIGURE 12. Rectosonography: cross-section of the small pelvis 1.5 years after Wertheim surgery performed in another hospital with subsequent radiation therapy. Bilaterally, near the pelvic wall, an extensive area of recurrent cancer leading to circular stenosis of the rectum appears.

recurrences even in a high location and under direct ultrasound guidance from the vagina. The possibility of rectosonographically controlled interstitial seed implantation with local recurrences — as it is applied to carcinoma of the prostate — should also be mentioned here.[10]

Finally it should be stated that by means of endosonography in cases of known histologic diagnosis, the extent and boundary of the tumor can be assessed. Endosonography should be used as a basic assessment for the staging of uterine malignomas. Additional information is now available before planning the individual therapy. Because of the objective pretherapeutical staging, the results of surgery and radiation treatment are now comparable.

Endosonographic follow-up investigations should also be obligatory in cases of high-risk patients for recurrences. Immediately after inspection and palpation, which is limited due to the length of the vagina or the length of the palpating finger, rectosonography should be applied for the investigation of structures located more cranially. Endosonography is a simple procedure with a high diagnostic value. Therefore, it should be performed before more complicated and invasive diagnostic methods like computer tomography or angiography are carried out. These methods could be limited to such cases where endosonography does not support the diagnosis of a malignant disease.

REFERENCES

1. **Bernaschek, G. and Janisch, H.,** Eine Methode zur Objektivierung des Parametrienbefundes beim Zervixkarzinom, *Geburtshilfe Frauenheilkd.,* 43, 489, 1983.
2. **Hötzinger, H., Engelmeier, K. H., Ries, G., Wischnik, A., and Sbornik, E.,** Zum Problem der Darstellung des Fundus uteri bei der Intrauterinsonographie, *Ultraschall,* 6, 189, 1985.
3. **Hötzinger, H.,** Durch Intrauterinsonographie optimierte intrakavitäre Strahlentherapie bei Korpuskarzinomen, *Strahlentherapie,* 160, 600, 1984.
4. **Hötzinger, H., Becker, H., and Becker, V.,** Intrauterine Ultraschalltomographie (IUT): Vergleich mit makroskopischen Präparatschnitten, *Geburtshilfe Frauenheilkd.,* 44, 219, 1984.
5. **Englmeier, K. H., Hötzinger, H., and Pöppl, S. J.,** Eine neue Methode zur individuellen Isodosengestaltung beim Korpuskarzinom, in *Gynäkologische Endosonographie,* Aktualisierter Kongreßband der Ersten Arbeitstagung Gynäkologische Endosonographie 1985 in Hamburg, Popp, L. W., Ed., Ingo Klemke, Quickborn, 1986, 171.
6. **Bernaschek, G., Tatra, G., and Janisch, H.,** Die rektale Sonographie — eine Erweiterung der Rezidivdiagnostik zervikaler Neoplasien, *Geburtshilfe Frauenheilkd.,* 44, 295, 1984.
7. **Bernaschek, G., Deutinger, J., Bartl, W., and Janisch, H.,** Endosonographic staging of carcinoma of the uterine cervix, *Arch. Gynecol. Obstet.,* 239, 21, 1986.
8. **Kölbl, H. and Bernaschek, G.,** Der Stellenwert der Zystosonographie beim Staging von gynäkologischen Malignomen, *Ultraschall Klin. Prax.,* 1 (Suppl. 1), 11, 1986.
9. **Bernaschek, G., Deutinger, J., Bartl, W., and Janisch, H.,** Erste Ergebnisse eines echographischen Staging beim Zervixkarzinom, *Wien. Klin. Wochenschr.,* 96, 286, 1984.
10. **Weigert, F., Hötzinger, H., and Atzinger, A.,** Die rektosonographische Differentialdiagnose lokaler Rezidive gynäkologischer Malignome von Narben und die gesteuerte Afterloadingtherapie von Rezidiven im kleinen Becken, in *Gynäkologische Endosonographie,* Aktualisierter Kongreßband der Ersten Arbeitstagung Gynäkologische Endosonographie 1985 in Hamburg, Popp, L. W., Ed., Ingo Klemke, Quickborn, 1986, 183.

Chapter 9

NORMAL ANATOMY OF THE FEMALE PELVIS AND PRINCIPLES OF ULTRASOUND DIAGNOSIS OF PELVIC PATHOLOGY

Davor Jurkovic and Biserka Funduk-Kurjak

NORMAL ANATOMY OF THE FEMALE PELVIS

The pelvis is a bony ring resembling a basin. Anatomically, it can be divided into the greater and lesser pelvis by an oblique line which passes through the prominence of the sacrum to the superior margin of the pubic symphysis.

By distension of the urinary bladder, gas-filled bowel loops are displaced from the lesser pelvis, permitting the visualization of the genital organs and anatomical structures within the lesser pelvis.[1,2] If gas in the restosigmoid colon disturbs visualization of the posterior aspect of the uterus, a water enema may be utilized to allow visualization of the whole lesser pelvis content. The quality of the ultrasound image remains unsatisfactory in the patients with the increased amount of mesenteric fat in the pelvis, and in such cases, other alternative imaging procedures will be offered.[3]

Knowledge of topographic anatomy and echoanatomy is a condition for evaluation by ultrasound. Echoanatomy is the result of distinguishing anatomic elements in the ultrasound image, but it demands knowledge of the anatomy as well as of the ultrasound method. In order to be able to recognize individual anatomic elements in the ultrasonic scan, various tissues must be distinguished. By using static equipment, it is possible to obtain a clear overview of the whole pelvic content,[4] including the anterior skeletal surface and pelvic musculature. The ultrasonic imaging of normal organs in the lesser pelvis has essentially been facilitated by the introduction of the gray scale in diagnosis.

The most significant advantage of real-time is the ease of maneuverability, whereby one can quickly change scan planes and rapidly survey the pelvis, getting a three-dimensional impression of the structure under investigation. Another advantage of real-time is the visualization of vascular pulsations and peristalsis, which may be helpful for the detection of the ovaries and prevents the misinterpretation of a fluid-filled bowel loop as an ovarian mass.

During the examination, the patient is lying supine, the probe is placed suprapubically, and parallel transverse and longitudinal scans are performed. Oblique scans are then employed for a better delineation of a particular structure.

It should be noted that the smaller scanning heads of real-time mechanical sector scanners represent an improvement over the larger, rectangular linear array probes, allowing easier accessibility to the sidewalls of the pelvis. As far as the frequency of the transducer is concerned, it is well known that it is always the rule in ultrasound to use the highest frequency transducer compatible with adequate penetration of the part being examined.[5] Most adult female pelvises, however, can be adequately scanned using a 3.5- or 5.0-MHz transducer with either a medium or long internal focus.

Accuracy of ultrasound in detection of pelvic abnormalities is estimated to be about 82 to 91%.[6] It depends upon proper examination technique and adequate distension of the urinary bladder, which serves as an acoustic window to visualize adjacent structures. Ultrasonic assessment of normal pelvic structures is described in the first part of this chapter, including the bones, muscles, blood vessels, ureter, urinary bladder, vagina, uterus, ovaries, uterine tubes, and rectosigmoid colon.

PELVIC SKELETON
Anatomy

The pelvis is a bony ring consisting of the bilateral symmetrical hipbones and sacrum. Each hipbone is composed of three parts: the ilium, ischium, and pubis, which unite at the acetabulum. The ilium is the most superior bone, the pubis the most anterior bone, and the ischium is the most inferior bone, being the strongest of them. Anatomically, the pelvis can be further divided into the greater and lesser pelvises by an oblique line termed the pelvic brim. The lesser pelvis communicates superiorly with the greater pelvis and is closed inferiorly by a group of muscles termed the pelvic diaphragm.

Ultrasound Image

Ultrasound enables visualization of the pelvic structures in any plane and offers the possibility of distinguish subtle differences in all soft tissues that have different densities and velocities of transmitted sound; but ultrasound waves are not able to penetrate bone. The anterior skeletal surfaces can be clearly distinguished so that the posterior boundary of the overlying soft tissues may be carefully analyzed. If scans are performed from the anterior, lateral, and posterior surfaces of the pelvis, the outer boundaries of the bones and the overlying soft tissues can be imaged. Gas-filled bowel presents difficulty in imaging because gas reflects sound back to the transducer, causing inadequate penetration. A better image is obtained with a full bladder which pushes away the intestine, or introduction of fluid per rectum if gas in the rectosigmoid colon limits visualization.[7]

PELVIC MUSCULATURE
Anatomy

In the greater pelvis, the iliopsoas muscle is a combination of the psoas major and the iliacus muscle. The first one is a thin, long muscle that originates in the paralumbar vertebral region and enters the greater pelvis anteriorly and laterally over the iliac crest. The second is a flat triangular structure arising posterior to the psoas major muscle. Both muscles have insertion on the femur. Within the lesser pelvis, the obturator internus muscle occupies a large part of the inner surface of the anterior and lateral pelvic walls and is surrounded by fascia. The levator ani muscle, together with coccygeus muscle, form the pelvic diaphragm.

Ultrasound Image

Muscles may be present within the pelvis, and their characteristic appearance must be known in order to avoid confusion with other structures, particularly ovaries. Three major groups of muscles are visualized on pelvic ultrasound examination. In the greater pelvis, the iliopsoas muscles can be seen, while in the lesser pelvis, the obturator internus and the levator ani muscles are consistently identified. The two other muscles of the lesser pelvis, the coccygeus and piriformis muscle, are located deep, posteriorly and cranially, and they are not routinely visualized on ultrasound examination.

Ventrolaterally to the ovaries the psoas muscle is seen with a very characteristic echogenic center. The long axis of the iliopsoas muscle is imaged in a longitudinal projection angled from the midline towards the hip. In the transverse section, the internal obturator muscle is demonstrated as a hypoechoic ovoid structure located ventrally to the ovaries. The levator ani muscle is seen on transverse scan at the level of the cervix and vaginal fornices. Other muscles forming the pelvic diaphragm are rarely seen because of their deep position. By extending the transverse sections laterally across the iliac bones and the lateral pelvic walls, the caput femoris and the gluteal muscles may be visualized.

PELVIC BLOOD VESSELS
Anatomy

The common iliac arteries arise from the bifurcation of the abdominal aorta at the level

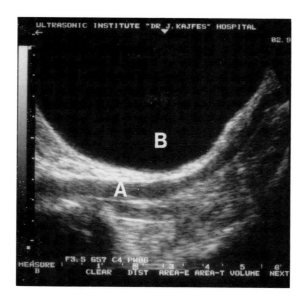

FIGURE 1.   External iliac artery is demonstrated in an oblique
scan on the lateral pelvic wall (A = artery, B = bladder).

of the fourth lumbar vertebral body and diverage laterally and caudally to enter the greater pelvis, coursing along the anterior medial aspect of the iliopsoas muscle. In the superior aspect of the greater pelvis, they are divided into external and internal iliac arteries. The external iliac artery remains within the greater pelvis, progressing through the inguinal canal to become the femoral artery. The internal iliac artery passes over the pelvic brim to descend into the lesser pelvis posterior and lateral to the ureter and ovary. The iliac veins (common, external, and internal) follow the same course as the arteries, except that they are more posteriorly and medially placed. The ovarian artery and vein enter the greater pelvis anterior to the common iliac artery and vein through the infundibulopelvic ligament and then descend into the lesser pelvis to reach the ovaries via the mesovarium.

Ultrasound Image

Pelvic vessels are clearly defined on ultrasound scan. They are sonographically demonstrated as tubular structures characterized by an anechoic lumen and hyperechoic walls. The internal iliac artery is seen by performing an oblique scan posteriorly and laterally to the ovaries. It can be easily distinguished from the internal iliac vein which is typically located posteriorly to the artery. If a real-time machine is used, pulsations of the artery are seen while diameter of the vein is constant. The external iliac artery and vein are also routinely imaged on an oblique scan directed through the bladder and to the contralateral pelvic wall. The external iliac vein can sometimes be compressed by an overfull urinary bladder so that only the artery is visualized (Figures 1 and 2).

The ovarian artery approaches the ovary from its lateral and posterior aspect, and being relatively thin, it is not regularly seen. However, meticulous scanning of the lateral peri-ovarian space will demonstrate in 60 to 70% of examined women the ovarian artery and vein which reach the ovaries via the mesovarium (Figure 3). Because of their small diameter and variable ovarian position, it is difficult to distinguish between artery and vein. Although there were several reports describing marked dilatation of the ovarian vessels at the peri-ovulatory phase of the cycle,[8] we were not able to confirm this in spite of systematic scanning of the patients during late follicular phase of the cycle until ovulation.

Recently, there were several reports describing blood flow characteristics in the pelvic vessels, but the clinical potential of these examinations remains to be clarified in the future.

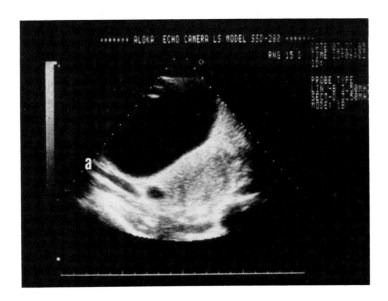

FIGURE 2. The right ovary shown in the sonogram contains a developing follicle and the internal iliac artery and vein passing laterally and posteriorly to the ovary (a = artery).

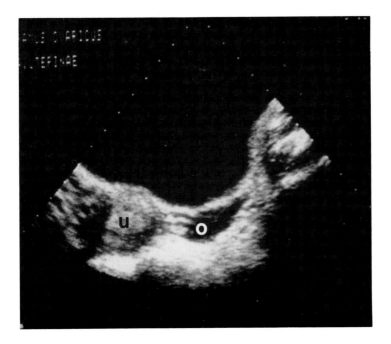

FIGURE 3. The right ovarian artery and vein reaching laterally to the ovary are demonstrated (u = uterus, o = ovary).

URETER
Anatomy

The ureters originate from the kidneys, lie anterior to the psoas muscles, and enter the pelvic course anterior to the common iliac artery and vein. After entering the lesser pelvis, they lie medial and anterior to the internal iliac vessels and continue caudally to insert into the trigone of the bladder.

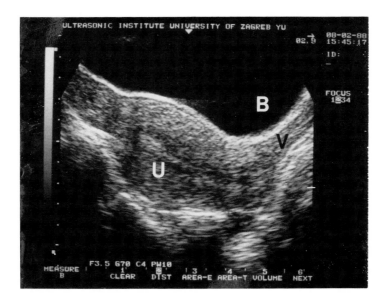

FIGURE 4.   Longitudinal scan of a normal uterus and vagina. The uterus is an-teverted and the fundus is more anterior than the cervix. The uterine fundus is larger than the cervix (B = bladder, U = uterus, V = vagina).

Ultrasound Image

On ultrasound examination, the ureter cannot be imaged within the greater pelvis, owing to its small size and overlying bowel. By contrast, the ureters can be routinely imaged in the lesser pelvis through a distended bladder.[4] The ureters are best seen by performing a longitudinal scan posteriorly to the ovaries, but may be also seen in transverse view. Any gross pelvic pathology of the uterus and ovaries may cause ureteral obstruction, so it is advisable to check its diameter during a routine examination.

On real-time examination, normal peristalsis can be seen in the ureter as a sparkling pattern of intermittent echoes. Within the urinary bladder, intermittent showers of echoes can be imaged as the urine passes from the ureter into the bladder.

URINARY BLADDER
Anatomy

The urinary bladder is the most anterior organ in the lesser pelvis, anchored inferiorly by the urethra and the trigone.

Ultrasound Image

On ultrasound scan, it is the most prominent organ, which appears as an anechoic structure with thin walls (Figures 4 and 5). Its shape depends, above all, on the quantity of urine in it, on the section level, and the obesity of the patient. If the bladder is not sufficiently full, it may hang from one or both sides of the uterus and imitate ovarian cysts.

In 60% of the patients, it is possible to observe dynamic movements within the bladder during examination. This so-called "jet phenomenon" was explained by the different os-molality and specific gravity of the fresh urine injected from ureters and fluid within the bladder[9] and can be potentially useful in diagnosis of unilateral kidney disease.

VAGINA
Anatomy

The vagina is anchored in the midline between the lower aspect of the urinary bladder

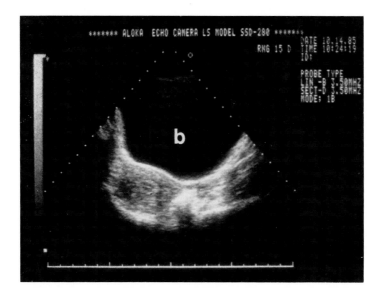

FIGURE 5.   Transverse sonogram of a normal uterus. The contour is clearly outlined and the texture displays homogenous and moderate echogenicity. The central cavity echo is clearly visible (b = bladder).

anteriorly and rectum posteriorly. The position of the vagina is not affected by bladder distension.

Ultrasound Image

On ultrasound examination, the vagina appears as a simple bright linear echo located below the bladder (Figure 4). This strong echo, measuring 7 to 10 cm in length, corresponds to the attached superficial layers of mucosa and is surrounded by the hypoechoic vaginal walls. If some fluid is present within the vagina, e.g., menstrual blood or urine, the linear echo is partially or completely absent, allowing its simple detection.

UTERUS
Anatomy

The uterus is the central organ in the female pelvis, clearly delineated and smooth. While the most common uterine position is midline and anteverted, the uterus may extend to the left or right, be retroverted, or be additionally anteflexed or retroflexed. The uterus is anchored at the superior aspect of the vagina and is situated between the caudal portions of the urinary bladder anteriorly and the rectum posteriorly. The uterine size and shape vary with age, parity, and time of menstrual cycle. In prepubertal age, the cervix occupies two thirds of the total uterine length, with the diameter of the uterine corpus less than the diameter of the cervix. During this period, the average uterine length is 2.5 cm, and the anteroposterior diameter is 1 cm. When menarche begins, the uterine corpus grows predominantly in width and thickness. In generative age, it is about 7 to 8 cm long, but in post menopause, the uterus undergoes atrophy and decrease in size to less than 6.5 cm in longitudinal and 2 cm anteroposterior dimension.

Ultrasound Image

The uterus can be accurately assessed by ultrasound. Uterine assessment includes its position, size, shape, contour, texture, and the appearance of the uterine cavity. Slight angulation of the uterine body either to the right or left is commonly seen in normal subjects.

The corpus is usually anteflected to the cervix. In cases of retroflection, the uterus is more difficult to assess and can be easily misinterpreted as a pathological finding by an inexperienced operator.[10] Uterine size and shape are mostly dependent on the patient's age and parity. Standards of uterine size have been described in numerous reports including the neonates,[11] premenarcheal girls,[12] and postpubertal[13] and postmenopausal[14] women. In girls up to 7 years of age, the uterine size is not influenced by age, and the cervix is relatively predominant over the corpus. Thereafter, the uterus increases steadily in size, and corpus gradually becomes larger than the cervix, as in postpubertal woman.[15] It is generally accepted that in normal nulligravidious women, the uterine size is up to 7 cm in longitudinal diameter and up to 4 cm in width and height. In multiparous women, all uterine diameters are, on average, 1.2 cm greater.[16] There are also slight variations in the uterine size during the cycle.[17]

The uterine contour is well defined, and the uterus is clearly separated from the adjacent pelvic structures. The texture of the myometrium can be clearly demonstrated by current gray scale equipment and is characterized by low to medium homogeneous echogenicity[18] (Figures 4 and 5). Recently, the sonographic appearance of the endometrial cavity in particular has been studied. Initial reports described the endometrium as a prominent central cavity echo, which was the only endometrial feature visible by instruments of relatively poor resolution capabilities. Further work has shown that phasic changes in the appearance of the endometrium can be recognized, and typical findings in the proliferative and secretory phase have been described.[19,20] The characteristic appearance of the preovulatory endometrium is well known as the "ovulation ring" and serves as an additional parameter for better prognosis and detection of ovulation.[21,22]

Comparison between the endometrium texture and thickness with other parameters, such as steroid hormone levels, the diameter of the dominant follicle, and histological findings, have indicated the usefulness of endometrium studies by ultrasound. It can serve as a guide in estimating the phase of the cycle and as a helpful parameter in *in vitro* fertilization procedures.[23-25]

OVARY

Anatomy

The ovary is a pare interperitoneal adnexal structure lying in the ovarian fossa on the lateral wall of the pelvis, bound by the external iliac vessels and the ureter. The ovary is suspended in the pelvic peritoneum by the mesovarium, the mesosalpinx, and by the broad ovarian and the infundibulopelvic ligaments. Usual position of the ovary is lateral to the superior aspect of the uterine body. In addition, ovarian position is affected by the position of the uterus, by urinary bladder distension, and by rectal fullness. The size of the ovary correlates closely with the endocrinologic status of the patients.

Ultrasound Image

In more than 99% of case, the ovaries are visible if current high-resolution real-time equipment is used[26] (Figures 6 and 7). The location of the ovaries is extremely variable in normal subjects because of their flexible attachment to the uterus and lateral pelvic wall. For this reason it is quite unusual to demonstrate both ovaries in one transverse section. If the uterus is inclinated to the right or left, one ovary is seen close to or even behind the uterus, while the contralateral one is positioned laterally at variable distance. In retroflected uterus cases, the ovaries are typically located anteriorly and superiorly to the uterine fundus. In such cases, pulsations of the internal iliac and ovarian arteries may be used as landmarks for assisting in ovarian identification.[27]

Normal ovaries are of fusiform shape, and their size varies according to the age of the patient. In women of generative age, the usual size of the ovary is 3 cm in transverse length,

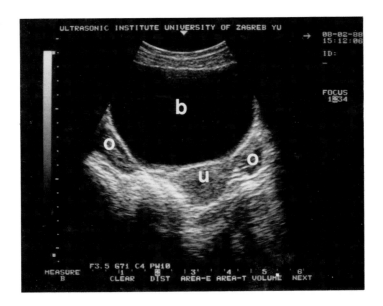

FIGURE 6. Transverse scan showing a normal uterus and both ovaries. The ovaries are of ovoid or fusiform shape and display a lower echogenicity as compared to the uterus. Small cysts affecting ovarian texture homogenicity can be seen almost regularly (b = bladder, u = uterus, o = ovaries).

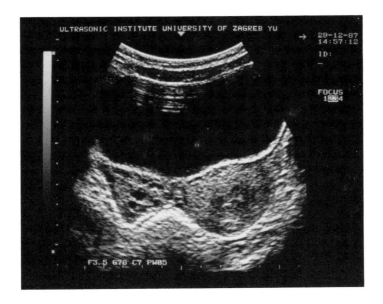

FIGURE 7. The oblique scan through the right ovary exhibits a normal shape and texture. A developing follicle is also demonstrated.

2 cm in anteroposterior length, and 1 cm in height. However, because of marked variability in ovarian shape and linear measurements, it would be more accurate to define ovarian volume according to the formula for a prolate elipse (V = 0.5233 × D1 × D2 × D3).[13] In premenarcheal girls, ovarian volume is relatively constant until 6 years of age, being below 1 ml.[15] From that age, the ovarian volume rises and reaches a mean value of 4 ml at 13 years. In the postpubertal group, the volume of the normal ovaries should be between

2 and 6 ml.[13] Postmenopausal ovaries, as previously shown in large series, are of similar size.[28] Ovarian size can also be estimated by calculating the ovarian surface or uterine to ovarian ratio.

The ovaries are generally hypoechoic as compared to the uterus because of the multiple small follicles present in the cortical area. The medulla and capsule exhibit a higher echogenicity as compared to the cortex. The growing follicle is easily demonstrated as a hypoechoic cystic structure within the ovarian substance, with a well-defined wall and a characteristic daily growth rate.

UTERINE TUBE
Anatomy

The uterine tubes are pair organs, about 12 cm long, and consist of three parts: intramural, isthmus, and ampula, which finishes with fimbrias. Fallopian tubes, together with broad ligaments, mesoalpinx, and ovaries, form the adnexal region. The Fallopian tubes extend serpinnously from the fundal aspect of the uterus to terminate finally at the ovaries.

Ultrasound Image

The broad ligament and the Fallopian tubes cannot be clearly distinguished by ultrasound under physiological conditions. When imaged, they are best seen in transverse view as a thin, moderately hypercechoic area no greater than 5 mm in maximum thickness,[29] arising from the uterine fundus. Abnormalities of the Fallopian tubes should be suggested if the area is thicker than usual, if it is tubular with an echo-free center, or if it is rounded.

RECTOSIGMOID COLON
Anatomy

In the lesser pelvis, the rectum begins where the pelvic mesocolon ceases and is placed in the midline directly posterior to the vagina. It is continuous with the sigmoid colon cranially, and at the level of the third sacral vertebra, extends caudally and finishes in the anal canal.

Ultrasound Image

On ultrasound examination, the rectosigmoid colon is sometimes visible behind the uterus, but its appearance is not characteristic, and it is possible to mistake it for a tumor in Douglas's pouch. The description of the colon has shown various patterns, depending upon the amount of gas, fluid, and feces present. When there is any doubt that a suspected mass might be a pseudotumor, particularly in the regions posterior or posterolateral to the uterus and ovaries, water should be introduced into the rectum to solve diagnostic problem.[30]

ULTRASOUND DIAGNOSIS OF PELVIC PATHOLOGY

VAGINAL ABNORMALTIES

The vagina is an easily accessible organ by pelvic examination, but ultrasound has proven to be very helpful in the initial evaluation of patients with vaginal masses, particularly in prepubertal girls. Successful ultrasound diagnosis of Gartner duct cysts, hemato- and mucocolpos, urine reflux, and solid masses have been reported.[31-33]

Vaginal obstruction is most commonly caused by an imperforate hymen, but is also seen in low vaginal atresia and in congenital anomalies caused by a failure of fusion of the Mullerian ducts. As these conditions are associated with a massive accumulation of fluid in the vagina, the ultrasound diagnosis is simple and accurate and can be made after a single examination. Differential diagnoses include fluid in the cul-de-sac, ovarian cysts, hematoma, or an abscess.

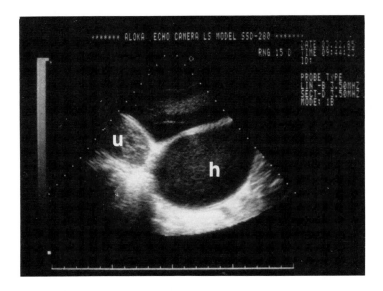

FIGURE 8.   Longitudinal sonogram of a patient with an imperforate hymen. The large cystic structure representing a hematocolpos (h) and the small uterus (u) is demonstrated.

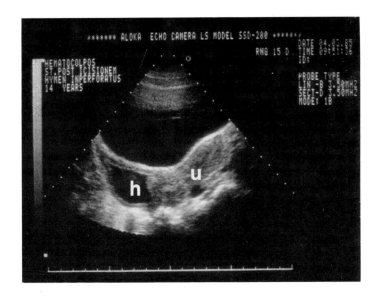

FIGURE 9.   Longitudinal sonogram of the same patient in Figure 8 after incision. The uterus (u), cervix, and dilated vaginal fornices (h) with some residual blood are visible.

The pathognomonic indication of vaginal fluid accumulation is the fusiform shape of the anechoic mass, which does not extend above the level of the uterine cervix, regardless of the patient's position (Figures 8 and 9). However, if muco- or hematometra has subsequently developed, fluid in the vagina is seen in continuity to the uterine cavity. Early diagnosis of vaginal obstruction by ultrasound is particularly useful in prepubertal girls because prognosis of mucocolpos is usually good. However, a poorer prognosis for future fertility can be expected in cases in which hematosalpinx and endometriosis have developed.[34,35]

Accumulation of fluid in the vagina may occasionally be seen in both children and adults due to urine reflex from the bladder. Asking the patient to void the bladder can solve diagnostic doubts in such cases.

The most common cystic lesions of the vagina are the Gartner duct cysts, which are usually incidental findings during pelvic sonography. These cysts are demonstrated as one or more well-defined cystic structures within the walls of the vagina, typically located along its anterolateral aspect.[31] Differential diagnosis of hematocolpos is important, but usually creates no difficulties.

Solid tumors of the vagina are extremely rare, and sonographic diagnosis has been described only in two cases of neurofibromas. Solid tumors in the vagina demonstrated by ultrasound more usually represent prolapsing submucosus leiomyoma.[37] In such cases, the sonogram demonstrates the typical appearance of these tumors. The differential diagnosis of solid tumors of the vagina always includes a tampon or other foreign bodies.

UTERINE ABNORMALITIES
Congential Uterine Anomalies

The incidence of congenital uterine abnormalities has been estimated to be between 0.1 to 12%.[38,39] As these conditions are associated with numerous complications in pregnancy (e.g., repeated spontaneous abortions, premature deliveries, premature rupture of membranes, abruptio placentae, rupture of the uterus, etc.), its diagnosis in a nonpregnant subject is particularly valuable. Moreover, uterine anomalies are highly associated with renal agenesis. Large series have shown an incidence of 48% of the specific genital anomalies in females with a congenital solitary kidney.[40] Until recently, hysterosalpinography was the only available imaging technique for identifying uterine anomalies, but now, however, it cannot be accepted as a satisfactory screening method, especially in the pediatric and adolescent female. Congenital uterine anomalies are usually classified in three groups: agenesis, failure of cavitation, and failure of fusion being the most common. Accurate ultrasound diagnosis of fusion anomalies in a pregnant patient during the first trimester and the first half of the second trimester usually poses no difficulties and has been extensively reported[41,42] (Figure 10). However, ultrasonic diagnosis of these conditions in a nonpregnant patient seems to be less accurate when static equipment is used.

If a high-resolution real-time mechanical sector is employed, one can attain such diagnostic accuracy that sonography can be considered as an ideal method for screening for uterine anomalies.[43] As uterine anomalies regularly affect the ultrasonic appearance of the endometrial cavity, clear visualization of the endometrium is a guide to diagnosis. The examinations should be regularly performed in the secretory phase of the cycle when the endometrium is strongly echogenic and naturally contrasts with the hypoechoic myometrium. After accurate delineation of the uterine position, scanning is performed in an entirely transverse uterine plane, starting from the level of the cervix and progressing superiorly by a slow continuous movement.

If there is a fusion anomaly present, one can clearly observe the splitting of the endometrial echo in the upper uterine portions. This is characteristic for the arcuate, subseptate, and bicornuate uterus (Figures 11 and 12). Differential diagnosis of septate uterus or uterus didelphis usually poses no difficulties, because in these cases one can easily see two separate cervical canals or the splitting of the entire uterine cavity, not only the upper portions. More information about the type of abnormality is obtained by assessment of the myometrium. In bicornuate uterus and uterus didelphis, this forms two separate horns, while in other anomalies it appears normal. However, any anomaly which has potential clinical significance should be confirmed by hysterosalpingography.

Uterine Fibroma

The most commonly acquired anomalies of the uterus are uterine fibroids or leiomyomata,

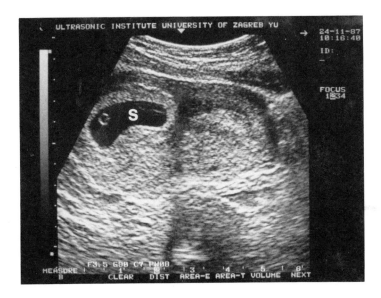

FIGURE 10.   Uterus bicornis bicollis. An 8-week gestational sac (s) containing a normally developing fetus is observed in the left horn. The right horn with a pronounced decidual reaction is also displayed.

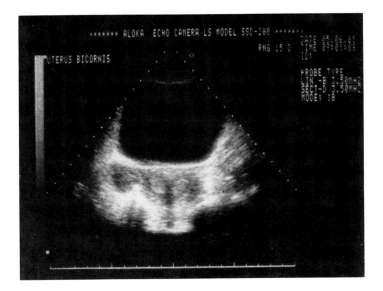

FIGURE 11.   Uterus bicornis unicollis. The transverse section displays two distinct uterine cavities and two separate uterine horns.

which are present in more than 20% of all women over 35.[44] The sonographic diagnosis of uterine fibroma is based on texture changes, distortion of the uterine contour, and uterine enlargement. The typical ultrasound image of fibroma is that of a hypoechoic intrauterine mass which affects the homogenicity of the normal uterine texture (Figures 13 and 14). Uterine enlargement is relatively constant, but is not a pathognomonic sign of uterine fibroma. The uterus can be generally enlarged and present globular contours; conversely, separate nodules can be seen with a lobular uterine contour. It has been shown that uterine enlargement

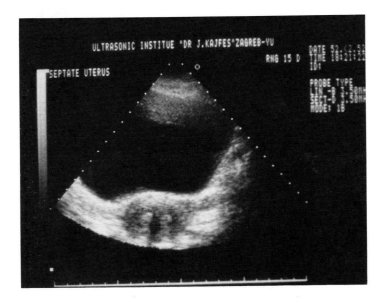

FIGURE 12.   Uterus septus. In the upper portion of the uterine cavity the separation of the unique endometrial echo is visible.

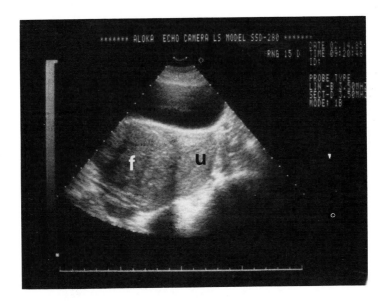

FIGURE 13.   Transverse sonogram showing a subserous myoma on the left (f) and the uterus (u) on the right.

occurs in 66% of cases of histologically proven fibromas, while contour distortion and textural changes are seen in 76 and 68% of cases, respectively.[45] Contour distortion seems to be the most sensitive parameter of tumor presence, unless it is large enough to be visualized as a distinctive mass. Nonetheless, the ultrasound diagnosis of fibroma is considered simple and accurate. The reported rate of specific histologic diagnosis by ultrasound was 65%.[46] The major cause of nonspecificity of sonographic findings is the presence of pedunculated tumors, which are sometimes hardly distinguished from solid adnexal mass (Figure 15).

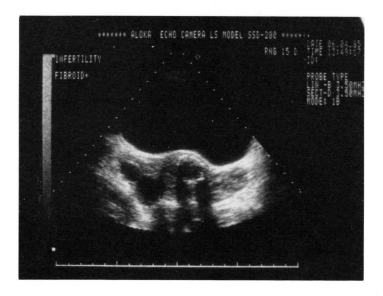

FIGURE 14.   Intramural myoma appearing as a cyst because of calcifications on the anterior surface of the tumor which can be accidentally misinterpreted as adenomyoma.

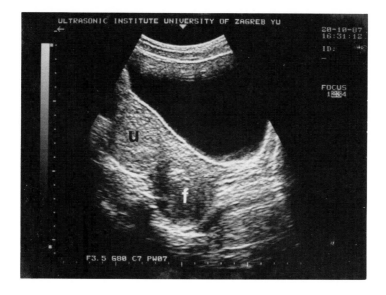

FIGURE 15.   Uterine sonogram demonstrating the uterine body (u) on the right and a subserous myoma on the left appearing as a solid adnexal tumor (f).

However, it should be remembered that leiomyomas are usually easily accessible for palpation, and the diagnosis of clinically significant tumors is in most cases made merely by palpation. Therefore, the need for ultrasound investigation of the fibroma can be easily reduced to cases in which either the palpatory findings are unclear or further information is required, e.g., in the obese patients, in difficult vaginal examination, in a combination of fibroma with other tumors, in a follow-up of smaller tumors to more precisely evaluate their growth, and for more accurate localization of myomatous knots.

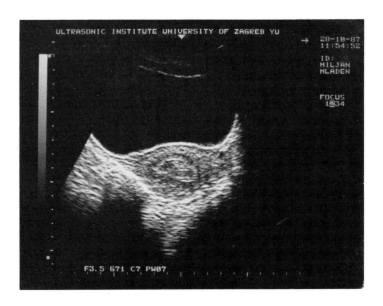

FIGURE 16. Transverse scan of the uterus in a postmenopausal patient with metrorrhagia. The endometrium appears thick and inhomogeneous. A case of stage 1 endometrial cancer.

Uterine Malignancies

The most common uterine malignancy is carcinoma of the cervix, but ultrasound is of limited value either for early detection of the disease or for the evaluation of advanced lesions.[47] Sonography is usually normal in the early stages of carcinoma of the cervix when the diagnosis is readily made by Pap smear or biopsy. In later stages, ultrasound can detect a cervical mass that may be smooth or lobulated and indistinguishable from a leiomyoma of the cervix. A particularly helpful ultrasonic finding is the demonstration of the tumor extension into the parametrium and lymph node involvement. Since it changes the clinical staging and substantially changes the therapeutic approach, findings should be confirmed by computer tomography, which is better than ultrasound at detecting pelvic wall extension.[48] Much better results are obtained with sonographic evaluation of endometrial adenocarcinoma. This malignant tumor is most common in nulliparous peri and postmenopausal women with vaginal bleeding. By using static gray scale equipment, Requard et al.[49] have shown that the sonographic demonstration of the uterine shape and echo pattern are helpful in pretreatment tumor staging. Of patients with stage I to II disease, 94% had a normal or bulbous uterus and a noraml or hypechoic pattern, while lobular uterus and mixed echo pattern were characteristic of stage III to IV. One more recent report has evaluated the potential of ultrasound as a screening test for endometrial carcinoma and has shown a 67% success rate as to the value of negative findings and an 83% success rate with positive findings. It has been concluded that although sonography cannot serve as a screening method for endometrial carcinoma because of low method sensitivity, the specificity is high, and in the case of suspicious findings, surgical investigation is definitely required[50] (Figure 16).

These results can be somewhat improved if one employs intrauterine radial scanning with a high-frequency probe instead of transabdominal scanning. By using this method, it is possible not only to detect disease, but also to define accurately the degree of myometrial invasion in more than 80% of cases.[51] As the extent of myometrial invasion indicates the probability of pelvic metastases, this method may be useful not only for tumor detection, but also for better staging of the disease. However, this method cannot be employed for screening and can be used only in highly specialized centers.

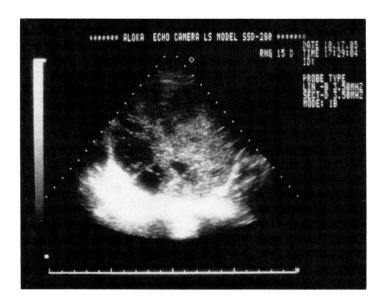

FIGURE 17. Extremely large uterine tumor with pronounced degeneration, necrosis, and hemorrhage. The diagnosis of uterine sarcoma was confirmed on laparotomy.

Other malignant uterine tumors are sarcomas, which are infrequently seen and represent 3% of the uterine tumors. The common sonographic appearance of these tumors is an enlarged uterus with an inhomogeneous texture. As secondary tumor changes often occur, large anechoic areas representing hemorrhage and necrosis are regularly seen.[52] Differential diagnosis to benign leiomyoma can be difficult, and sonography is most helpful in the demonstration of the growth of previously detected leiomyoma in a postmenopausal patient (Figure 17).

Intrauterine Contraceptive Device

As far as sonography of the uterus is concerned, ultrasonic localization of an intrauterine contraceptive device (IUD) should be described. Using an IUD is a popular method of contraception, being the second most effective method of preventing pregnancy. Sonographic demonstration of an IUD is, in most cases, an accidental finding during routine scanning, but in certain situations, accurate detection of an IUD is of particular clinical importance.

Although, the sonographic appearance of an IUD depends on the type used, common characteristics of each type are a strong echo activity and posterior shadowing[53] (Figure 18). By using these criteria, the IUD can be defined in almost all cases when present within the uterus. Occasionally, differential diagnosis of the IUD includes air, swab, or intrauterine synechia (Figures 19 and 20).

Sonography can reliably detect complications with IUDs, like partial expulsion, embedment, and partial or complete uterine perforation. As malplacement of an IUD is recognized as a major cause of the complications listed above, some authors have reported that IUD placement under ultrasonic control could reduce the rate of complications.[54] However, when the IUD cannot be visualized by ultrasound, radiography should be employed to exclude the possibility of pelvic localization. Another advantage of sonography is a reliable diagnosis of method failure by demonstration of an early gestational sac (Figure 21), and the detection of pelvic inflammatory disease, which is often associated with IUD presence (Figure 22).

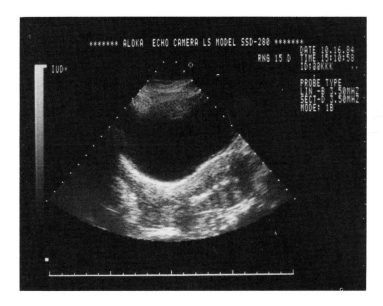

FIGURE 18. Sonogram of the uterus, showing a correctly placed IUD (Lippes Loop).

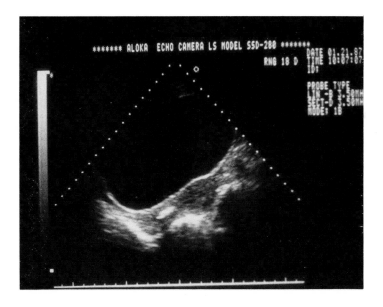

FIGURE 19. Longitudinal sonogram of the uterus, showing a strong echo in the cervical canal.

THE OVARIAN AND OTHER ADNEXAL MASSES

Polycystic Ovarian Disease

Polycystic ovarian disease (POD) is a complex endocrinological disorder characterized by bilateral symmetrical ovarian enlargement and microcystic changes in the internal structure of the ovaries. It regularly results in chronic anovulation and is associated with numerous clinical signs, e.g., hirsutism, obesity, menstrual irregularities, and infertility. POD is clinically diagnosed by the analysis of hormonal levels, which are, however, extremely variable and are not disturbed exclusively by the presence of ovarian disease.

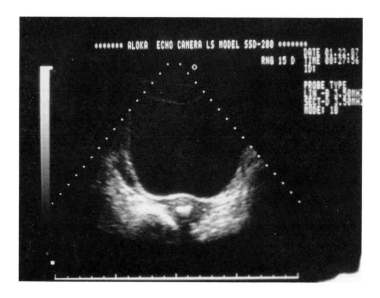

FIGURE 20. The transverse scan demonstrates a wide and strong echo at the same level. A case of intrauterine synechia caused by vigorous curettage.

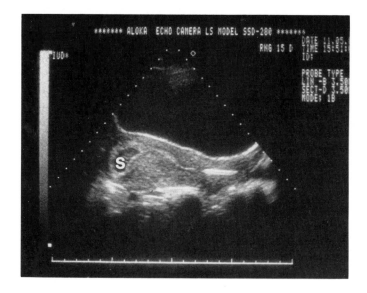

FIGURE 21. Longitudinal scan through the uterus, demonstrating a 6-week pregnancy with an intrauterine contraceptive device partially expelled into the cervical canal.

Ultrasound demonstration of ovarian enlargement and characteristic morphologic appearance are important in accurate diagnosis of POD. Typical ultrasonic appearance of this condition is a bilateral ovarian enlargement with numerous small cysts that range from 2 to 6 mm in size (Figures 23 to 24).

Although ovarian enlargement has been clearly demonstrated by using static equipment, intraovarian cysts can be seen only by using real-time machines. In approximately 20% of patients, a polycystic pattern cannot be demonstrated, but the ovaries appear hypoechoic,

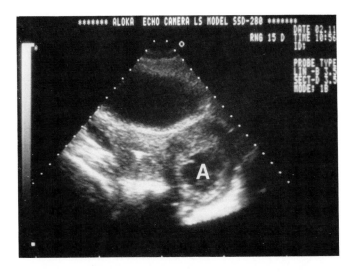

FIGURE 22.   Transverse scan shows the IUD within the uterus and a large inhomogeneous adnexal mass on the left (A). The mass represents tubo-ovarian abscess — a relatively common complication of intrauterine contraception.

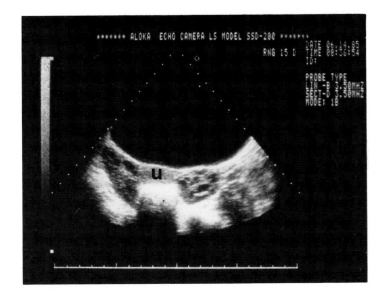

FIGURE 23.   Stein-Leventhal syndrome. Transverse sonogram of a patient with amenorrhea and hirsutism. Both ovaries are enlarged and polycystic. The uterus (u) is small, and the transverse uterine diameter is smaller than the longitudinal ovarian diameter.

and many thick echoes arranged along parallel lines can be seen.[55,56] However, in 25 to 29% of cases, POD does not cause ovarian enlargement, and ultrasonic demonstration of normal-sized ovaries does not necessarily imply the absence of the disease.[57] The accuracy of ultrasonic diagnosis of POD can be improved if the criteria, which include assessment of ovarian stroma, are included in the diagnosis. According to Franks et al.,[58] the increased stroma is an important feature, since it helps to distinguish the polycystic ovaries from the multifollicular appearances. These may be seen as a temporary feature of normal pubertal

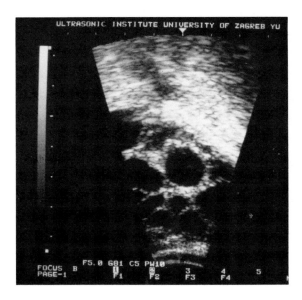

FIGURE 24.   Transvaginal sonogram of a polycystic ovary showing an enlarged ovary filled with numerous small cysts measuring
less than 1 cm in size.

development or in weight loss-related amenorrhoea. Such "multicystic ovaries" do not
contain increased stroma and appear to be normal ovaries which are receiving abnormal
gonadotrophin stimulation.

In summary, being an entirely noninvasive method, ultrasound provides high diagnostic
accuracy of the disease and can be considered the best method in this field.

Ovarian and Other Adnexal Masses

A more common problem in clinical practice is sonographic diagnosis of adnexal masses.
Clinicall detected adnexal mass represents one of the most frequent indications for ultrasound
examination in gynecology. Accuracy of ultrasound in the evaluation of pelvic masses has
been reported to be as high as 91 to 97%.[56] When ultrasonic findings were compared with
histomorphology after surgery, in the majority of cases sonographic data about the presence,
size, location, and internal consistency of a mass correlated well with pathological findings.[59,60]

Although there were several attempts to establish characteristic sonographic patterns of
certain adnexal masses, particularly in cases of ovarian cystadenoma[61] and dermoid cysts,[62]
other authors described less encouraging experiences.[63,64] So, it is generally accepted that
ultrasonography does not reveal information about the histology of a tumor and, consecu-
tively, cannot provide a definitive clinical diagnosis. Accordingly, the most rational approach
presumes meticulous analysis of the morphologic characteristics of the mass, including its
origin, size, texture, and relationships to the other pelvic organs. Criteria for the sonographic
assessment of adnexal masses have been developed by Fleischer et al.[59] and interpreted
together with relevant clinical data, enabling a considerable reduction of diagnostic possibilities.

In clinical practice, adnexal tumors are most commonly divided into four categories
based on the complexity of tumor appearance. Every category has a relative specificity and
should always be viewed within the framework of other clinical findings.

A completely cystic adnexal mass represents the first category and is defined according
to the following criteria: anechoic cyst content, well-defined walls of varying thickness, and
posterior acoustic enhancement. The most common type of adnexal mass which meets these
criteria is the functional ovarian cyst. These cysts originate from the unruptured follicle or

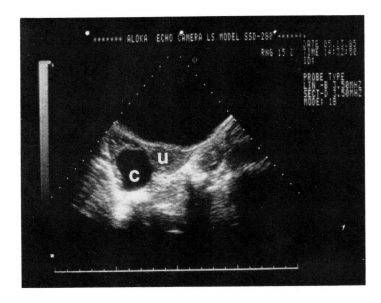

FIGURE 25.   Follicular cyst in the right ovary. Normal preserved ovarian parenchyma is visible on the upper cyst pole (u = uterus, c = cyst).

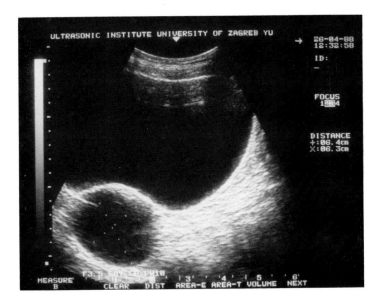

FIGURE 26.   Large cyst in the left ovary. The cyst is simple and unilocular, with thin and well-defined borders and no internal echoes. A case of physiological ovarian cyst.

from the corpus luteum and are unilateral with a smooth and thin wall. Their size rarely exceeds 10 cm, and normal ovarian tissue can occasionally be seen along the part of the cyst wall (Figures 25 and 26). Their main characteristic is quick regression, and the ultrasonic examination can therefore be repeated within a few days. Paraovarian cysts which develop from Gartner's duct have the same appearance as functional cysts and are infrequently distinguishable from them. Paraovarian cysts can measure only 2 to 3 cm, but more often are found to be quite large. They can be diagnosed ultrasonically if the ovary and the cyst are detected on the same side and if both are clearly separated from the uterus.

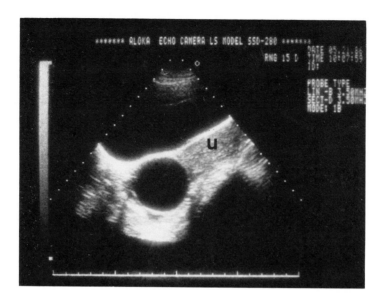

FIGURE 27. Tubo-ovarian abscess (right). Unilocular cystic structure appearing as a follicular cyst at first sight (u = uterus).

Large endometriomas can also present an entirely cystic pattern and sometimes cannot be distinguished from functional cysts. They are usually situated in the posterior or posterolateral areas of the uterus, and it is not uncommon for them to be bilateral. Examination of the rectovaginal septum, which is very often affected by endometriosis, sometimes reveals small cysts and might be a helpful sign for differential diagnosis.

Hydrosalpinx and tubo-ovarian abscess often appear as a cystic mass. A smaller hydrosalpinx usually assumes a fusiform shape, but if large, it is of a rather round shape (Figure 27). A tubo-ovarian abscess can be differentiated from hydrosalpinx by the demonstration of ovarian tissue incorporated within the abscess wall. Besides clinical history, examination of the cyst wall is sometimes of help in differentiating physiological cysts from other cystic masses. Careful examination will reveal slight irregularities of the inner border in cases of hydrosalpinx or tubo-ovarian abscess, which are not seen in physiological cysts. Wall thickness is regularly greater in nonphysiological cysts and is also a helpful sign for differential diagnosis. Ovarian neoplasms, such as cystadenoma or cystic teratoma, may appear as entirely cystic tumors at first sight, but a detailed examination will regularly reveal the solid part of the tumor and help to correct the diagnosis.

The second morphological group of adnexal masses comprises predominantly cystic tumors containing internal echoes such as septa, solid tissue, or any other echogenic material. The most common adnexal mass in this group is ovarian cystadenoma. Serous and mucinous cystadenomas are the most common ovarian epithelial neoplasms, having a very specific ultrasonic appearance. They are usually large with echogenic linear internal septa. The septa are more pronounced in the mucinous type, while in the serous type, papillary projections and wall thickening are occasionally observed (Figures 28 to 30). As a general rule, the distinction between benign and malignant cystadenomas on the basis of the ultrasonic image is uncertain. Identification of the irregular solid part of the tumor or of an extension of solid tissue through the cyst wall can sometimes be used as the key to detect malignant tumors.

Dermoid cysts account for approximately 25% of all ovarian tumors. The sonographic appearance of these tumors is extremely variable, but a cystic mass containing a cone of solid tissue with a highly echogenic focus and posterior shadowing is a pathognomonic finding (Figures 31 to 34). Dermoid cysts are most frequently seen in childhood and in early reproductive age, but can also be occasionally found in older patients.

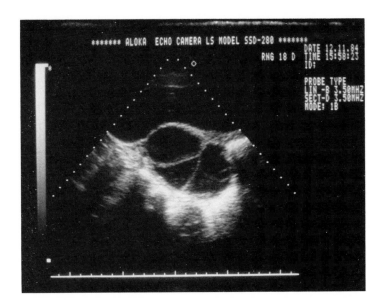

FIGURE 28.   Mucinous cystadenoma exhibiting the characteristics of a complex, predominantly cystic ovarian mass.

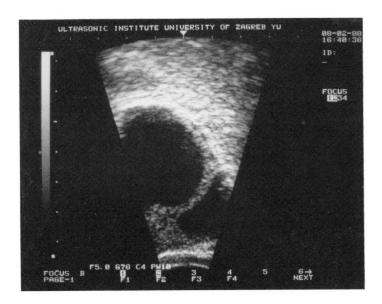

FIGURE 29.   Middle-sized mucinous cystadenoma with well-defined septa on transvaginal scan.

Other gynecological disorders exhibiting a complex predominantly cystic appearance include tubo-ovarian abscesses, which can contain echoes or fluid levels representing the layering of purulent debris, endometriomas containing echogenic blood clots, and tubal ectopic pregnancy.

Complex tumors with a dominant solid component include most of the masses listed in the previous category such as dermoid cysts, ectopic pregnancy, and endometriosis. Cystadenomas with a more pronounced solid part are also demonstrated in a significant number of cases. The proportion of malignant cystadenomas is much higher in this group than in

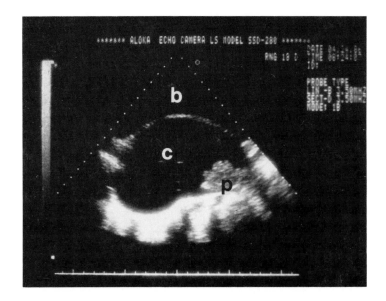

FIGURE 30.   Papillary serous cystadenoma. The sonogram shows a large, complex, predominantly cystic mass (c) and papillary proliferations within the cystic tumor (p).

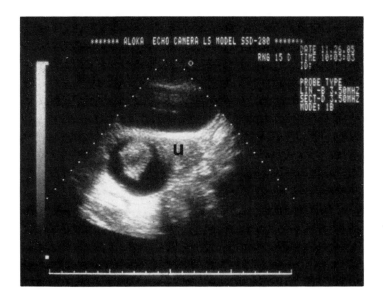

FIGURE 31.   Dermoid cyst. The transverse sonogram displays a complex, predominantly solid tumor on the left. Note the strong echogenicity of the solid tumor parts (u = uterus).

the previous one. Most ovarian neoplasms, e.g., endometrioid carcinoma, clear cell carcinoma, dysgerminoma, granulosa cell, and Sertoli-Leydig cell tumors, exhibit a solid, partly cystic ultrasonic appearance (Figures 35 to 39).

Solid ovarian tumors are included in the fourth category. The most common tumor types being solid are malignant teratoma and adenocarcinoma (Figures 40 to 42). Since solid ovarian tumors are rare, one should also consider nonovarian causes of solid adnexal masses

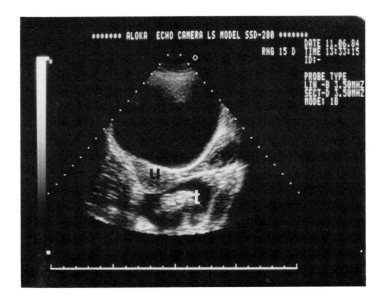

FIGURE 32.   Dermoid cyst detected in a 15-year-old patient (u = uterus, t = dermoid).

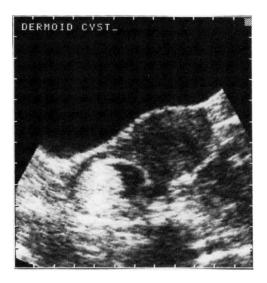

FIGURE 33.   Typical ultrasonic appearance of the dermoid cyst in a characteristic position above the uterus.

such as subserous leiomyoma, hematoma, or chronic ectopic pregnancy. Nongenital metastatic tumors can also be demonstrated as solid adnexal masses.

A particular problem in this field remains to be the diagnosis of ovarian cancer. Malignant tumors represent 25% of all gynecological malignancies, but are the first as a cause of death and represent the fourth most common cause of cancer deaths in women. These neoplasms may be clinically occult for a prolonged period of time, with 70% presenting in stage III or IV. As the extent of disease, besides the biology of the tumor, is a major determinant of survival rate, an early diagnosis of the presence of a tumor and accurate staging of the disease by sonography is extremely important.

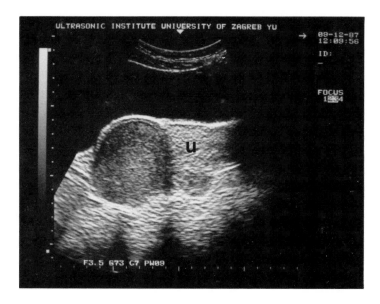

FIGURE 34. A dermoid tumor of completely solid appearance on the transverse echogram (u = uterus).

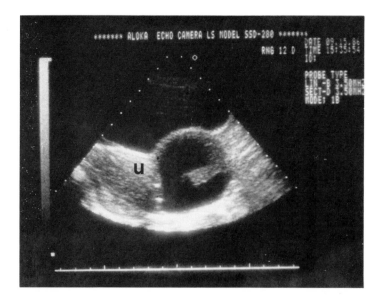

FIGURE 35. Bizarre appearance of the adnexal tumor in a case of ovarian carcinoma (u = uterus).

Ultrasonography is capable of detecting a primary pelvic tumor in almost all patients with advanced disease,[65] but it served poorly when characterization of the mass and tumor staging were attempted.[66] It has been reported that certain sonographic features like thick septa and solid nodules are highly suggestive of malignancy, and the likelihood of malignancy increases proportionally to the amount of solid echogenic material within the tumor.[67,68] However, such sonographic features were encountered in up to 30% of histologically benign ovarian cysts; conversely, in 10 to 16% of proven malignancies, there were no sonographic signs of malignancy.[69] Therefore, a significant overlap in ultrasonic characteristics of benign

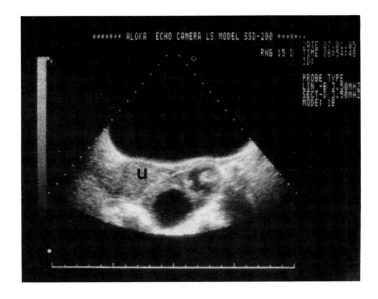

FIGURE 36.   Cystadenocarcinoma detected in the initial stage of tumor development. Note marked texture inhomogenicity and irregular shape of the tumor (u = uterus).

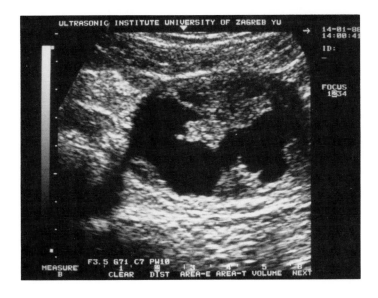

FIGURE 37.   Solid-cystic tumor with marked texture irregularities. The diagnosis of malignancy was confirmed after surgery.

and malignant tumors can be expected, and the only means by which a diagnosis can be made with certainty is by microscopic evaluation.

Furthermore, significant efforts have been made to perform clinical staging of ovarian tumors, but the results obtained were not encouraging. Specifically, the sensitivity of ultrasound in detecting adenopathy, omentum, bowel and mesentery, and peritoneal involvement was 29, 27, 37, and 16%, respectively. Sonography has been useful only for ascites detection, with an 87% sensitivity rate and a 99% specificity rate.[70,71]

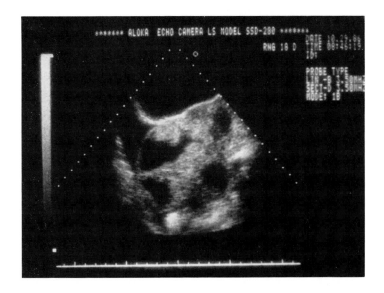

FIGURE 38.   Large solid-cystic mass representing an ovarian cancer.

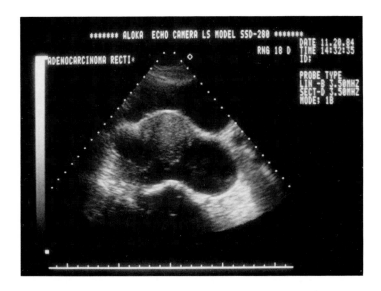

FIGURE 39.   Multiple large cysts posterior to the uterus in a patient who was operated on because of adenocarcinoma of the rectum 6 months before.

Recently, Goswamy et al.[26] have reported good results considering real-time ultrasound as a screening test for ovarian cancer. Recognizing the age of the patients as the only obvious risk factor, they performed screening on a large group of women over 45. In 15 patients in whom morphologically abnormal and enlarged ovaries were observed, subsequent patho-histological examination revealed various ovarian abnormalities in all cases, with no false positive results. In one case, definitive diagnosis was clear cell carcinoma stage I, and in five cases, benign cystadenomas. Although these results indicate the high specificity of sonographic findings, even in the early stage of ovarian malignancy, further work is required to estimate the rate of false negative diagnosis before the definitive acceptance of sonography as a valuable screening test.

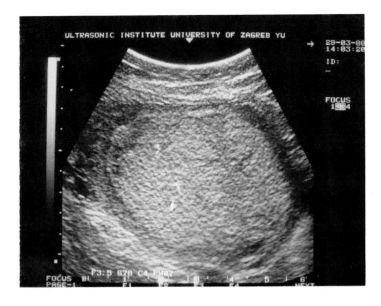

FIGURE 40. Thecoma of the ovary demonstrated as a large, completely solid tumor on ultrasonogram.

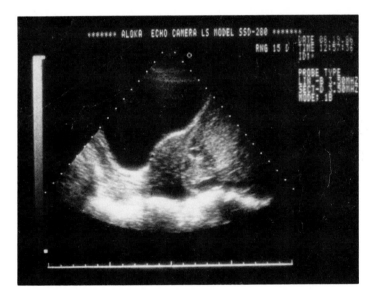

FIGURE 41. Longitudinal sonogram showing the uterus and a large solid tumor in the left adnexal region.

Endometriosis

In terms of incidence, endometriosis is the third most important gynecologic disease, after inflammation and myoma. Endometriosis is a disease with a markedly progressive course leading to subfertility and sterility. The results of treatment are better in the early stages of the disease, and every diagnostic method which can contribute to its earlier detection is therefore advantageous.

The ectopic endometrium is subject to the same cyclic changes as the endometrium in the cavum uteri. Cyclic bleeding leads to the formation of hemorrhagic cysts filled with

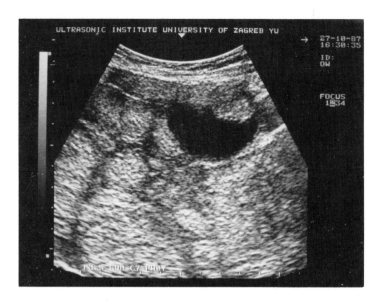

FIGURE 42.   Malignant teratoma of the left ovary. Note the pronounced echogenicity of the completely solid tumor detected in a young patient.

thick, dark blood wherever endometriosis develops. Bleeding leads to extremely strong adhesions which become even stronger because of accompanying inflammation. All of this causes the formation of conglomerated tumors very similar to those in inflammations, carcinoma, or ectopic pregnancy.

The boundaries of these cystic tumors are at first clear, and the adjoining uterus is clearly visible. In the further course of the disease, conglomerated tumors are formed, presenting ultrasonic characteristics such as unclear boundaries, irregular contours, and mixed solid-cystic structure. In the course of time, the uterus is included into the image of the conglomerates and is no longer visible as a separate organ (Figures 43 to 45). At this stage, the ultrasonic image is very similar to that of inflammation. Since the adhesions in endometriosis are extremely strong, this is also evident on the ultrasonic image through the appearance of very pronounced echogenic structures which do not usually appear in such marked form in other pelvic diseases.

Ultrasonic diagnosis of endometriosis suffers from similar limitations, as in the case of an ovarian neoplasm. When the disease is present as a discrete pelvic mass, although sonographic findings are nonspecific, a characteristic clinical history or a physical examination are both helpful and may promote the correct diagnosis.[72]

The major problem is the diagnosis of the much more common diffuse form of the disease. This form is characterized by numerous small cysts which can be found at almost any location within the pelvis, but because of their small size, they cannot be visualized by current equipment, being below the resolution limits. As the largest concentration of endometriotic cysts is usually around the attachments of the uterosacral ligaments to the cervix and in the rectovaginal septum, it has been suggested that an increased background echogenicity of the pelvis may serve as an ultrasonic sign of disease.[73] Other possibly helpful signs are a poor definition of the pelvic structures due to associated adhesions, and the presence of irregular cystic spaces through the myometrium, which represent concomitant adenomyosis in up to 36% of cases.[74] Unfortunately, recent correlation of sonographic findings in 37 patients with laparoscopically proven endometriosis showed that sonography correctly identified only 10.8% of cases. So, it seems that ultrasound is of limited value in diagnosis of endometriosis, particularly in cases where no large endometriomas are present.[75]

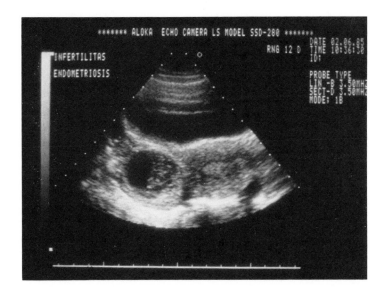

FIGURE 43. Large endometrioma (right) with pronounced internal echoes. Such a finding cannot be distinguished from a tubo-ovarian abscess, and the diagnosis was made on laparotomy.

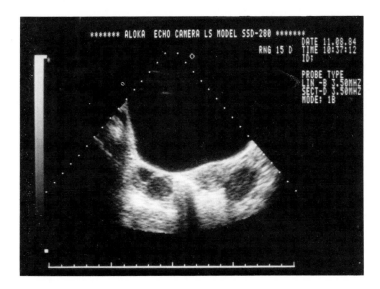

FIGURE 44. Endometriomas in the ovaries. Note the irregular shape of the cyst and internal echoes.

Pelvic Inflammatory Disease

Inflammations are deemed to be among the most frequent diseases in women during the generative period, inflammations of the adnexa in particular. Cyclic and acyclic bleeding, abortion, and delivery contribute to this pathology.

Morphologic changes are the basis for diagnosis by ultrasound; they depend in turn on the development of the disease. The inflammation is usually ascending, so that it first spreads from the vagina, cervix, and endometrium and develops in the Fallopian tube. Initial in-

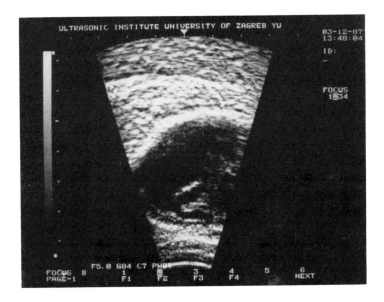

FIGURE 45.   Endometrioma in the right adnexal region with clearly visible internal echoes as seen by transvaginal probe.

flammatory changes in the tube — endosalpingitis and salpingitis — involve edema and inflammatory infiltration of the wall. The inflammatory process may develop in several known forms:

1.   The conglomerated adnexal mass appears after the spreading of the inflammation to the tubal serosa, particularly with the overflowing of the inflammatory exudate through the abdominal orifice of the tube, and within the formation of adhesions with the ovary, the uterus, the intestines, and the omentum. The edema and the exudate in such a conglomerated tumor may present a variegated but, where interpretation is concerned, frequently unclear image.
2.   Due to inflammatory changes, adhesions often occur in the region of the abdominal orifice of the tube, which dilates into a retor-like fluido- or pyosalpinx.
3.   The pyo-ovarium, caused by the spreading of inflammation from the tube, is very rarely isolated.
4.   Piercing of the wall frequently occurs between the pyosalpinx and the pyo-ovarium, which unite into one pus-filled cavity — the tubo-ovarina abscess.
5.   With the collection of pus in Douglas's pouch, inflammation is formed.

The common characteristic of all forms of inflammatory processes in the adnexa is the formation of stronger or weaker adhesions. Under the influence of therapy, the conglomerated tumors decrease and sometimes completely disappear. However, they often leave behind permanent changes in the form of adhesions, tubo-ovarian cysts, fluidosalpinx, or cystic degeneration of ovaries, the formation of which is explained, in inflammation cases, by the impossibility of ovulation due to adhesions on their surface.

The ultrasonic visualization of inflamed adnexa depends on pathoanatomic changes. Each of the listed changes has a corresponding ultrasonic image, although it is not always quite clear.

The conglomerated tumor formed by adhesion is usually unclearly delineated and of irregular form. Since adhesions are also formed with the uterus, usually it cannot be visualized as a separate formation. Because of exudation and suppuration, the tumor, which is mainly

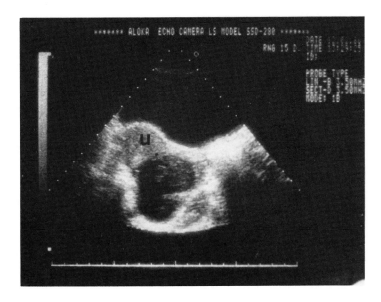

FIGURE 46. Sonogram demonstrating a tubo-ovarian abscess (left) with internal low-level echoes (u = uterus).

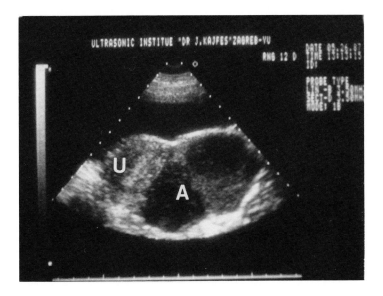

FIGURE 47. Acute pelvic infection. Note the formation of a complex mass (A) left to the uterus (U) which can hardly be outlined.

solid, contains occasional accumulations of liquid which give it a mixed solid-cystic appearance.[76] Such an ultrasonic image is not specific of inflammation since endometriosis, ovarian carcinoma, or ectopic pregnancy can produce a similar image.

The tube, widened into a hydro- or pyosalpinx, appears on the ultrasonic scan as an oval, cystic formation, usually with one septum which corresponds to the bend of the tube. The abscess, usually a tubo-ovarian one, may present a fluid-fluid level which divides the thicker pus with debris from the rest of the exudate.[77] It is impossible to distinguish between ovarian and tubo-ovarian abscesses by ultrasound (Figure 48).

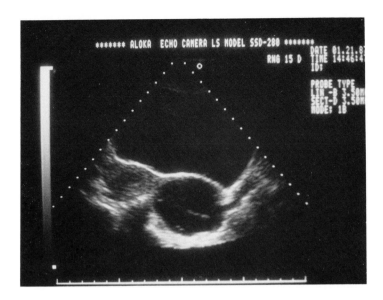

FIGURE 48.   Tubo-ovarian abscess (left). Unilocular cystic structure appearing as a follicular cyst at first sight; however, wall irregularities and thickness are pathognomonic of an abscess and cannot be observed in cases involving a simple cyst.

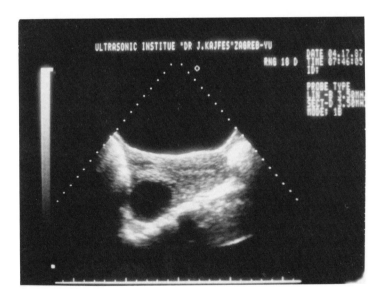

FIGURE 49.   Abscess in the cul-de-sac. The longitudinal scan displays a cystic structure posterior to the uterus.

Douglas's abscess appears on the ultrasonic scan as an anechoic area behind the uterus. It can be mistaken for another liquid (blood, exudate) or for a cyst in Douglas's pouch (Figure 49).

Adhesions in chronic adnexitis are visible on the ultrasonic scan as changes in the position of the known pelvic organs. Hydrosalpinx and the tubo-ovarian cysts are visualized as cystic formations with some septa. Changes in the ovary, when cystic degeneration because of obstructed ovulation occurs, are typical (Figure 50).

The ultrasonic diagnosis of pelvic inflammatory disease is not specific, but it can be

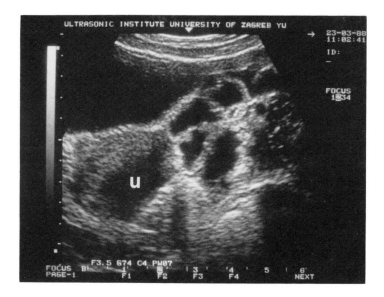

FIGURE 50. Transverse sonogram demonstrating complex cystic-solid strutures in the left adnexal region in a patient with chronic pelvic inflammatory disease. The adhesion led to bowel loop fixation in the lesser pelvis. (u = uterus).

useful together with other information.[78] Endometriosis, carcinoma, and ectopic pregnancy may produce a similar image. Awareness of this fact, and careful evaluation, can make this field of ultrasonic diagnostics very advantageous:

1. In combination with other case history data, and clinical and laboratory investigations, it can be of help in establishing the primary diagnosis.
2. During the course of the disease, it can help in the guided evacuation of smaller, palpatorily unclear collections of inflammatory exudates and pus, as well as in direct drug administration.
3. Along with clinical palpatory control, it can yield more objective data on the progression or regression of the inflammatory process.
4. It helps in establishing chronic changes and also in determining the indication for surgery.

REFERENCES

1. **Donald, I., MacVicar, J., and Brown, T. G.,** Investigation of abdominal masses by pulsed ultrasound, *Lancet,* I, 1888, 1958.
2. **Morley, P. M. and Barnett, E.,** The ovarian mass, in *Principles and Practice of Ultrasonography in Obstetrics and Gynecology,* Sanders, R. C. and James, A. E., Eds., Appleton-Century-Crofts, New York, 1985, 739.
3. **Bree, R. L. and Schvab, R. E.,** Contribution of mesentric fat to unsatisfactory abdominal and pelvic ultrasonography, *Radiology,* 140, 773, 1981.
4. **Kurtz, A. B. and Rifkin, M. D.,** Normal anatomy of the female pelvis: ultrasound with computed tomography correlation, in *Principles and Practice of Ultrasonography in Obstetrics and Gynecology,* Sanders, R. C. and James, A. E., Eds., Appleton-Century-Crofts, New York, 1985, 99.
5. **Wells, P. N. T.,** *Biomedical Ultrasonics,* Academic Press, London, 1977, 43.
6. **Kurjak A.,** *Atlas of Ultrasonography in Obstetrics and Gynecology,* Mladost, Zagreb, 1986, 246.

7. **Cochrane, W. J.,** Ultrasound in gynecology, *Radiol. Clin. North Am.,* XIII, 457, 1975.
8. **Hackeloer, B. J.,** Analysis of five-year experience in follicular demonstration, in *Ultrasound and Infertility,* Christie, A. D., Ed., Chartwel-Bratt, Bromley, 1981, 125.
9. **Kremer, H., Dobrinski, W., and Mikyska, M.,** Ultrasonic in vivo and in vitro studies on the nature of the ureteral jet phenomenon, *Radiology,* 142, 175, 1982.
10. **Athey, P. A.,** Uterus: abnormalities of size, shape, contour and texture, in *Ultrasound in Obstetrics and Gynecology,* Athey, P. A. and Hadlock, F. P., Eds., C. V. Mosby, St. Louis, 1985, 167.
11. **Nussbaum, A. R., Sanders, R. C., and Jones, M. D.,** Neonatal uterine morphology as seen on real-time U.S., *Radiology,* 160, 641, 1986.
12. **Ivarsson, S. A., Nilsson, K. O., and Person, P. H.,** Ultrasonography of the pelvic organs in prepubertal girls, *Arch. Dis. Child.,* 58, 352, 1983.
13. **Sample, W. F., Lippe, B. M., and Gyepes, M. T.,** Grey scale ultrasonography of the normal female pelvis, *Radiology,* 125, 477, 1977.
14. **Miller, E. L., Thomas, R. H., and Lines, P.,** The antrophic postmenopausal uterus, *J. Clin. Ultrasound,* 5, 261, 1977.
15. **Orsini, L. F., Salardi, S., and Pilu, G.,** Pelvic organs in premenarcheal girls: real-time ultrasonography, *Radiology,* 153, 113, 1984.
16. **Fleicher, A. C., Entman, S. S., Porrath, S. A., and James, A. E.,** Sonographic evaluation of uterine malformations and disorders, in *Principles and Practice of Ultrasonography in Obstetrics and Gynecology,* Sanders, R. C. and James, A. E., Eds., Appleton-Century-Crofts, New York, 1985, 531.
17. **Piiroinen, O.,** Ultrasonic localization of IUDs, *Acta Obstet. Gynecol. Scand.,* 51, 203, 1972.
18. **Gross, B. H. and Callen, P. W.,** Ultrasound of the uterus, in *Ultrasonography in Obstetrics and Gynecology,* W. B. Saunders, Philadelphia, 1983, 243.
19. **Hall, D. A., Hann, L. E., and Ferrucci, J. T.,** Sonographic morphology of the normal menstrual cycle, *Radiology,* 185, 233, 1979.
20. **Sakamoto, C. and Nakano, H.,** The echogenic endometrium and alterations during menstrual cycle, *Int. J. Gynecol. Obstet.,* 20, 255, 1982.
21. **Hackoeler, B. J.,** The role of ultrasound in female infertility management, *Ultrasound Med. Biol.,* 10, 35, 1984.
22. **Christie, A. D., Ed.,** *Ultrasound and Infertility,* Chartwel-Bratt, Bromley, 1981, 24.
23. **Glissant, A., De Mouzon, J., and Frydman, R.,** Ultrasound study of the endometrium in vitro fertilization cycles, *Fertil. Steril.,* 44, 786, 1985.
24. **Kurjak, A. and Jurkovic, D.,** Demonstration of the uterime endometrial changes during the menstrual cycle, in *Proc. 4th Meet. World. Fed. for Ultrasound In Medicine and Biology,* Gill, R. W. and Dadd, M. J., Eds., Pergamon Press, Sydney, 1985, 224.
25. **Fleischer, A. C., Kalemeris, G. C., and Entman, S. S.,** Sonographic depiction of the endometrium during normal cycles, *Ultrasound Med. Biol.,* 12, 271, 1986.
26. **Goswamy, R. K., Campbell, S., and Whitehead, M. I.,** Screening for ovarian cancer, *Clin. Obstet. Gynecol.,* 10, 621, 1983.
27. **Hackeloer, B. J. and Nitsche-Debelstain, S.,** Ovarian imaging by ultrasound: an attempt to define a reference plane, *J. Clin. Ultrasound,* 8, 497, 1980.
28. **Campbell, S., Goessens, L., Goswamy, R., and Whitehead, M. I.,** Real-time ultrasonography for determination of ovarian morphology and volume. A possible early screening test for ovarian cancer, *Lancet,* I, 425, 1982.
29. **Kirkpatrick, R. H., Nikrui, N., and Wittenberg, J.,** Gray scale ultrasound in adnexal thickening: correlation with laparoscopy, *J. Clin. Ultrasound,* 7, 115, 1979.
30. **Saks, A.,** Ultrasonic diagnosis in gynecology, in *Diagnostic Ultrasound in Developing Countries,* Kurjak, A., Ed., Mladost, Zagreb, 1986, 241.
31. **Scheible, F. W.,** Ultrasonic features of Gartner's duct cysts, *J. Clin. Ultrasound,* 6, 438, 1978.
32. **Schaffer, R. M., Taylor, C., and Haller, J. O.,** Nonobstructive hydrocolpos: sonographic appearance and differential diagnosis, *Radiology,* 149, 273, 1983.
33. **Siegberg, R., Tenhunen, A., and Ylostalo, P.,** Diagnosis of mucocolpos and hematocolpos by ultrasound: two case reports, *J. Clin. Ultrasound,* 13, 421, 1985.
34. **Schifrin, B. S., Erez, S., and Moore, J. G.,** Teenage endometriosis, *Am. J. Obstet. Gynecol.,* 116, 973, 1973.
35. **Sailer, J. F.,** Hematometra and hematocolpos: ultrasound findings, *Am. J. Roentgenol.,* 132, 1010, 1979.
36. **McCarty, S. and Taylor, K. J. W.,** Sonography of vaginal masses, *Am. J. Roentgenol.,* 140, 1005, 1983.
37. **Walzer, A., Flynn, E., and Koenigsberg, M.,** Sonographic appearance of a prolapsing submucous leiomyoma, *J. Clin. Ultrasound,* 11, 101, 1983.
38. **Woolf, R. B. and Allen, W. B.,** Concomitant malformations: the frequent, simultaneous occurrence of congenital malformations of the reproductive and urinary tracts, *Obstet. Gynecol.,* 2, 336, 1953.

39. **Green, L. K. and Harris, R. E.,** Uterine anomalies: frequency of diagnosis and associated obstetric complications, *Obstet. Gynecol.,* 47, 427, 1976.
40. **Collins, D. C.,** Congenital unilateral renal agenesis, *Ann. Surg.,* 95, 715, 1932.
41. **Kurtz, A. B., Wappner, R. J., and Rubin, C. S., et al.,** Biocornuate uterus: unilateral pregnancy and pelvic kidney, *J. Clin. Ultrasound,* 8, 353, 1980.
42. **Jones, T. B., Fleicher, A. C., and Daniel, J. F., et al.,** Sonographic characteristics of congenital uterine abnormalities and associated pregnancy, *J. Clin. Ultrasound,* 8, 435, 1980.
43. **Kurjak, A. and Jurkovic, D.,** The value of ultrasound in initial assessment of gynecological patients, *Ultrasound Med. Biol.,* 12, 637, 1987.
44. **Silverberg, S. H.,** Principles and practice of surgical pathology, John Wiley & Sons, New York, 1983, 1323.
45. **Gross, B. H., Silver, T. M., and Jaffe, M. H.,** Sonographic features of uterine leimyomas: analyses of 41 proven cases, *J. Ultrasound Med.,* 2, 401, 1983.
46. **Walsh, J. W., Taylor, K. J. W., Wasson, J. F., et al.,** Grey-scale ultrasound in 204 proved gynecologic masses: Accuracy and specific diagnostic criteria, *Radiology,* 130, 391, 1979.
47. **Bejzian, A. and Caretero, M.,** Ultrasonic evaluation of pelvic masses in pregnancy, *Clin. Obstet. Gynecol.,* 20, 325, 1977.
48. **Coulam, C. B., Julian, C., and Fleicher, A. C.,** Clinical efficacy of CT and US in gynecologic tumors, *Appl. Radiol.,* 11, 79, 1982.
49. **Requard, C. K., Wicks, J. D., and Mettler, F. A.,** Ultrasonography in the staging of endometrial carcinoma, *Radiology,* 140, 781, 1981.
50. **Chambers, C. B. and Unis, J. S.,** Ultrasonographic evidence of uterine malignancy in the postmenopausal uterus, *Am. J. Obstet. Gynecol.,* 154, 1194, 1986.
51. **Obata, A., Akamatsu, N., and Sekiba, K.,** Ultrasound estimation of myometrial invasion of endometrial cancer by intrauterine radial scanning, *J. Clin. Ultrasound,* 13, 397, 1985.
52. **Lawson, T. L. and Albarelli, J. N.,** Diagnosis of gynecologic pelvic masses by grey scale ultrasonography: analyses of specificity and accuracy, *Am. J. Roentgenol.,* 128, 1003, 1977.
53. **Callen, P., Filly, R. A., and Munyer, T. P.,** Intrauterine contraceptive devices: evaluation by sonography, *Am. J. Roentgenol.,* 135, 797, 1980.
54. **Mahran, M., Thomas, S., and Saleh, A.,** Ultrasonically guided procedures in ginecology, in *Diagnostic Ultrasound in Developing Countries,* Kurjak, A., Ed., Mladost, Zagreb, 1986, 306.
55. **Swanson, M., Sauerbrei, E. E., and Coopeberg, P. L.,** Medical implications of ultrasonically detected polycystic ovaries, *J. Clin. Ultrasound,* 9, 219, 1981.
56. **Parisi, L., Tramonti, M., Derchi, L. E., et al.,** Polycystatic ovarian disease: ultrasonic evaluation and correlations with clinical and hormonal data, *J. Clin. Ultrasound,* 12, 1221, 1984.
57. **Tabbakh, G. H., Lofty, I., and Azab, I.,** Correlation of the ultrasonic appearance of the ovaries in polycystic ovarian disease and the clinical, hormonal and laparoscopic findings, *Am. J. Obstet. Gynecol.,* 154, 892, 1986.
58. **Franks, S., Adams, J., Mason, H., and Polson, D.,** Ovulatory disorders in women with polycystic ovary syndrome, *Clin. Obstet. Gynecol.,* 12, 605, 1985.
59. **Fleischer, A. C., James, A. E., Millis, J. B., and Julian, C.,** Differential diagnosis of pelvic masses by gray scale sonography, *Am. J. Roentgenol.,* 131, 469, 1978.
60. **Mettler, F. A. and Wicks, J. D.,** Preoperative sonography of malignant ovarian neoplasms, *Am. J. Roentgenol.,* 137, 79, 1981.
61. **Walsh, J. W., Rosenfield, A. R., and Jaffe, C. C.,** Prospective comparison of ultrasound and computed tomography in the evaluation of gynecologic pelvic masses, *Am. J. Roentgenol.,* 131, 955, 1978.
62. **Guttman, P. H.,** In search of the elusive benign cystic ovarian teratoma: application of the ultrasound "tip of the iceberg" sign, *J. Clin. Ultrasound,* 5, 403, 1976.
63. **Sandler, M. A., Silver, T. M., and Karo, J. J.,** Gray-scale ultrasonic features of ovarian teratomas, *Radiology,* 131, 705, 1979.
64. **Laing, F. C., Van Dalsen, V. F., and Marks, W. M.,** Dermoid cysts of the ovary: their ultrasonographic appearances, *Obstet. Gynecol.,* 57, 99, 1981.
65. **Palling, M. R. and Shawker, T. H.,** Abdominal ultrasound in advanced ovarian carcinoma, *J. Clin. Ultrasound,* 9, 435, 1981.
66. **Weinreb, J. C., Brown, C. E., and Ouwe, T. W.,** Pelvic masses in pregnant patients: MR and US imaging, *Radiology,* 159, 717, 1986.
67. **Meine, H. B., Farrant, P., and Guha, T.,** Distinction of benign from malignant ovarian cysts by ultrasound, *Br. J. Obstet. Gynecol.,* 85, 893, 1978.
68. **Moyle, J. W.,** Sonography of ovarian tumors: predictability of tumor type, *Am. J. Roentgenol.,* 141, 985, 1983.
69. **Morley, P. M. and Barnett, E.,** The use of ultrasound in the diagnosis of pelvic masses, *Br. J. Radiol.,* 43, 602, 1970.

70. **Wicks, J. D., Mettler, F. A., Hilgers, R. D., and Ampuero, F.,** Correlation of ultrasound and pathologic findings in patients with ephitelial carcinoma of the ovary, *J. Clin. Ultrasound,* 12, 397, 1984.
71. **Khan, O., Cosgrove, D. O., Fried, A. M., and Savage, P. E.,** Ovarian carcinoma follow-up: US versus leparotomy, *Radiology,* 159, 111, 1986.
72. **Coleman, B. G., Arger, P. H., and Mulhern, C. B.,** Endometriosis: clinical and ultrasonic correlation, *Am. J. Roentgenol.,* 132, 747, 1979.
73. **Birnholz, J. C.,** Endometriosis and inflammatory disease, *Semin. Ultrasound,* 4, 184, 1983.
74. **Walsh, J. W., Taylor, K. J. W., and Rosenfield, A. T.,** Gray scale ultrasonography in the diagnosis of endometriosis and adenomyosis, *Am. J. Roentgenol.,* 132, 87, 1979.
75. **Friedman, H., Vogelzang, R. L., and Mendelson, E. B.,** Endometriosis detection by US with laparoscopic correlation, *Radiology,* 157, 217, 1985.
76. **Bowie, J. D.,** Ultrasound of gynecologic pelvic masses: the indefinite uterus and other patterns associated with diagnostic error, *J. Clin. Ultrasound,* 5, 323, 1977.
77. **Uhrich, P. C. and Sanders, R. C.,** Ultrasonic characteristics of pelvic inflammatory masses, *J. Clin. Ultrasound,* 4, 199, 1976.
78. **Swayne, L. C., Love, M. B., and Karasick, S. R.,** Pelvic inflammatory disease: sonographic-pathologic correlation, *Radiology,* 151, 751, 1984.

Chapter 10

ECTOPIC PREGNANCY

Asim Kurjak and Sanja Kupesic-Urek

INTRODUCTION

The term ''ectopic pregnancy'' refers to the implantation of the ovum in any place outside the uterine cavity. Approximately 95% of ectopic pregnancies are tubal, mainly occurring in the ampullary and isthmic parts of the oviduct. The remaining 5% occur in the ovary, the abdomen, the retroperitoneal space, the broad ligaments, or a rudimentary horn.

Ectopic pregnancy is responsible for 6.5% of all maternal deaths in the U.S. The incidence ranges from 0.3 to 1% of all pregnancies and in the U.S., it increased from 17,800 to 42,000 from 1970 to 1978. The death rate decreased by 75% during this period.[1] The causes of tubal pregnancy include all the factors which may impede or delay the normal transport of the developing zygote into the endometrial cavity. The inflammatory disease of the tube is the most important factor implied in the tubal pregnancy. A nearly threefold increase of ectopic pregnancy incidences during last 2 decades is largely attributed to the widespread use of antibiotic therapy. Pelvic inflammatory disease treated with antibiotics results in the reducible incidence of sterility, but more women with open malfunctioning tubes are exposed to the danger of ectopic pregnancy.[2,3] The fertilized ovum implanted beneath the tubal epithelium establishes a fluid-filled gestational sac lined with trophoblastic tissue within the wall of the tube. The ectopic gestation progresses until 6 or 12 weeks and, because of its inadequate blood supply or increasing size, causes rupture of the tube. The gestational sac within the oviduct of a ruptured ectopic pregnancy in many cases is surrounded by blood or fluid secondary to erosion of adjacent vessels. When the ovum is aborted slowly, hemorrhage is slight. If the end of the tube is occluded, hematosalpinx will result. Usually, the separation of the decidua from the tubal wall results in fetal death. Rupture or extrusion of a tubal pregnancy into the peritoneal cavity with reimplantation within the bowel, broad ligaments, parietal peritoneum, or uterus results in abdominal pregnancy. In that way, abdominal pregnancy can be divided in two groups: primary abdominal pregnancy, which occurs when fertilized ovum escapes through the open end of the tube, and secondary, one that occurs during the process of tubal or ovarian abortion or rupture. Cervical pregnancy can also be included in extrauterine pregnancies. The cervical endometrium is not prepared for the adequate nidation because it does not follow typical progestational changes. The placenta is attached to the cervical myometrium, and abortion always occurs after the 3rd month. In cases with chronic tubal pregnancy, the bleeding is slow. It is characterized with chronicity of symptoms (amenorrhea, vaginal bleeding, temperature elevation, adnexal mass), hemodynamic stability, and a high incidence of false negative pregnancy tests.

DIAGNOSTIC PROCEDURES

The diagnostic procedures in the evaluation of extrauterine pregnancy can be divided in two groups: noninvasive (clinical history and examination, hCG radioimmunoassay, ultrasonography) and invasive diagnostic modalities (culdocenthesis, laparoscopy, intrauterine curettage).

The most common presenting symptoms of ectopic pregnancy are lower abdominal pain (90%), vaginal bleeding (80%), and amenorrhea (70%).[4] Pain may be mild and intermittent or persistent and severe. In cases with adequate placental endocrine function, uterine bleeding is usually absent; but when endocrine support of decidua becomes inadequate, the uterine mucosa will bleed. Free intraperitoneal bleeding causes peritoneal irritation, and diffuse abdominal pain may be present.[5] The patient may also present a picture of shock correlated to the rupture through the wall of the tube and ovary. Some other studies[1,6] reported a palpable adnexal mass or fullness in 48 to 80% of ectopic pregnancies. These anamnestic and clinical findings are suspected signs of ectopic pregnancy, which may be presented either individually or in a number of combinations. They are nonspecific and can be attributed to pelvic inflammatory disease, dysfunctional uterine bleeding, spontaneous abortion, and functional cyst.[7] The urinary pregnancy test is sensitive to a level of 1 to 15 IU/l of human chorionic gonadotropin. This glycoprotein produced by placental trophoblastic tissue doubles every 48 h, beginning with the 8th d after conception. The urinary pregnancy test becomes positive at a 4- to 5-week menstrual age and can be false positive in patients with proteinuria, hematuria, gynecologic neoplasms, tubo-ovarian abscess, and in patients taking some drugs (aspirin, methadone, or tranqulizers).[8] The recent radioimmunoassay pregnancy test is specific and detects the beta subunit of hCG, since alpha subunit is shared by other hormones, such as follicle stimulating hormone or luteinizing hormone. Because of its exquisite sensitivity, it becomes positive from the 10th d of postconception in all cases of ectopic pregnancies except those in which threre is no remaining functioning trophoblastic tissue. Some radioimmunoassays are even quantitive and can be used to ascertain proper growth of an intrauterine pregnancy or to warn when the amount of hCG increases at an abnormal rate, like in abnormal pregnancies such as missed abortion or ectopic pregnancy. Kadar et al.[9] established that 93.5% of normal gestations produce more than 6,500 mIU/ml of hCG by the time that the well-defined intrauterine sac has been demonstrated by ultrasound examination. This "discriminatory zone" lies between 6,000 and 6,500 mIU/ml. Therefore, the absence of an intrauterine gestation sac associated with hCG value below the discriminatory zone is highly suggestive of an ectopic pregnancy. Kadar et al.[10] examined the use of multiple nomograms for doubling time of hCG in order to improve the diagnosis of ectopic pregnancy. Multiple nomograms identified that 79% of women with ectopic pregnancies had rising levels of hCG. The suggestion that multiple nomograms should be adopted in clinical practice leads to difficulties because they are highly applicable and about 19% of women could not be adequately categorized. During the last 15 years, diagnostic ultrasound has become helpful in providing additional diagnostic information on those patients suspected of having an ectopic pregnancy. A scheme involving the use of β-hCG assays and ultrasound examination seems to be a rational decision for those patients whose condition is stable.[11,12] Since laparoscopy and culdocenthesis are invasive procedures, they are performed only in selected cases or under certain clinical conditions. Culdocenthesis is considered positive when blood aspirated from the posterior cul-de-sac has failed to clot within 10 to 15 min. It is positive in approximately 85 to 97% of patients with ectopic pregnancy. It has the advantage of being quick, safe, and less expensive, but it results in patient discomfort. Culdocenthesis should be reserved only for patients in whom free fluid in the cul-de-sac is ultrasonically visible.[3,13] Laparoscopy is indicated in many cases, especially in patients before the 6th week of pregnancy whose ultrasound examination could not differentiate between intrauterine and extrauterine pregnancy, but in whom hCG could be detected in blood. Ollendorf et al.[14] examined the value of curettage in the diagnosis of ectopic pregnancy. They concluded that it might be associated with any histologic type of endometrium. It depends on whether hormonally active trophoblastic tissue is present or on absence or presence of significant uterine bleeding. There is no special, single method of choice which could lead us to the diagnosis of ectopic pregnancy, so we still need to combine methods (Table 1).[15] Huhges[16] reported that 10% of patients with an extrauterine pregnancy were sent home, often having had a curettage because of suspected incomplete or missed abortion.

TABLE 1
Diagnostic Procedures in Extrauterine Pregnancy

Noninvasive	Invasive
Clinical history and examination	Intrauterine curettage
hCG radioimmunoassay	Culdocentesis
Ultrasonography	Laparoscopy

ULTRASONIC FINDINGS

During the last 10 years, high-resolution real-time and B mode gray scale scanners have become widely used because of their accuracy and speed in routine work. This technique is considered to have a primary role in the diagnosis of ectopic pregnancies. However, a considerable number of intra- and extrauterine features in other pelvic pathologies unfortunately have an ultrasonic appearance similar to that seen in patients with ectopic pregnancy. This, indeed, represents a potential error, sometimes resulting in misdiagnosis and mismanagement.[17,18] Kobayashi described the ultrasonic appearance of extrauterine pregnancy by using bistable-B-scan ultrasonography. All the reported cases were either ruptured tubal or abdominal pregnancies. In Kobayashi's series, the true positive rate was 76%, the false negative rate was 24%, and the false positive rate was 28%.[19] The ultrasonic criteria for ectopic pregnancy were divided into uterine findings (absence of an intrauterine pregnancy, diffuse amorphous uterine echoes, and uterine enlargement) and extrauterine findings (irregular echomass beside uterus and an ectopic fetal head). During the last 10 years, high-resolution real-time and B mode gray scale scanners have become widely used, owing to their accuracy and speed in routine work, as well as to the provided possibility of visualizing fetal heart activity. The criteria employed by Robinson et al.[20,21] were divided into primary role (demonstration of an empty uterus) and seocndary role (presence of an adnexal mass, determination of its nature, presence of free fluid in the pelvis) in the assesment of the patients having an ectopic pregnancy (Figures 1 and 2). By identifying an intrauterine gestation, the opportunity of an ectopic pregnancy has been virtually excluded. Simultaneous extrauterine pregnancy is possible in approximately 1 in 30,000 pregnancies. Coexistent intrauterine and ectopic pregnancy result in heterotopic pregnancy. The incidence of combined extra- and intrauterine gestation grows to 1 in 8000 pregnancies, largely due to the therapeutic practice of pharmacologic induction of ovulation, which has increased the incidence of multiple gestations.

The diagnosis of heterotopic pregnancy is very difficult, and the ultrasonic finding of an intrauterine gestational sac and fetus associated with a gestational sac and fetus in the adnexa is a confirmation of it.[22] Recent reports by Reece et al.[23] and Hann et al.[24] show an incidence of 1 per 7963 and 1 per 6778 (Figure 3).

The ultrasonic diagnositic criteria for ectopic pregnancy, reported by Maklad and Wright,[25] may be divided into two groups: ruptured and unruptured extrauterine pregnancies (Table 2). In Maklad's series, the true positive rate was 92.3%; one case was false negative and two cases were false positive.

Strict criteria used for defining a normal intrauterine pregnancy are normal size, shape, and position of the gestational sac within the uterine cavity, "double sac" appearance, and a fetal pole with confirmation of its heart motion (Figure 4). The critical time for the demonstration of a normal intrauterine pregnancy is 5 weeks of menstrual age (3 weeks after conception). The "double sac" sign is a feature created by two concentric echogenic rims from the concentric decidua capsularis and decidua parietalis. That sign is difficult to obtain in 5- to 6-week pregnancies.[26] Cardiac activity can be detected by using combined B × A mode technique as early as 6 weeks.[27]

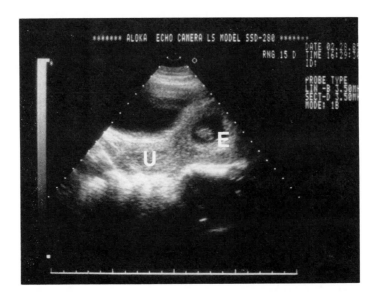

FIGURE 1. Transverse sonogram showing the enlarged uterus (U) with a strong uterine cavity echo in a patient with severe pain in the lower abdomen. The large gestational sac with visible fetal pole is also demonstrated in the right adnexal region (E).

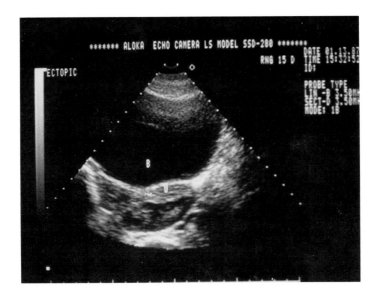

FIGURE 2. Longitudinal sonogram of a patient with suspected ectopic pregnancy showing the uterus (U) and a large amount of free fluid in the pouch of Douglas. The diagnosis of ruptured tubal ectopic pregnancy was confirmed at laparotomy.

Sometimes in pregnant patients with demonstrable circulating hCG, the uterus is presumably empty, but ectopic pregnancy does not occur. These results always require careful interpretation in patents with irregular cycles, those who stopped usage of oral contraceptive therapy, or in those with blighted ova.

A moderately enlarged uterus is detected in the unruptured extrauterine pregnancy due to the effect of circulating gestational hormones.

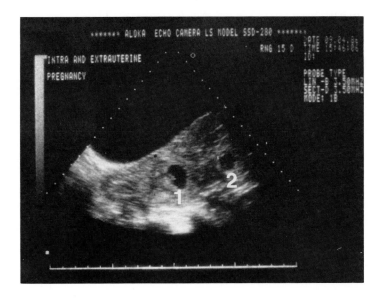

FIGURE 3. A case of combined intra- and extrauterine pregnancy at the 7th week of amenorrhea. An oblique sonogram demonstrates a normal intrauterine pregnancy (1) and another gestational sac-like structure in the right adnexal region (2). In both sacs the fetal pole and heart motions were identified, enabling the diagnosis of heterotopic pregnancy.

TABLE 2
Ultrasonic Diagnostic Criteria in Extrauterine Pregnancy

Unruptured		Ruptured	
Intrauterine findings	**Extrauterine findings**	**Intrauterine findings**	**Extrauterine findings**
Absence of GS[a]	Echodense ring-like structure (GS) outside the uterus	Absence of GS	Parauterine mixed, solid cystic oval mass
Uterine enlargement		Uterus with or without enlargement	
Abnormal echopattern	Detection of fetal echoes and fetal activity inside GS	Uterus with or without abnormal echo pattern	Echo-free area in the cul-de-sac
	Oval, fluid-filled adnexal mass containing GS (distended Fallopian tube)		

[a] GS = gestational sac.

The intrauterine echoes in ectopic pregnancy can be classified into three different ultrasonic samples: "linear" configuration (the decidua is lost from the uterine cavitiy; Figure 5), "cluster" configuration (small pieces of decidua accompanied with blood are retained within the uterine cavity; Figure 6), and the "pseudogestational sac" configuration (Figure 7) (Table 3).

In about 20.5% of patients with a demonstrated extrauterine pregnancy, an intrauterine "pseudogestational sac" can be seen ultrasonically.[28] It can perfectly mimic the normal gestation sac. Small pseudosacs represent a collection of fluid exudate from the decidualized endometrium, while larger ones usually contain blood, the result of bleeding from edematous

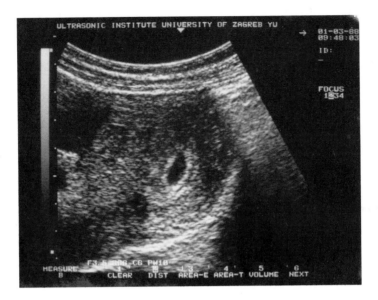

FIGURE 4.   Normal appearance of a 6-week gestational sac in a case of an un-
eventful intrauterine pregnancy. Visualization of two concentric echogenic rims
surrounding the gestational sac that represent decidua capsularis and decidua parietalis ("double sac" sign) enables reliable diagnosis of intrauterine pregnancy even
in the absence of visible fetal pole.

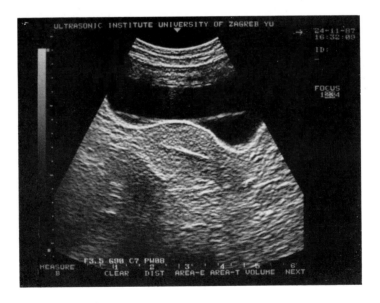

FIGURE 5.   Linear echo of the uterine cavity in a case of an unruptured tubal
pregnancy.

and devitalized decidua. Demonstration of a fluid-debris level within the endometrial cavity
is important in order to confirm the absence of intrauterine pregnancy.[29,30] Smaller pseudosacs
present great diagnostic problems because of a very small sonolucent area equivalent to a
normal 5-week gestational sac or an early blighted ovum. In clinically stable patients,
repeating the scan in a few days shows the disappearance of the pseudosac or the evolution

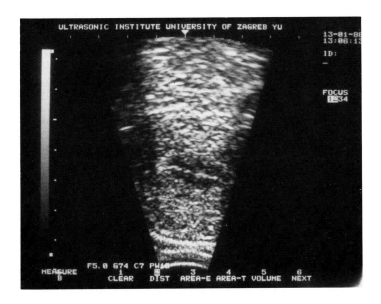

FIGURE 6. Thick endometrium as seen on transvaginal scan in a case of ectopic pregnancy.

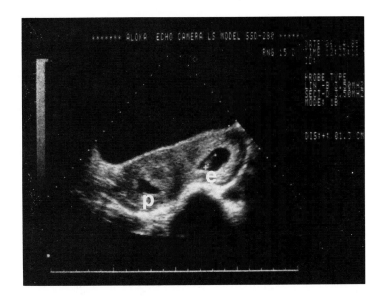

FIGURE 7. Large pseudogestational sac in a patient at the 7th week of amenorrhea with clinical signs of ectopic pregnancy. It has a gestational sac-like appearance, but neither the fetal pole or "double sac" sign are seen (p). On the right to the uterus, ectopic gestational sac with a live embryo is also demonstrated (e).

of "double decidual sac". Larger pseudosacs have sizes which are equivalent to those of a 10-week pregnancy, but usually show low-level echoes from the blood clot.[31-33]

From January 1982 to December 1987, 110 women with ectopic pregnancy were examined (Figures and 8 and 9). In this group, the pseudogestational sac was identified utlrasonically in 15 (13.6%): 11 with developing ectopic pregnancy in which an ectopic gestational sac containing a live fetus inside the sac had been recognized between 7 and 9

TABLE 3
Differential Echographic Parameters of Gestational Sac and Pseudogestational Sac
(at 5th to 6th Week of Amenorrhea)

Echographic variable	Pseudogestational sac	Gestational sac
Location	Center of the uterus	Eccentric
Shape	Irregularly ovoidal	Spheroidal
Contour	Thin (0.1—2 cm)	Thick (>0.2 cm)
	One	Double sac
	Hyperechoic	Hyperechoic
Center of the sac	Hypoechoic	Homogeneously transonic

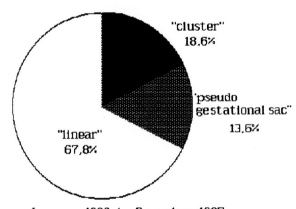

FIGURE 8.   Intrauterine ultrasonic findings in 110 cases of ectopic pregnancy.

weeks of pregnancy, while 4 were tubal abortions. In three cases of tubal abortion, the fluid of the pseudogestational sac was extracted from the uterine cavity with a thin catheter controlled by a real-time ultrasound machine. The cytologic examination ascertains blood fluid including endometrial cells, leukocytes, and histiocytes. Abramovich[34] reported that the most important criterion in differentiating a pseudogestational sac from a gestational one was the detection of its exact location. Ultrasonic appearance of the pseudogestational sac involves a very central, symmetrical intrauterine sac or ring. On the other hand, a 5-week gestational sac ultrasonically appears as an assymmetrical eccentric sac or ring (Figure 10). After 6 weeks of pregnancy, the sac tends to occupy the central part of the uterine cavity. The pseudogestational sac is detectable in several clinical conditions such as hematometra, vaginal bleeding, normal menstruation, and after curettage of the endometrial cavity. In these cases, the pseudogestational sac is always located in the middle of the uterine cavity.

Nowadays, a real diagnostic improvement of ectopic pregnancy is the direct recognition of the ectopic gestational sac with demonstrable fetal heart movements. Pedersen[35] has demonstrated extrauterine fetal cardiac action in 4 of 103 patients, and Robinson was able to demonstrate the presence of fetal heart movements in 6 of 100 patients suspected of having ectopic pregnancy. Fetal heart activity inside the ectopic gestational sac has been

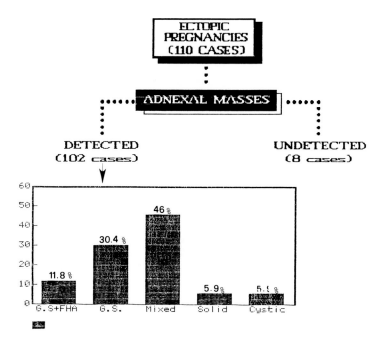

FIGURE 9.   Extrauterine ultrasonic findings in 110 cases of ectopic pregnancy.

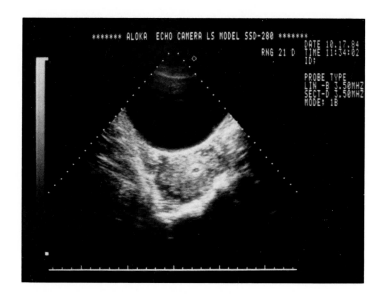

FIGURE 10.   Transverse scan through the uterus, demonstrating a gestational sac at 5 weeks. Note its eccentric position and a uniformly thick echodense ring around the sac representing the rapidly proliferating cyto- and synciciotrophoblast.

presented only in 12 (11.8%) out of 102 cases with detected adnexal masses (Figures 11 to 13).

Ultrasound findings in the adnexa include a well-defined gestational sac which appears as a uniform band of sonodensity (chorion) surrounding an echo-free area (amniotic cavity), adnexal rim sign, or a diffusely echogenic mass (Figures 14 to 16).

Sometimes adnexal masses cannot be seen at all. In our study, which included 110

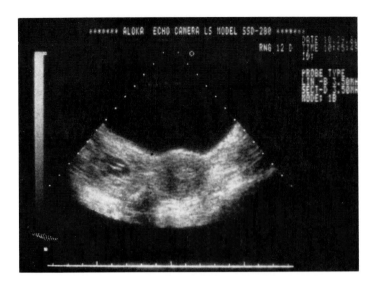

FIGURE 11. Transabdominal transverse scan showing extrauterine pregnancy with an embryo at 8 weeks of gestation left of the empty uterus.

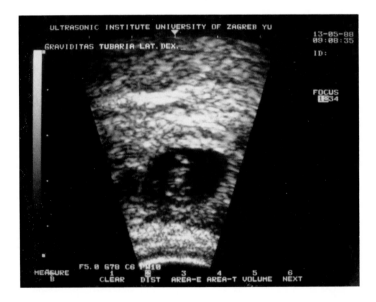

FIGURE 12. Transvaginal scan showing a gestational sac with a normal live embryo at 8 weeks. The diagnosis of left tubal pregnancy was confirmed at laparotomy.

ectopic pregnancies, adnexal masses were detected in 102 (92.7%) and undetected in 8 (7.3%) cases.[4] Adnexal rim sign represents tubal gestational sac without fetal contents. It could be mixed up with hemorrhagic cyst or tubo-ovarian abscess.[36] The absence of the embryo inside the extrauterine gestational sac, the blighted ovum, is nearly as frequent as in spontaneous abortions (50 to 90%), which could explain the ultrasonic failure to visualize the poorly developed extrauterine sac.[37] The first moment of tubal abortion is a partial separation of the trophoblast from the tubal wall, leading to the death of the embryo. This collection of blood between the placental and the tubal wall, called ''subchronic tubal hemorrhage'', can ultrasonically be described as echo-free space partially involving the

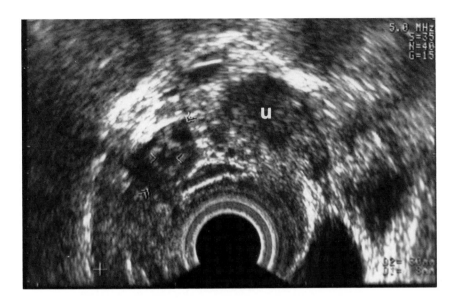

FIGURE 13.   Transvaginal sector scan showing the empty uterus (u) and gestational sac with a live embryo located in the right tube (arrows) at the 7th week of amenorrhea.

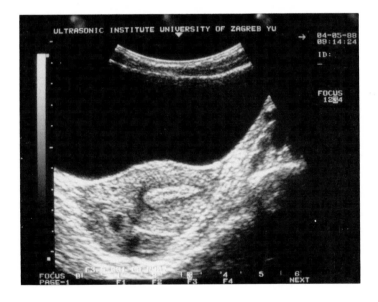

FIGURE 14.   Enlarged uterus with a strong uterine cavity echo in a patient with pain in the lower abdomen. The small retrouterine gestational sac is also visible, but the embryo was not identified.

collapsed ectopic gestational sac. Sonographic appearance of a "collapsed gestational sac" as an echodense adnexal ring-like structure with a thick wall (0.5 to 2 cm) and a clossed chorionic cavity (0.5 to 1 cm) is highly suggestive of an early tubal abortion (Figure 17). Diffusely echogenic adnexal mass could be simulated by hematosalpinx. These discrete, diffusely echogenic adnexal masses can be detected in 85% of patients with an ectopic pregnancy.[38] Shoenbaum et al.[39] showed that these sonolucent masses can be caused by corpus luteum, hematocele, endometriosis, inflammatory changes, and ovarian or uterine

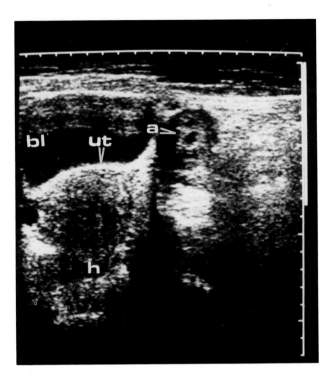

FIGURE 15.   Transabdominal transverse sonogram demonstrating the enlarged uterus (ut), free fluid in the pouch of Douglas (h), and an empty gestational sac in the left adnexal region (a).

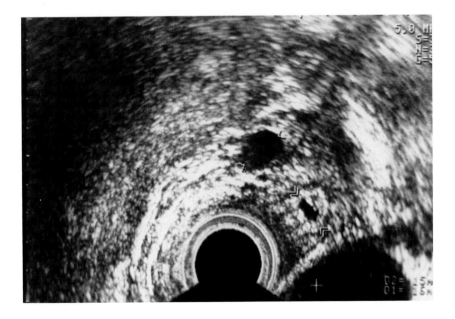

FIGURE 16.   Transvaginal scan showing the small, irregular and empty gestational sac in the right adnexal region (arrows).

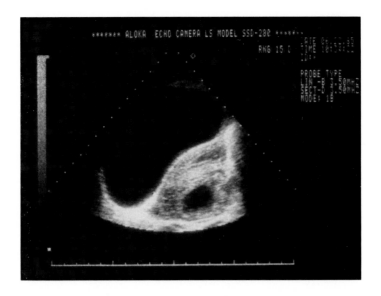

FIGURE 17.   An echodense adnexal ring-like structure located posterolaterally to the uterus represents an early tubal abortion.

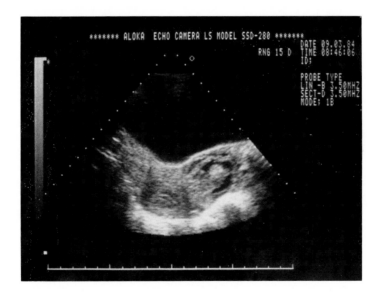

FIGURE 18.   The large, inhomogeneous, predominantly solid tumor on the left represents hematocele in a case of ectopic pregnancy.

tumors. The ectopic gestation may be aborted, ruptured, or chronic and be described as large, complex, predominantly cystic abdominal masses (Figure 18).

In our own experience, the incidence of ectopic gestational sacs was 31 (30.4%) out of 102 women with detected adnexal masses; 10 women presented with blighted ectopic gestational sacs, and 21 with collapsed ectopic gestational sacs. In our case, the incidence of mixed masses was 46%, while that of the solid and cystic masses was 5.9 and 5.3%, respectively.

An ultrasonic feature that may distinguish an abdominal pregnancy in the first trimester

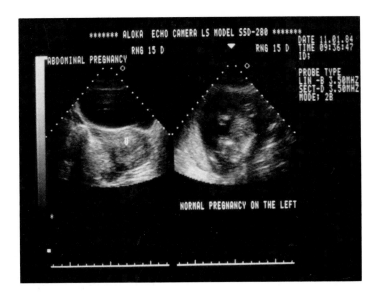

FIGURE 19.   A case of advanced abdominal pregnancy. The uterus is small and empty, while the normal 18-week-old fetus is seen in the left upper part of the abdominal cavity.

from an unruptured tubal pregnancy includes the incomplete myometrial mantle around the sac. In the second and third trimesters, the most specific sonographic appearances are visualization of the uterus in an eccentric position separated from the fetus, unsuccessful visualization of the uterine wall between the fetus and maternal urinary bladder, fetal parts are very close to the maternal abdominal wall, and visualization of the extrauterine placental tissue.[40,41] The echo-free area beside the uterus in the cul-de-sac occurs when hemorrhage into the peritoneal cavity is extensive. Robinson reported that a very small amount of fluid (2 to 3 ml) in the pouch of Douglas could be identified[42,43] (Figure 19).

A transvaginal ultrasound probe may provide superior visualization of the pelvic anatomy and improve the diagnosis of ectopic pregnancy (Figure 20).

Intracavitar fluid collection, blood clots, or retained products of concept may be performed by this method. In the presence of pelvic fluid, the Fallopian tube can be visualized as a tortuous structure nearly 1 cm length. Intraluminal fluid or a gestational sac should also be presented by transvaginal sonography, so the early and reliable diagnosis of tubal gestation is one of the major strengths of this examination.[44-47]

CONCLUSION

The clinical conclusion should not be based only on ultrasound, because one false negative diagnosis in ectopic pregnancy may result in a tragic and dramatic event. Diagnostic ultrasound should be used in conjunction with urinary pregnancy tests or radioimmunoassay of beta subunits hCG. An empty uterus in addition to an adnexal mass and/or the presence of free fluid in the cul-de-sac, together with a positive urinary pregnancy test, gave a true positive rate for extrauterine pregnancy of 95%. An empty uterus with positive biochemistry, but in the absence of an adnexal mass or free fluid, is only suggestive of an ectopic pregnancy. The ultrasonic finding of a living fetus outside the uterus is an absolute sign of ectopic pregnancy, while a negative serum beta subunit hCG assay actually excludes it. It is believed that a scheme involving serum hCG assays and mechanical sector real-time sonography should result in detection of the vast majority of patients with ectopic pregnancy and stable

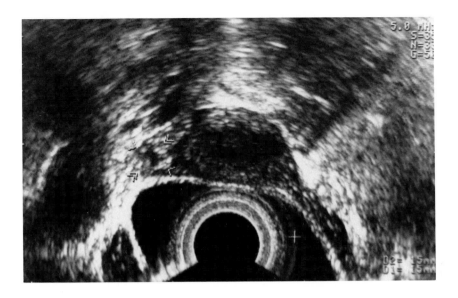

FIGURE 20.   Illustration of an early ectopic pregnancy by transvaginal probe at the 6th week of amenorrhea. The gestational sac is located close to the uterus (arrows), but the fetal pole is not visible.

condition. The combined introduction of these two modalities, in addition to the education of women, will contribute to a decreased mortality and morbidity from ectopic pregnancy.

REFERENCES

1. **Rubin, G., Peterson, H., and Dorfman, S.,** Ectopic pregnancy in the United States 1970 through 1978, *JAMA,* 249, 1725, 1983.
2. **Kleiner, G. and Roberts, T.,** Current factors and causation of tubal pregnancy: a prospective clinical pathologic study, *Am. J. Obstet. Gynecol.,* 99, 21, 1967.
3. **Jurkovic, D., Kurjak, A., Alfirevic, Z., and Klobucar, A.,** Ultrasound diagnosis of combined intrauterine and extrauterine pregnancy, *J. Clin. Ultrasound,* 16, 259, 1988.
4. **Volpe, G. and Volpe, P.,** Ultrasound in ectopic pregnancy, in *Ultrasound in Developing Countries,* Kurjak, A., Ed., Mladost, Zagreb, 1986.
5. **De Cherney, A. H., Minkin, M. J., and Spangler, S.,** Contemporary management of ectopic pregnancy, *J. Reprod. Med.,* 26, 519, 1981.
6. **Schwartz, R. O. and Di Pietro, D. L.,** Beta hCG as a diagnostic aid for suspected ectopic pregnancy, *Obstet. Gynecol.,* 56, 197, 1980.
7. **Athey, P. A. and Hadlock, F. P.,** Ectopic pregnancy, in *Ultrasound in Obstetrics and Gynecology,* Athey, P. A. and Hadlock, F. P., Ed., C. V. Mosby, St. Louis, 1985.
8. **Jacobsen, E. and Rothe, D.,** False positive hemaglutination inhibition tests for preegnancy with introovarian abscess, *Int. J. Gynecol. Obstet.,* 17, 307, 1980.
9. **Kadar, N., De Vore, and Romero, R.,** Discriminatory hCG zone: its use in the sonographic evaluation for ectopic pregnancy, *Obstet. Gynecol.,* 58, 156, 1981.
10. **Kadar, N. and Romero, R.,** Observations on log human chorionic gonadotropin-time relationship in early pregnancy and its practical implications, *Am. J. Obstet. Gynecol.,* 157, 73, 1987.
11. **Laing, F. C. and Jeffrey, R. B.,** Ultrasound evaluation of ectopic pregnancy, *Radiol. Clin. North Am.,* 20, 383, 1982.
12. **Catwright, P. and Di Pietro, D.,** Ectopic pregnancy: change in serum hCG concentration, *Obstet. Gynecol.,* 63, 76, 1984.
13. **Weckstein, L. N., Boucher, A. R., and Tucker, H.,** Accurate diagnosis of early ectopic pregnancy, *Obstet. Gynecol.,* 65, 393, 1985.

14. **Ollendorf, D. A., Moshe, B., and Gerbie, B. A.,** The value of curettage in the diagnosis of ectopic pregnancy, *Am. J. Obstet. Gynecol.,* 157, 71, 1987.
15. **Joupilla, P.,** Ultrasound-evaluation as a method of choice in the diagnosis of ectopic pregnancy, in *Progress in Medical Ultrasound,* Kurjak, A., Ed., Excerpta Medica, Amsterdam, 1980, 173.
16. **Hughes, G. J.,** The early diagnosis of ectopic pregnancy, *Br. J. Surg.,* 66, 789, 1979.
17. **Langer, A. and Iffy, L., Eds.,** *Extrauterine Pregnancy,* John Wright-PSG, Littleton, MA, 1986.
18. **Romero, R., Taylor, K. J. W., Kadar, N., and Hobbins, J. C.,** The diagnosis of ectopic pregnancy, in *Gynecology and Ultrasound,* Steel, W. B. and Cohrane, W. J., Eds., Churchill Livingstone, Edinburgh, 1984, 123.
19. **Kobayashi, M., Hellman, L. M., and Fillisti, L. P.,** Ultrasound — an aid in the diagnosis of ectopic pregnancy, *Am. J. Obstet. Gynecol.,* 103, 1131, 1969.
20. **Robinson, H. P.,** The current status of sonar in obstetrics and gynecology, in *Recent Advances in Obstetrics and Gynecology,* Stalworthy, J. and Bourne, G., Eds., Churchill Livingstone, Edinburgh, 1977, 239.
21. **Robinson, H. P.,** Normal development in early pregnancy, in *Handbook of Clinical Ultrasound,* De Vilieger, M., Kazner, E., and Kossott, G., Eds., John Wiley & Sons, New York, 1978, 121.
22. **Yagel, S., Hurwitz, A., Ron, M., and Palti, Z.,** Ultrasonic demonstration of heterotopic pregnancy, *J. Clin. Ultrasound,* 11, 502, 1983.
23. **Reece, E. A., Petrie, R. H., and Sirmans, M. F.,** Combined intrauterine and extrauterine gestations. a review, *Am. J. Obstet. Gynecol.,* 146, 323, 1983.
24. **Hann, L. E., Bschman, D. M., and McArdle, C. R.,** Coexistent intrauterine and ectopic pregnancy: a reevaluation, *Radiology,* 152, 151, 1984.
25. **Maklad, N. F. and Wright, C. H.,** Grey scale ultrasonography in the diagnosis of ectopic pregnancy, *Radiology,* 126, 221, 1978.
26. **Robinson, H. P. and De Crespigni, L. C.,** Ectopic pregnancy, *Clin. Obstet. Gynecol.,* 10, 407, 1983.
27. **Robinson, H. P.,** Detection of fetal heart movements in the first trimester of pregnancy using pulsed ultrasound, *Br. Med. J.,* 466, 1972.
28. **Marks, W. M.,** The decidual cast of ectopic pregnancy: a confusing ultrasonographic appearance, *Radiology,* 133, 451, 1979.
29. **Mueller, C. E.,** Intrauterine pseudogestational sac in ectopic pregnancy, *J. Clin. Ultrasound,* 7, 133, 1979.
30. **Spirt, B. A., O'Hara, K. R., and Gordon, L.,** Pseudogestational sac in ectopic pregnancies: sonographic and pathologic correlation, *J. Clin. Ultrasound,* 9, 338, 1981.
31. **Nyberg, A. A., Laing, F. C., and Filly, R. A.,** Ultrasonographic differentiation of the gestational sac of early intrauterine pregnancy from the pseudogestational sac of ectopic pregnancy, *Radiology,* 146, 755, 1983.
32. **Philippe, E., Bilenki, I., and Warter, A.,** Pathology of ectopic pregnancy, in *Extrauterine Pregnancy,* Langer, A. and Iffy, L., Eds., John Wright-PSG, Littleton, MA, 1986, 107.
33. **Weiner, C. P.,** The pseudogestational sac in ectopic pregnancy, *Am. J. Obstet. Gynecol.,* 139, 959, 1981.
34. **Abramovich, H., Auslender, R., Lewin, A., and Faktor, J. H.,** Gestational-pseudogestational sac: a new ultrasonic criterion for differential diagnosis, *Am. J. Obstet. Gynecol.,* 3, 377, 1983.
35. **Pedersen, J. F.,** Ultrasonic scanning in suspected ectopic pregnancy, *B. J. Radiol.,* 1, 53, 1980.
36. **Brown, T. W.,** Analysis of ultrasonographic criteria in the evaluation of ectopic pregnancy, *Am. J. Radiol.,* 131, 967, 1978.
37. **Poland, B. J., Dill, F. J., and Styblo, C.,** Embryonic development in ectopic human pregnancy, *Teratology,* 14, 315, 1976.
38. **De Cherney, A. H., Minkin, M. J., and Spangler, S.,** Contemporary management of ectopic pregnancy, *J. Reprod. Med.,* 26, 519, 1980.
39. **Schoenbaum, S., Rosendorf, L., Kappelman, N., and Rowan, T.,** Gray scale ultrasound in tubal pregnancy, *Radiology,* 127, 757, 1978.
40. **Allibone, G. W., Fagan, C. J., and Porter, S. C.,** The sonographic features of intra-abdominal pregnancy, *J. Clin. Ultrasound,* 9, 383, 1981.
41. **Lawson, T. L.,** Ectopic pregnancy: the criteria of accuracy of ultrasonic diagnosis, *Am. J. Roentgenol.,* 131, 153, 1978.
42. **Volpe, G., D'Addario, V., Daminani, L., and Volpe, P.,** L'ecografia in tempo reale nella diagnosi della gravidanza ectopica, in *Esperienze di Ultrasonografia in Ostetricia e ginecologia,* Bios-Cosenz, Ed., Rome, 1982, 499.
43. **Volpe, G. and Kurjak, A.,** Controversies and perspectives in the ultrasonic assessment of ectopic pregnancy, *Acta Med. Iugosl.,* 1988, accepted for publication.
44. **Feichtinger, W. and Kemeter, P.,** transvaginal sector scan sonography for needle guided transvaginal follicle aspiration and other applications in gynecologic routine and research, *Fertil. Steril.,* 45, 722, 1986.
45. **Timor-Tritsch, I. E. and Rottem, S.,** Transvaginal sonography in the management of infertility, in *Ultrasound and Infertility,* Kurjak, A., Ed., CRC Press, Boca Raton, FL, 1988, in press.

46. **Timor-Tritsch, I. E. and Rottem, S.,** Transvaginal study of the fallopian tube, *Obstet. Gynecol.,* 70, 426, 1987.
47. **Rottem, S. and Timor-Tritsch, I. E.,** Think ectopic, in *Transvaginal Sonography,* Elsevier, New York, 1988, 125.

Chapter 11

ULTRASOUND AND INFERTILITY

Asim Kurjak and Davor Jurkovic

INTRODUCTION

Ultrasound plays an important role in the diagnosis and treatment of infertility. Since Kratochwil's first demonstration of ovaries by ultrasound,[1] this method has become recognized as an integral part of diagnostic investigation in gynecology. By using modern real-time gray scale equipment, it is possible to diagnose various pathologic conditions within the female lesser pelvis. Simple ultrasound examination may provide the clinician with important information about female genital organs and help to detect pathology that may be responsible for fertility problems. Some of the causes of infertility detectable by ultrasound are listed in Table 1. The list includes congenital uterine anomalies, uterine fibroids, and adenomyosis. Any of these anomalies may be responsible for fertility problems. Congenital uterine anomalies are frequently associated with infertility and habitual spontaneous abortion. Nowadays, it is well documented that ultrasound is an acceptably accurate method for diagnosis of these anomalies[2,3] (Figures 1 and 2). Therefore, hysterosalpingography should be indicated only for a more detailed analysis of a structural defect, and ultrasound is preferred as a screening method.

Ultrasonic visualization of a uterine fibroid provides fast and simple detection of the cause of infertility. Infertility is the only symptom in a considerable proportion of patients with a uterine fibroid. Large nodes in the posterior uterine wall dislocate the tubes and diminish their motility, so that the acceptance and transport of fertilized ova is impossible. Nodes situated close to the ostia tubae uterine can cause mechanical obstruction of the tubes, and submucosal myomas interfere with the nidation (Figures 3 and 4).

Adenomyosis is characterized by ingrowths of the endometrium into the myometrium. It is usually asymptomatic, but there may be uterine bleeding, pain, and infertility. The characteristic ultrasonic finding involves the disrupted homogenicity of the uterine texture by irregular cystic spaces.[4] Adenomyosis may also be the cause of uterine enlargement, and its differentiation from myoma may be difficult.

Disease of the tubes is the cause of infertility in most cases. A normal Fallopian tube cannot be visualized by ultrasound, except in the presence of ascites. The tubes are most often affected by infection, and in such cases they can be visualized.[5]

Chronic inflammatory changes are frequently associated with infertility. Several kinds of chronic changes may occur, even after one episode of acute pelvic inflammatory disease. Pelvic adhesions develop first, fixing pelvic structures to one another and to the adjacent bowel and omentum. If a pyosalpinx occurs, it may evolve into a hydrosalpinx in which purulent exudate is replaced by serous fluid. Pelvic sonograms may be confusing in such cases.[6] While the adhesions themselves are invisible, they may lead to the fixation of bowel loops and omentum in the pelvis, which may in turn be mistaken for pelvic cysts and masses (Figure 5). The chronic residua of tubo-ovarian and pelvic abscesses, such as a hydrosalpinx, inflammatory cysts, or adhesions, may produce complex patterns of pelvic fluid loculations, often markedly expanding the pouch of Douglas and encompassing the uterus (Figure 6). Without conventional clinical findings or serial sonographic changes, the ultrasound examination is not specific. An echo-free tubular pelvic structure may not represent the expected hydrosalpinx, but instead a dilated distal ureter. Complex residua of abscesses and inflammatory cysts may be indistinguishable from cystic neoplasms, endometriosis, or chronic ruptured ectopic pregnancy.[7]

TABLE 1
The Causes Of Infertility Detectable By Ultrasound

Uterus
  Congenital anomalies (aplasia, hypoplasia, bicornuate
    uterus, septate uterus, etc.)
  Fibroma
  Adenomyosis
  Endouterine synechia
Fallopian tubes
  Pyosalpinx, hydrosalpinx
Ovaries
  Polycystic ovaries
  Chronic infections (tubo-ovarian abscess)
  Tumors
Endometriosis

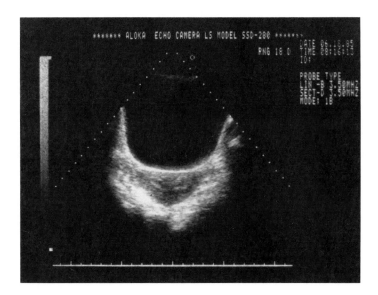

FIGURE 1.   Transverse sonogram in a case of arcuate uterus. Note typical splitting
of the endometrial echo in the upper parts of the uterine cavity.

Functional cysts frequently coexist with chronic pelvic inflammatory disease (Figure 7). However, the cysts usually resolve, whereas chronic pelvic inflammatory disease does not. Normal fluid-filled bowel loops may even masquerade as abscesses. The role of sonography in chronic pelvic inflammatory disease is to document the appearance of sequelae, to gauge the effectiveness of therapy, and to help to elucidate the causes of infertility.

Ultrasound examination of the ovaries is essential for the elucidation of any infertility case. Besides the monitoring of growth and development of Graafian follicles, some ovarian abnormalities are discovered by routine procedures. The most common finding is polycystic ovaries. The ovaries are enlarged and filled with numerous cysts less than 10 mm in diameter which represent immature follicles[8] (Figure 8). Sometimes the cysts are situated along the border of the ovary. The syndrome of polycystic ovaries, amenorrhea, and hirsutism is referred to as the Stein-Leventhal syndrome. However, it is unusual for all of these features to be present in patients with polycystic ovaries.

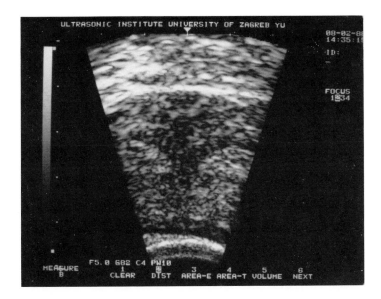

FIGURE 2.   A case of septate uterus. Two endometrial echoes are visible, separated by thin, hypoechoic uterine septum.

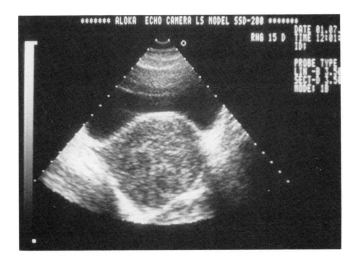

FIGURE 3.   Typical sonographic appearance of fibroma uteri. The uterus is enlarged, its contour is irregular, and normal homogenicity of myometrium is disturbed.

Large cystic tumors of the ovaries can cause infertility. By disturbing normal anatomic relations within the pelvis, the tumor dislocates the tubes or causes their mechanical obstruction. Infertility and ectopic pregnancy are the most common complications (Figure 9).

The association of infertility and endometriosis is well documented. Many attempts have been made to diagnose and define the extent of endometriosis. It has generally been accepted that ultrasound is useful in the detection of large endometrioma, but it is impossible to define the extent of the disease with accuracy[9] (Figures 10 and 11).

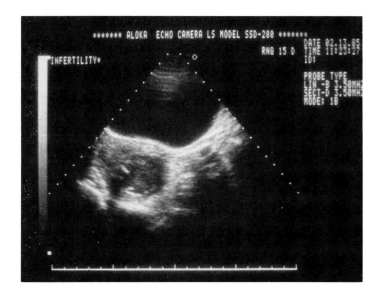

FIGURE 4.   Another example of fibroma uteri with marked calcification of the tumor, which produces characteristic posterior shadowing on the sonogram.

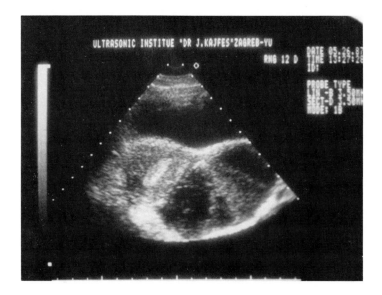

FIGURE 5.   The large echogenic tumor on the right represents a tubo-ovarian abscess occupying the pouch of Douglas and fixed bowel loops in a patient suffering from chronic pelvic infection.

MONITORING THE GROWTH AND DEVELOPMENT OF GRAAFIAN FOLLICLES

In any assessment of the ovarian function, the techniques used should be noninvasive, have a high degree of patient acceptability, and provide readily accessible information to the clinician. Although radioimmunoassays for steroid hormones are available, their levels indirectly reflect the changes within the ovary and give no information about the number or nature of the follicles which may be developing.

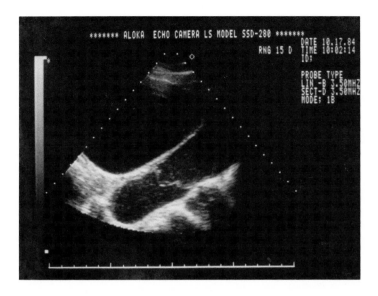

FIGURE 6.   Bilateral hydrosalpinx in a case of chronic pelvic inflammatory disease appearing as large, irregular, hypoechoic tumors.

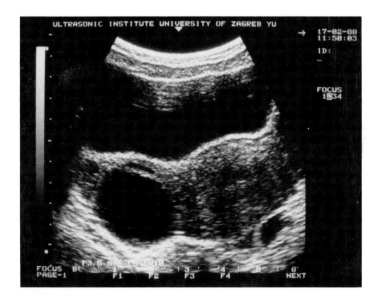

FIGURE 7.   Large cyst in the left ovary. The cyst is simple, unilocular, with thin and well-defined borders and no internal echoes. A case of physiological ovarian cyst.

Recently, ultrasound has provided a new method for the evaluation of ovarian function with reference to both follicular development and corpus luteum function. The first systematic investigations with ultrasonic demonstration of follicular development during the spontaneous and stimulated cycles were performed in 1977.[10] Since then, numerous authors have confirmed the initial observations that ultrasound provides a simple and noninvasive insight into physiologic changes during the menstrual cycle and accurate and reproducible studies of follicular size during the late follicular phase.[11,12]

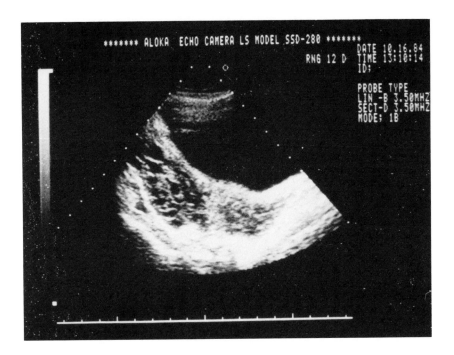

FIGURE 8.   A case of polycystic ovarian disease in a patient suffering from primary infertility. The ovary is markedly enlarged and filled with numerous small, immature follicles measuring less than 10 mm in size.

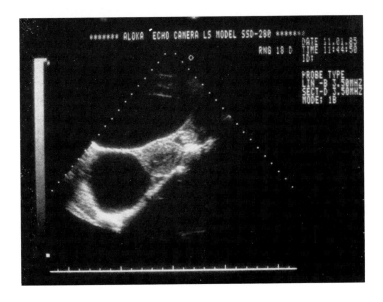

FIGURE 9.   Large cystic ovarian tumor on the right which should be recognized as a possible cause of tubal obstruction in infertile patients.

Static B mode gray scale scanners were for a long time considered to provide the best visualization of anatomical details within the lesser pelvis, but recent improvements in real-time mechanical sector resolution capabilities bring up the fact that their imaging capabilities gradually match those of static machines. Examinations with real-time sector probes are much more simple and less time consuming if compared with the static machines, and the

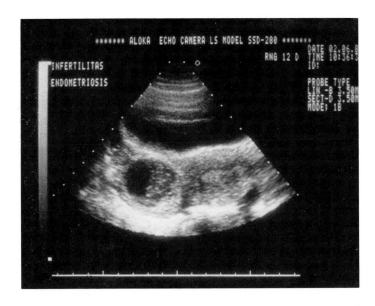

FIGURE 10. Endometrioma on the right with pronounced internal echoes. Such a finding cannot be distinguished from a tubo-ovarian abscess, and the diagnosis was made on laparotomy.

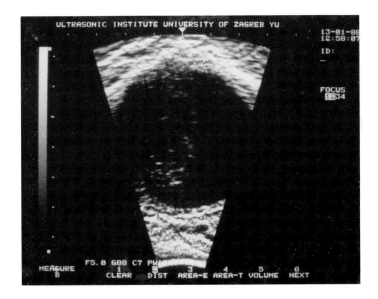

FIGURE 11. Transvaginal scan of the large endometriotic cyst in the left ovary. Note the presence of internal echoes which represent blood clots within the cyst.

ultrasonic findings are less operator dependent. These obvious advantages of real-time machines made them the currently preferred mode of pelvic sonographic imaging.

Recently, it has been shown that transvaginal sonography offers numerous advantages over transabdominal sonography, and this new method will most probably completely rule out transabdominal scanning for the purpose of monitoring follicular growth and ovulation.[13] The major advantage of transvaginal scanning is the superior quality of the image due to high frequency (5 to 10 MHz) of the probes used, without the need to fill the urinary bladder.

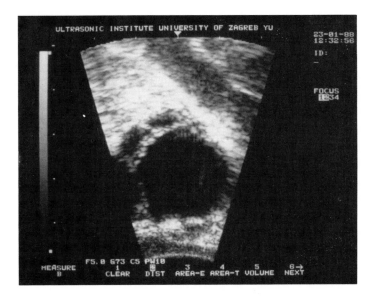

FIGURE 12.   Mature preovulatory follicle demonstrated by transvaginal scanning. The dominant follicle is clearly seen, and few immature follicles located around its periphery are also demonstrated.

That makes examination more accurate and more convenient to the patients who are submitted to daily serial examinations (Figure 12).

ULTRASOUND ASSESSMENT OF SPONTANEOUS CYCLES

Monitoring of follicular growth and ovulation by ultrasound should be started on day 9 or 10 of a regular-day menstrual cycle. Depending on the cycle length, serial examinations may be attempted a few days earlier or later. The best results could be achieved if all examinations in each particular patient are performed by the same observer. At 3 to 5 d before ovulation, i.e., days 8 to 10 of a regular 28-d cycle, the dominant follicle can be identified as an anechoic cystic structure with well-defined borders, measuring 8 to 10 mm in size, and being significantly larger than other follicles still present within the ovaries. During the next several days, the preovulatory follicle undergoes fast growth, and 1 d before ovulation, it reaches a diameter of 20 mm[14,15] (Figures 13 to 15).

The basic ultrasonic parameter for the assessment of follicular maturation is the diameter of the dominant follicle. The size of the follicle is measured by means of a built-in digital caliper system. By positioning two bright calipers on the inner walls of the follicle, as it would be seen on the frozen image on the screen, the diameter is automatically displayed (Figure 16).

Even though the basic technique of the measurement is the same, there are significant differences in the size of the preovulatory follicle between various reports. That can be partly attributed to the differences among the equipment used and experience, but the major source of the wide range of values lies in the number of planes in which the measurements were performed. Early reports were based either on single maximal, two- or three-diameter measurements. Nowadays, most authors are estimating the follicle size by calculating mean diameter from linear measurements taken in three orthogonal planes.[16]

In a view of the fact that the shape of the follicle is rarely round, but more commonly ovoid or elongated, that approach gives the most reliable information about actual follicular size. By performing measurement of three diameters, one can easily calculate the volume of the follicular fluid. It does not represent an improvement over the mean diameter estimation

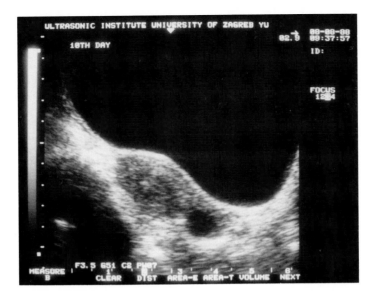

FIGURE 13. Transverse sonogram of the right ovary, showing a developing follicle. The follicle appears as a small and round cystic structure with well-defined walls and clear fluid within.

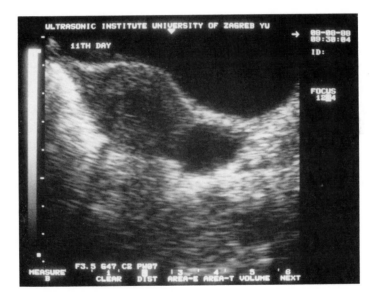

FIGURE 14. The small increase of follicle size can be recognized on the sonogram on the following day.

for the assessment of follicular growth, but it can be useful in certain situations (e.g., before aspiration of follicular fluid for *in vitro* fertilization).

The daily growth rate of the preovulatory follicle is between 2 and 3 mm and parallels rising estradiol levels (Figure 17). On the basis of previous studies which showed that more than 90% of circulating estradiol is produced by the preovulatory follicle,[17] Hackeloer et al.[18] compared the ultrasonic follicular measurements with endocrinologic parameters of follicular growth and maturity. Their results showed that there was a clear-cut correlation

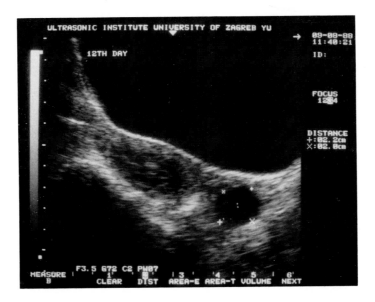

FIGURE 15.   Mature preovulatory follicle on the 12th d of the menstrual cycle. The mean diameter of the follicle is 20 mm, and the follicular wall is smooth, suggesting luteinization of the granulosa cells.

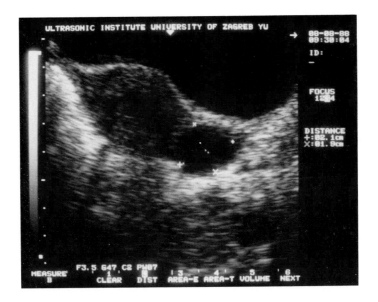

FIGURE 16.   Technique of ovarian follicles measurement. Three diameters are usually measured by placing the calipers on the inner wall of the follicle.

between the diameter of the growing follicle and peripheral estradiol levels estimated by radioimmunoassay either when the mean values of both parameters or paired data were analyzed for days from −5 to 0. Synchronous analysis of luteinizing hormone (LH) profile in the same study showed a regular coincidence of midcycle LH surge with the maximal diameter of the preovulatory follicle. Those data clearly show that on the basis of morphologic studies of the growing follicle, it is possible to collect information about its functional capability. It could be helpful for interpreting the peripheral target organ and plasma steroid level changes, particularly in cases of abnormal cycles, which will be discussed later.

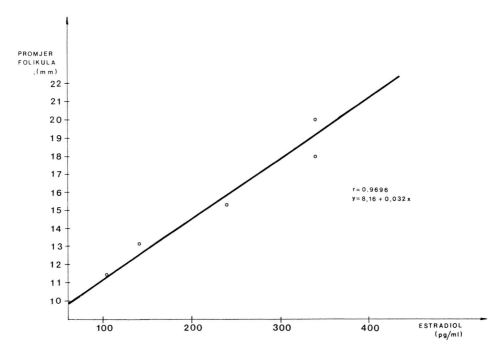

FIGURE 17. Correlation diagram showing the mean values of the follicle size and mean estradiol concentrations on cycle days −5 to −1.

The most common indication for the ovarian scanning during the spontaneous cycles is better prediction of ovulation in patients who are undergoing artificial insemination. However, the accurate prediction and detection of ovulation carries critical importance in the success of that procedure. Although ultrasound scanning is particularly reliable for the detection of ovulation, prediction of ovulation, based on the diameter of the dominant follicle alone, is not sufficiently accurate.[19] As mentioned previously, the mean diameter of the preovulatory follicle 1 d before ovulation is about 20 mm, but the range of values is wide, being between 16 to 25 mm. For that reason, several authors have tried to define minor morphological changes in the appearance of the preovulatory follicle that are suggestive of imminent ovulation.

Bomsel-Helmereich et al.[20] obtained clear evidence that the ultrasonic appearance of triangular intrafollicular echogenic structure, regularly seen adjacent to the inner wall of the follicle, represents dissociated cumulus oophorus (Figure 18). According to their results, echo of the cumulus oophorus can be demonstrated in the preovulatory follicle only after its dissociation and can, therefore, be used as a reliable sign that LH surge has already occurred. Although that finding indicates forthcoming ovulation, its use in the assessment of the ovarian function is limited by the relatively low visualization rate of 15 to 20%.[21] However, there are a few reports which claim much higher visualization rates of the cumulus oophorus, but to obtain such results, exceptionally good equipment, meticulous examination of the entire follicular surface, and vast experience are required.

To summarize, the presence of a well-defined echo of the cumulus oophorus allows accurate prediction of ovulation within the next 24 h, but a negative finding does not imply its absence and should be critically accepted. Another very consistent ultrasonic feature in the preovulatory follicle is related to the morphology of the follicular wall, and it was first reported by Picker at al.[22] in 1983. It has been described as a line of decreased echogenicity around the follicle and may be seen within 24 h before ovulation. The finding was explained by the histological studies of the preovulatory follicle after LH surge, which showed edem-

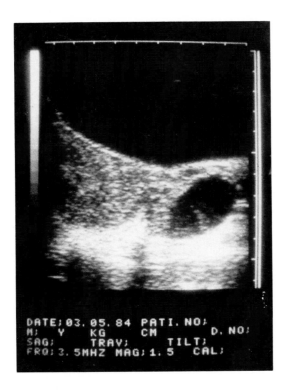

FIGURE 18. The real-time scan of the mature preovulatory follicle demonstrates a triangular echo of dissociated cumulus oophorus.

atous thecal tissue and separation of granulosa and theca cell layers. As ovulation approaches, separation is progressive and causes folding of the granulosa cell layer, which can be demonstrated sonographically as a crenation of the follicular wall. Massive separation and folding of the granulosa occur just a few hours before ovulation, and for that reason it is rarely seen with the usual one-per-day frequency of examinations.[22]

The process of ovulation and follicular rupture has also been demonstrated by ultrasound.[23] There were no significant changes either in the size or morphology of the follicle before the sudden decrease in its size that denotes escape of follicular fluid in the periovarian region. It took between 7 to 35 min until complete collapse of the follicle. As early as 1 h after rupture, the corpus hemorrhagicam may be visualized. Sonographically demonstrated, early corpus luteum may have varying appearance, and that can occasionally cause difficulties in diagnosis of ovulation. The most common feature includes complete collapse of the follicle and the presence of a small residual cyst with thick walls. It is usually filled with echogenic blood clots. In such cases, diagnosis of ovulation is relatively simple and reliable (Figure 19). In about 20% of cases, the follicle is almost of the same or of slightly decreased size. It loses its tense appearance and is also filled with echongenic material. That represents a reaccumulation of the fluid and blood within the ruptured follicle and is accepted as clear ultrasonic evidence of ovulation, too. The most controversial finding is the presence of a cyst of the same or even larger size with tense walls and some internal echoes. This finding is highly suggestive of defective ovulation and will be discussed in detail later.

Although the main morphological changes related to the menstrual cycle concern the ovaries, important findings are also demonstrated in uterine mucosa.

In the immediate postmenstrual phase, the endometrium is seen as a thin, highly echoic linear echo (Figure 20). During the 2nd week of the proliferative phase, it is becoming

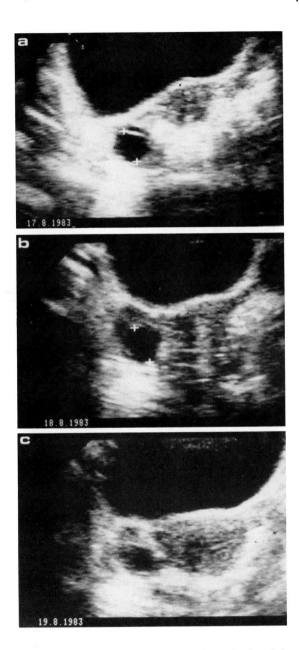

FIGURE 19.   Illustration of sonographic diagnosis of ovulation by serial daily scanning. On the two first figures, the growth of the preovulatory follicle is demonstrated. Ovulation is seen as a marked reduction in the size of the preovulatory follicle, which lost its tense appearance.

gradually thicker and is characterized by a thin and well-defined boundary with the myometrium. A marked linear middle echo represents the attached superficial endometrial layers. The endometrium is hypoechoic as compared to the echogenicity of the myometrium (Figure 21). That can be explained by the presence of edematous fluid which separates the stroma cells of the superficial layer.[24] In the preovulatory phase of the cycle, the endometrium is 3.5 to 7 mm thick as measured by ultrasound. A day before ovulation there is an obvious increase in its echogenicity, particularly in the basal portions. Middle echo is less pronounced, but still present[25] (Figure 22).

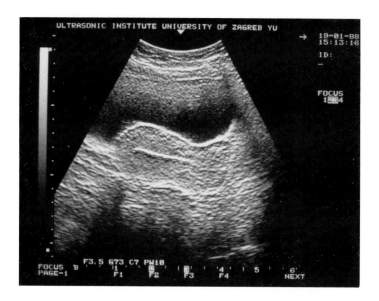

FIGURE 20.   Longitudinal sonogram of the uterus in the early proliferative phase
of the cycle showing a strong uterine cavity echo. The strong echo represents the
thin endometrium with attached superficial layers.

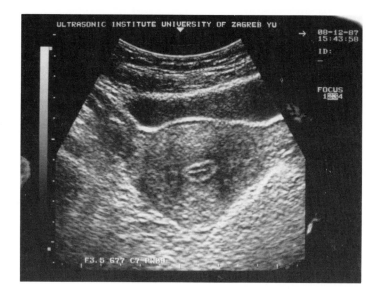

FIGURE 21.   The endometrium in the late proliferative phase. The endometrium
is hypoechoic as compared to the myometrium, and its boundary with the latter is
well defined. The central echo of the attached superficial layers is also clearly
visible.

In the midluteal phase, the endometrium is thick and homogeneous. The endometrial
surfaces do not adhere to each other as in the proliferative phase, and the linear echo is,
therefore, lost. The endometrium is highly echogenic and clearly visible[26] (Figure 23).

This ultrasonically obtained information about the morphological characteristics of endometrium correspond well to the classic histological descriptions. The accuracy of endo-

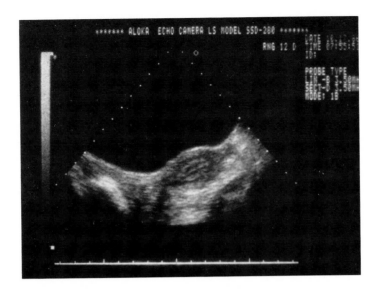

FIGURE 22. Typical appearance of the preovulatory endometrium exhibiting increased basal layer echogenicity.

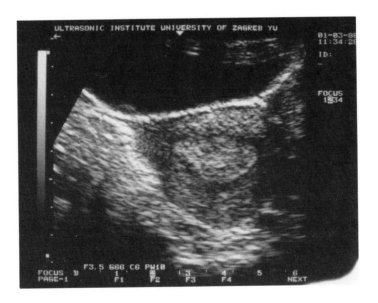

FIGURE 23. Echogenic endometrium in the secretory phase. The endometrium is thick, and the central echo is lost.

metrial thickness measurement by ultrasound has been proven by comparing the ultrasonically and histologically estimated endometrial size, which showed an excellent correlation.

The characteristic ultrasonic appearance of the preovulatory endometrium resembles the ultrasonic finding of an early gestational sac, and it is well-known as the "ovulation ring". For a long time it has served as an additional parameter for detection of ovulation.[28]

Assessment of endometrial changes during ultrasound monitoring of follicular growth provides additional data about the functional capability of the growing follicle. It could be particularly useful for better prediction of ovulation, fast and simple orientation about the phase of the menstrual cycle, and detection of certain cycle abnormalities.

During the luteal phase of the cycle, the corpus luteum can be seen in approximately 60% of patients. However, the corpus luteum morphology has a low specificity, and demonstration of its characteristics is only of academic interest because it does not offer any relevant clinical information.

Ultrasound detection of disturbed ovulation is based on well-defined morphological criteria for normal follicular growth and ovulation in comparison to radioimmunoassay of pituitary and ovarian hormones in peripheral blood. Even in their early report, which actually established the important role of sonography for the study of ovarian function, Hackeloer et al.[10] described 3 cases of apparently abnormal follicular maturation, confirmed by hormone assays, in a group of 15 healthy volunteers. The significance of sonographically observed follicle maturation and ovulation abnormalities has been confirmed in numerous subsequent reports. Polan et al.[29] have found in 5 of 14 women (38%) suffering from the secondary infertility various cycle abnormalities. The common ultrasonic finding in that group of patients was the demonstration of the significantly smaller size of the preovulatory follicle, with asynchronicity between its morphological characteristics and serum levels of ovarian steroids and LH. Elevated progesterone levels in the luteal phase and biphasic basal body temperature curve were seen in all patients with abnormal ultrasonic findings. Based on these results, the authors have pointed out the inadequacy of standard criteria for the ovulatory cycle. That can partly explain the failure of achieving pregnancy in patients who apparently respond well to the ovarian stimulation or in patients in whom numerous unsuccessful artificial inseminations were attempted.[29]

A similar conclusion could be drawn from the report of Couts et al.[30] who found cycle abnormalities in 13 out of 25 investigated cycles in a group of patients with unexplained infertility. A regular finding in the luteal phase of abnormal cycles was the presence of intraovarian cyst with acoustic characteristics markedly different from normal corpus luteum. Luteal progesterone levels were significantly lower, if compared to the normal corpus luteum.

Among the ultrasonically detectable cycle abnormalities, the diganosis of luteinized unruptured follicle (LUF) syndrome is most extensively reported. The term "luteinized unruptured follicle" was introduced by Jewelewicz in 1975.[31] The main characteristic of this condition is complete luteinization of the follicle without ovulation and oocyte release. Etiology of LUF syndrome still remains unexplained. Actually, it seems that ovulation abnormality may be caused by primary oocyte abnormality,[32] abnormalities in prostaglandin synthesis,[33] and defective midcycle LH surge.[34]

Frequency of LUF syndrome is, according to the reported data, extremely variable in potentially fertile women and is estimated to be between 6 and 47%.[35,36] In endometriotic patients, reported incidence of LUF was 11 to 33%.[37,38] In patients with the infertility of unknown reason, LUF syndrome was found in 60% of cases.[39] A particularly high incidence was also reported in patients with chronic pelvic infection, being up to 52%.[40] Obvious differences in estimated frequency of this condition can be partly attributed to the heterogenicity of investigated patients, different criteria for the normal ovulatory cycle, and nonuniform timing of laparoscopy.

Ultrasound diagnosis of LUF syndrome is based on the daily observation of normal follicular development and the normal diameter of the preovulatory follicle. During the period of expected ovulation, the follicle remains the same size or slightly increases and maintains its tense appearance. Luteinization of the unruptured follicle is seen as progressive accumulation of strong echoes, predominantly located in the periphery of the cyst[41] (Figure 24).

Although ultrasound diagnosis of LUF syndrome is considered to be relatively simple and accurate, the comparison of sonographic and laparoscopic findings gives some other facts.

Negative ultrasonic findings of LUF correlated well with laparoscopy without false

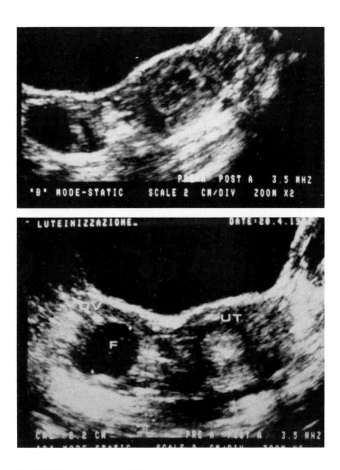

FIGURE 24.   A case of LUF syndrome. The upper part of the figure shows
an apparently normal preovulatory follicle that reached a mean size of 20
mm. In spite of that, ovulation failed to occur, and luteinization of the
unruptured follicle is seen as an accumulation of low-level echoes around
the periphery of the follicle.

negatives, but false positive findings of the disease were found in 17% of cases.[32] This
tendency of sonography to overestimate frequency of the LUF syndrome may be explained
by sonographic findings in normal ovulatory cycles. The ruptured follicle may be filled with
fluid within several hours after ovulation, without significant decrease in its diameter. It
may give the false impression of defective ovulation on repeated ultrasonic examination the
following day.[23] Diagnostic error may also occur in the presence of intraovarian cyst or
hydrosalpinx. Such structures can be misinterpreted as unruptured follicle, particularly if
examinations are started later in the follicular phase, on day 11 or 12.

ULTRASOUND MONITORING OF INDUCED OVULATION

The role of sonography in induced ovulation could be summarized as follows: detection
of the number of developing follicles, assessment of adequacy of follicular response and
detection of ovulation, assistance of human chorionic gonadotropin administration timing,
and detection of complications. The technique of ultrasound examinations is the same as in
the spontaneous cycles. It is equally important to repeat examinations every day starting
from the 9th of cycle, and all examinations should be performed by the same observer. The
follicle growth rate in the stimulated cycle is similar to the spontaneous cycle, and the
diameter of the dominant preovulatory follicle is insignificantly larger.[42,43] Detection of the

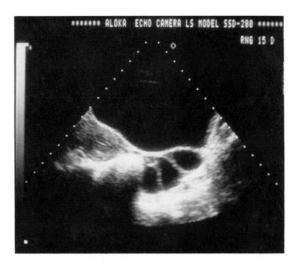

FIGURE 25.   Transverse sonogram performed on the 12th d of
the cycle in a patient receiving clomiphene stimulation. The right
ovary contains three follicles of almost the same size.

number of developing follicles helps in the interpretation of peripheral plasma estradiol levels
and may prevent the occurrence of multiple pregnancies when vast follicles are demonstrated.[44] However, there is a poor correlation between the peripheral estradiol levels and
the diameter of the dominant follicle in stimulated cycles.[45] It could be easily explained by
the presence of multiple follicles which contribute to overall estradiol production. Much
better results were obtained when either the number of follicles larger than 10 mm or the
total follicular volume were compared to the plasma estradiol.[46] An important limitation of
these correlations is the variable responsiveness of the follicles to stimulation in terms of
estrogen production capacity and distortion of follicular shape due to mutual follicle compression. In spite of described limitations, there is a common attitude that ultrasound is helpful
for interpreting estradiol concentrations. Peripheral estradiol levels may reflect either the
production of a single, large preovulatory follicle or of multiple immature follicles. By
sonographic visualization of the ovaries, that diagnostic problem is effectively solved (Figures
25 and 26). Furthermore, sonographic studies offer the advantage of easy orientation about
therapy success, particularly in cases with poor follicular development. A typical finding in
such cases is the demonstration of single or multiple follicles exhibiting a slow or irregular
growth pattern. Ultrasound can also provide data about the insufficient ovulation, regardless
of the successful initiation of follicular growth and maturity. In both clomiphene- and
menopausal gonadotropin (hMG)-stimulated cycles, the defective ovulation is characterized
by the presence of either luteinized or nonluteinized follicular cysts that fail to decrease in
size after spontaneous LH surge or hCG administration.[47,48] LUFs resemble the ultrasonic
appearance of LUF syndrome in spontaneous cycles, with the same diagnostic limitations
as extensively discussed before.

Human menopausal gonadotropin therapy requires the use of serial estradiol estimations
and sonographic examinations to estimate the optimal time of hCG administration. Optimal
estradiol concentrations are usually between 1000 and 1500 pg/ml. Although, there were
several reports of successful hCG timing when the dominant follicle reached 18 mm or more
in size, further experience indicated that follicle size alone cannot serve as a reliable parameter
of follicular maturity.[49,50]

It can be simply explained by the fact that the largest follicle does not always represent
the most mature one in terms of estrogen synthesis and oocyte maturity. Optimal timing of

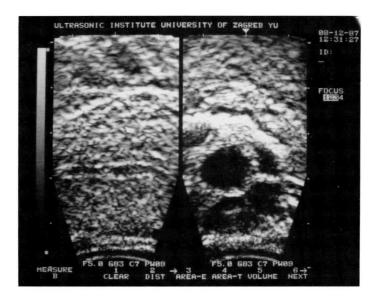

FIGURE 26.   Multiple follicles as seen on transvaginal scan on the 10th d of the cycle in a case of ovulation induction (right). The endometrium shows the characteristics of the late proliferative phase of the cycle (left).

hCG remains a particularly important part of ovulation induction, because either premature or late application can be atetrogenic and, therefore, actively inhibit ovulation.[51] Because of that, simultaneous biochemical and biologic assessments of follicle maturation are necessary for optimal result.

The most important complication of ovulation induction is hyperstimulation. It is characterized by multiple follicular growth and the development of luteal cysts after ovulation. Ovarian enlargement is always present in such cases and can be well documented by ultrasound (Figure 27). Sonographic measurement of ovarian size is quite superior to clinical estimations and enables better distinction between the patients who developed mild or moderate hyperstimulation.[52] However, mild to moderate hyperstimulation is regarded as acceptable sequelae of ovulation induction and does not cause significant complications, except increased probability of multiple pregnancy.

On the contrary, severe hyperstimulation represents a potentially life-threatening condition. It is characterized by marked ovarian enlargement (over 10 cm in diameter) and the presence of peritoneal and pleural effusions with symptoms of cardiovascular and renal failure. The development of severe ovarian hyperstimulation can be suspected in the patients who develop numerous small follicles of similar size as early as day 8 or 9 of the cycle. Clear evidence of continuous ovarian enlargement over the next few days indicates a high risk of ovarian hyperstimulation syndrome development.[53] If such a finding is accompanied by high estradol levels above 2000 pg/ml, hCG injection should be withheld to avoid full expression of symptoms (Figure 28).

In conclusion, ultrasound monitoring of follicular growth and ovulation has become an important method in the management of female infertility. Potential benefits of the use of sonography in the assessment of spontaneous and induced cycles have been well documented during the last several years. A new technical achievement, the transvaginal probe, will probably contribute to the further expansion of ultrasound diagnostics in this field. The use of the transvaginal probe alleviates the need for the full bladder technique and provides a high-resolution image of the ovaries. This makes examinations more simple and convenient than before. Moreover, ultrasound examination thus becomes a logical extension of clinical

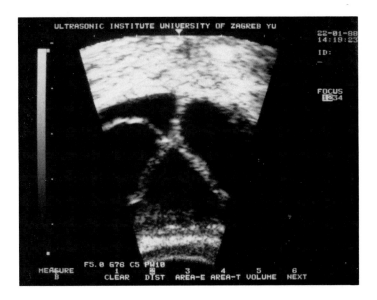

FIGURE 27. Moderate hyperstimulation as seen on transvaginal sonogram in a patient receiving human menopausal gonadotropin for ovulation induction. The ovary is enlarged and filled with several large follicles.

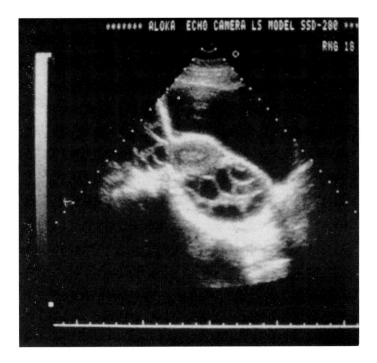

FIGURE 28. A case of severe hyperstimulation after ovulation induction with hMG. Both ovaries are very large in size as compared to the uterus and filled with numerous follicles of varying size.

examination, and this will undoubtedly result in a better understanding of ovarian physiology and the further refinement of therapeutic approaches.

ULTRASONICALLY GUIDED PUNCTURE OF OVARIAN FOLLICLES FOR *IN VITRO* FERTILIZATION

In comparison with other available imaging modalities such as radiography, computed tomography, or nuclear magnetic resonance, ultrasound has proven to be superior as a puncture guide. Punctures are performed by using small, hand-held transducers, and needle point position can be visualized continuously during the procedure. In experienced hands, ultrasonically guided punctures are so safe, accurate, and simple to perform that some authors strongly advocate that an ultrasonically guided biopsy should be considered as an integral part of ultrasound examination when additional information about the nature of the tumor is necessary.

Interest for interventional ultrasound in gynecology has dramatically increased since Lenz and Lauritsen[55] described the technique of ultrasonically guided transabdominal aspiration of human oocytes for an *in vitro* fertilization program. This technique is now accepted by the majority of authors as the alternative to laparoscopy for collecting oocytes from the ovaries in patients with tubal infertility. Together with the increased diagnostic capabilities of modern ultrasonic equipment, which allows clear visualization of normal and abnormal lesser pelvis anatomy, and recently developed technique of ultrasound monitoring of follicular growth and ovulation, ultrasonically guided follicular puncture helped to ascertain an important role of diagnostic ultrasound in the diagnosis and management of female infertility.

TECHNICAL REMARKS

Modern real-time ultrasonic equipment is an absolute prerequisite for successful oocyte collection. The machine should be equipped with either an electronic or, preferably, a mechanical sector probe. Probe frequency should be 2.5 to 4.0 MHz. The sector probe affords easy accessibility to the lateral pelvic walls, great maneuverability, and clear visualization of deep-lying structures in the female pelvis. Because of this, sector probes have numerous advantages over large linear array probes, which are not suitable for the successful performance of the procedure. Furthermore, with a sector probe it is easier to hit the needle with the incident beam nearer to 90°, where the needle reflects ultrasound better than if it is hit by the scanner pulses at a grazing angle.

The probe should be mounted with a needle steering device which enables oblique needle steering into the image plane. If a steering device is used, one can predict needle route upon a marker line on the screen as the needle is guided via the puncture channel directly into the follicle. This is very convenient when puncture is done by less experienced personnel.

Recently, specially designed high-frequency (5 to 10 Mhz) puncture vaginal probes became commercially available. These sector probes mounted with steering devices are characterized by a large field of view (240 to 270°) and an excellent visualization of pelvic organs.[56] A significant advantage of these probes is the shortening of the puncture route and the elimination of the full-bladder technique, which will be discussed later.

A 20- to 25-cm-long stainless steel needle with stylet should be used. There is no general agreement about the outer diameter of the needle which enables a high recovery rate and minimizes risk of complications. Most groups are using 1.2- to 1.6-mm-outer-diameter needles with virtually no difference in the rate of the successful aspirations and complications. The use of needles with outer diameters of 1.0 mm or less results in a decreased oocyte recovery rate and is not justifiable.[57,58]

Aspiration of follicular fluid can be performed either by means of simple plastic syringes with the appropriate fitting or by means of a collection set connected to a vacuum aspirator.

If plastic syringes are applied, it is important to obtain those especially designed for tissue culture. Syringe volume should be at least 10 ml to allow the complete aspiration of the largest follicles. Vacuum aspiration of oocytes doesn't offer any significant advantage over syringe aspiration and is relatively more complicated and more expensive. A vacuum aspirator which builds up and releases the suction pressure immediately is necessary. A collection set consists of flexible polyethylene connectors which connect the needle and aspirator with a collection tube or flask.

Punctures should be performed by clinicians who possess considerable skill and knowledge of the use of diagnostic ultrasound in gynecology. Besides an operator, two assistants, preferably nurses, are indispensable for the successful performance of the procedure. The number of trained assistants mostly depends on the organization of the whole *in vitro* fertilization program at the department.

A meticulous ultrasound examination should be made in the beginning of the treatment cycle, before ovarian stimulation therapy is started. This examination is of particular importance to define ovarian position, estimate feasibility of the puncture, and to recognize the eventual presence of intraovarian cysts which can alter patient response to stimulation or can be later misinterpreted for the growing follicles. Detection of intraovarian cysts is very important if diameter of the dominant follicle is used as the basic parameter for hCG application timing. It also helps to avoid puncture of the cysts during follicular puncture. All follicles should be aspirated first to prevent possible contamination of the needle or collecting system with cyst content.

Ultrasound monitoring of follicular growth usually starts on the 9th or 10th d of the menstrual cycle and doesn't depend on the stimulation regiment which is employed. In our own experience, ultrasound monitoring of follicular growth should be performed even in the cases when timing of the puncture is based mostly on hormonal parameter changes. Examinations are performed daily, preferably by the clinician who is supposed to make the puncture in that particular patient. There are two major reasons for such an approach. During several days, the operator becomes familiar with the lesser pelvis anatomy of the patient and is able to acquire a clear three-dimensional impression of ovarian position and the location of each particular follicle within it. He can also accurately define relations between the ovaries and other adjacent pelvic structures, like blood vessels, ureters, or fixed bowel loops, which helps in definitive selection of the most appropriate puncture route and avoidance of puncturing any of these structures, causing possible complications.

Most patients will tolerate puncture well if only slight sedation and analgesia are applied. Reported premedication is somewhat different between the various centers, but most authors claim that good results can be achieved by intravenous administration of 10 mg of diazepam and 100 mg of pethidin or 30 mg of pentazoizin just before the puncture. However, there are some patients who may experience intolerable pain during the puncture that can be obviated by doubling the dose. In 3 to 5% of cases general anesthesia is required.

TRANSABDOMINAL-TRANSVESICAL PUNCTURE ROUTE

This is the first and the most commonly used route for ultrasonically guided oocyte collection. Transabdominal ultrasonically guided puncture is a relatively simple procedure and can be easily performed in most cases. In comparison to other ultrasonically guided punctures of abdominal structures, the puncture conditions in gynecology are almost ideal. When the needle is placed into the fluid-filled bladder, it can be clearly seen, which enables easy orientation about its position and direction. Because of that, transabdominal follicle puncture can be performed in a slightly modified way, i.e., ultrasonically monitored or "free hand" puncture. This technique presumes that the needle steering device is not used and the probe and the needle can be moved independently, each held with the other hand (Figures 29 and 30).

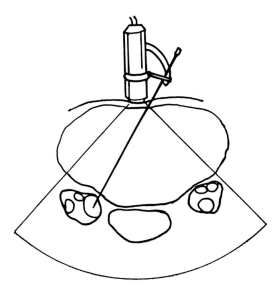

FIGURE 29. Schematic drawing illustrating transabdominal follicle puncture guided by ultrasound. The needle steering device is used, and the follicle is focused in the puncture line on the screen.

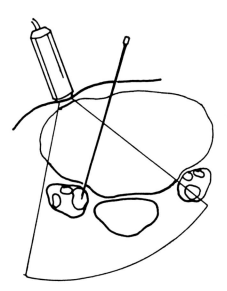

FIGURE 30. Scheme illustrating "free hand" follicle puncture. The follicle and needle are visualized simultaneously in the scanning plane.

However, this technique is more difficult to learn, and one should have a clear impression of the scanning plane at every moment during the puncture and also be able to move the probe and the needle simultaneously, so that the needle never leaves the scanning plane. In comparison to guided puncture, "free hand" puncture offers several important advantages. The operator can move the probe and the needle freely and is not limited by the steering device and a fixed puncture angle. This provides an optimal visualization of any follicle to be punctured and easy avoidance of other structures like thick adhesions or bowel loops.

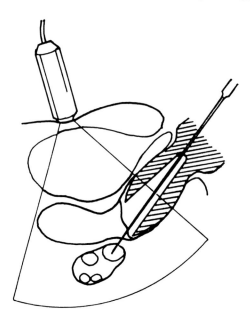

FIGURE 31.   Illustration of transvaginal follicle puncture. The probe is placed over the lower abdomen of the patient, and the needle and follicle are visualized in one scanning plane.

TRANSVAGINAL ROUTE

The transvaginal route is the second described technique for collecting oocytes for *in vitro* fertilization and is used mostly for the puncture of the ovaries which are lying retrouterine, deep in the pouch of Douglas.[59] In that case, it is not possible to reach the ovaries by the transabdominal approach.

The major advantage of this route is easy puncture of low retrouterine-located ovaries and is often combined with the transabdominal-transvesical route. However, as the needle is not passing through the fluid-filled bladder, the visualization of the needle, as well as the needle direction, are much more difficult. If the ovaries are placed more than 2 cm from the vaginal fornices, this route should not be employed (Figure 31).

In such conditions, the puncture is painful, and as the needle is passing through a poorly visualized and highly vascularized area, the probability of complications is much higher. Some authors have suggested the use of the transvaginal-transvesical route in such cases. The needle is introduced through the anterior vaginal fornix into the bladder, and then through the posterior bladder wall into the follicle. It is not clear whether such an approach offers any advantage over transabdominal puncture, and experience with this technqiue is very limited.

Recently, the introduction of a specially designed vaginal puncture probe has opened new possibilities to increase the efficiency of ultrasonically guided oocyte collection. The high-frequency sector probe with mounted steering device is introduced into the vagina. Contact with vaginal wall is provided by an antiseptic gel. Extensible vaginal walls enable placement of the probe close to the ovary, and the follicle is focused in a guide line on the screen. This provides for maximal shortening of the puncture route and easy and accurate placement of the needle point into the follicle[60,61] (Figure 32).

Important advantages of this technique are the elimination of bladder filling and the superior visualization of the pelvic anatomy, which also contributes to the accuracy and safety of the puncture. Although experience with the vaginal probe is still limited, its use is in considerable expansion and will probably be the premier method for ultrasonically

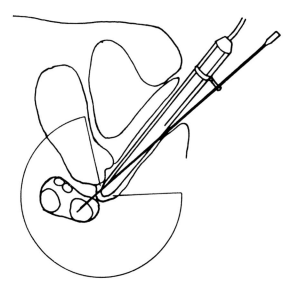

FIGURE 32.   Schematic drawing of follicle puncture by using a transvaginal probe. The probe is mounted with the steering device that facilitates accurate needle guidance.

controlled follicle puncture in the future. Increasing experience will help to elucidate some still controversal points, like the possibility of puncturing extremely high ovaries and the incidence of complications.

TRANSURETHRAL ROUTE

The perurethral route for oocyte aspiration was first described by Parson et al.[61] in 1985. The patient with full urinary bladder is also placed in lithotomy position. The needle is introduced through the urethra into the bladder, and sterilization of the abdominal wall or the probe is unnecessary.

The transurethral approach is well suited for puncture of relatively high ovaries and is the best method for puncturing the ovaries which are located above the top of the full bladder. Another advantage is that there are no skin wounds. However, there is always the possibility of urethral injury during the needle introduction (Figure 33). Moreover, there are no data about whether stretching of the urethra during angulation of the needle towards the lateral pelvic wall can cause long-term consequences on the urethral sphincter competence. Another disadvantage, as indicated in Parsons' original report, is the transient dysuria which occurs regularly after perurethral puncture.

COMPLICATIONS

In approximately 50% of patients after transabdominal-transvesical follicle puncture, small blood clots can be found in the urine after bladder catherization. This small amount of blood usually originates from superficial skin vessels. It is found in the urine because of leakage of blood through the needle route and is more commonly seen in patients who have undergone previous surgery. Blood leakage is seen during the puncture as a stream of echogenic particles which are falling down from the anterior bladder wall. Although it can give the impression of severe bleeding, it is without any significance in most cases. As reported by Lenz,[55] moderate hematuria can be expected in approximately 5% of cases and spontaneously resolves within 24 h.

In a recent report, Feichtinger and Kemeter[56] have analyzed the occurrence of complications after 371 transabdominal-transvesical follicular punctures, and have found 14 patients

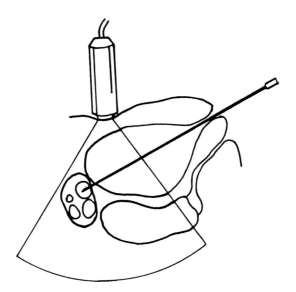

FIGURE 33.   Illustration of transurethral route for oocyte aspiration. Note that the angle between the needle and the ultrasound probe is nearly 90°.

with moderate hematuria lasting no more than 1 d, which is similar to Lenz's report. Furthermore, they describe seven cases of bowel puncture and two cases of iliac vein puncture which were mistakenly punctured for a follicle, but without any complications. In two cases, patients developed cystitis after the puncture, and in three cases, patients complained of severe pain which could not be explained by any pathological finding.

Experience with tranvaginal puncture using a high-frequency probe suggests that this technique for oocyte collection also carries minimal risk to the patient. In a study group that included 50 patients, no severe complications were observed. In 6% of patients, slight vaginal bleeding developed after the procedure which was easily stopped by applying moderate pressure to the puncture site. It is very important that there were no signs of bacterial contamination in the culture media.[65]

Reported experience with other puncture routes is still too limited to estimate the true risk of complications. However, there is common a impression that, if properly done, ultrasonically directed follicle puncture can be considered a low-risk procedure. but further comparative trials are required to confirm it.

During the past couple of years, since ultrasonically guided follicular puncture has been introduced into routine clinical practice, there is still present controversy about the most efficient way of collecting oocytes for *in vitro* fertilization. As the first successful *in vitro* fertilization programs were established by using the laparoscopic technique of collecting oocytes, this was adopted by many centers and proven a good and reliable method for the purpose. Initially reported experience with ultrasonically guided puncture demonstrated less successful results as compared to laparoscopy in terms of oocyte recovery rate and number of clinical pregnancies. However, with increased experience, subsequent reports show that there is no significant difference in the overall success rate between various centers, regardless of the technique of oocyte collection. A prospective comparison between laparoscopic and ultrasound groups in the same center, as reported by Lewin et al.,[63] confirmed these results.

In conclusion, ultrasound is proven to be as effective as laparoscopy for oocyte collection at present, and oocyte collection technique has no major influence on the final result of the procedure, i.e., clinical pregnancy rate. At this point, ultrasonically directed puncture offers some advantages over laparoscopy, which is making ultrasound puncture more and more popular.

By performing ultrasonically guided puncture, it is possible to organize the *in vitro* fertilization program as a complete outpatient procedure. This approach significantly reduces costs and is more acceptable for the patients. The technique of ultrasonically guided puncture is relatively simple and less invasive as compared to laparoscopy. Only slight sedation and analgesia are required, and there is rarely a need for general anesthesia. Besides, it can be easily repeated if successful fertilization doesn't occur.

REFERENCES

1. **Kratochwil, A., Urban, G., and Friedrich, G.,** Ultrasonic tomography of the ovary, *Ann. Chir. Gynaecol. Fenn.,* 61, 211, 1972.
2. **Athey, P. A.,** Uterus: abnormalities of size, shape contour and texture, in *Ultrasound in Obstetrics and Gynecology,* Athey, P. A. and Hadlock, F. P., Eds., C. V. Mosby, St. Louis, 1985, 167.
3. **Kurjak, A. and Jurkovic, D.,** The value of ultrasound in the initial assessment of gynecological patients, *Ultrasound Med. Biol.,* 13, 401, 1987.
4. **Gross, B. H. and Callen, P. W.,** Ultrasound of the uterus, in *Ultrasonography in Obstetrics and Gynecology,* Callen, P. W., Ed., W. B. Saunders, Philadelphia, 1983, 243.
5. **Green, B.,** Pelvic ultrasonography, in *Diagnostic Ultrasound,* Sarti, D. A. and Sample, W. F., Eds., Hall, Boston, 1980, 502.
6. **Swayne, L. C., Love, M. B., and Karasick, S. R.,** Pelvic infammatory disease: sonographic-pathologic correlation, *Radiology,* 151, 751, 1984.
7. **Spirtos, H. J., Bernstine, R. L., and Crawford, W. L.,** Sonography in acute pelvic inflamatory disease, *J. Reprod. Med.,* 27, 312, 1982.
8. **Swanson, M., Sauerbrei, E. E., and Coopberg, P. L.,** Medical implications of ultrasonically detected polycystic ovaries, *J. Clin. Ultrasound,* 9, 219, 1981.
9. **Friedman, H., Vogelzang, R. L., Mendelson, E. B., Nieman, H. L., and Cohen, M.,** Endometriosis detection by US with laparoscopic correlation, *Radiology,* 157, 217, 1985.
10. **Hackeloer, B. J., Nitschke-Debelstein, S., Daume, E., Sturm, G., and Bucholz, R.,** Ultraschalldarstellung von ovarderaenderungen bei gonadotropin stimulierung, *Geburtshilfe Frauenheilkd.,* 37, 185, 1977.
11. **Fleischer, A. C., Darnell, J., Rodier, J., Lindsay, A., and James, A. E.,** Sonographic monitoring of ovarian follicular development, *J. Clin. Ultrasound,* 9, 275, 1981.
12. **O'Herlihy, C., de Crespigny, L., and Robinson, H. P.,** Monitoring ovarian follicular development with real-time ultrasound, *Br. J. Obstet. Gynecol.,* 87, 613, 1980.
13. **Feichtinger, W. and Kemeter, P.,** Transvaginal sector scan sonography for needle guided transvaginal follicle aspiration and other applications in gynecologic routine and research, *Fertil. Steril.,* 45, 722, 1985.
14. **O'Herlihy, C., de Crespigny, L., Lopata, A., Johnston, I., Hoult, I., and Robinson, H.,** Preovulatory follicular size: a comparison of ultrasound and laparoscopic measurements, *Fertil. Steril.,* 34, 24, 1980.
15. **Funduk-Kurjak, B. and Kurjak, A.,** Ultrasound monitoring of follicular maturation and ovulation in normal menstrual cycles and ovulation induction, *Acta Obstet. Gynecol. Scand.,* 61, 329, 1982.
16. **Ritchie, W. G. M.,** Ultrasound in the evaluation of normal and induced ovulation, *Fertil. Steril.,* 43, 167, 1985.
17. **Baird, D. T. and Fraser, I. S.,** Blood production and ovarian secretion rate of estradiol and estrone in women throughout the menstrual cycle, *J. Clin. Endocrinol. Metab.,* 38, 1009, 1974.
18. **Hackeloer, B. J., Fleming, R., Robinson, H. P., Adam, A. H., and Coutts, J. R. T.,** Correlation of ultrasonic and endocrinologic parameters of human follicular development, *Am. J. Obstet. Gynecol.,* 135, 122, 1979.
19. **Buttery, B., Trounson, A., McMaster, R., and Wood, C.,** Evaluation of diagnostic ultrasound as a parameter of follicular development in an in vitro fertilization program, *Fertil. Steril.,* 39, 458, 1983.
20. **Bomsel-Helmreich, O., Bessis, R., Vu, N., and Huyen, L.,** Cumulus oophorus of the preovulatory follicle assessed by ultrasound and histology, in *Ultrasound and Infertility,* Christie, A. D., Ed., Chartwel-Bratt, Bromley, 1981, 105.
21. **Kerin, J. F., Edmonds, D. K., Warnes, G. M., Cox, L. W., Seamark, R. F., Matthews, C. D., Young, G. B., and Baird, D. T.,** Morphological and functional relationships of graafian follicle growth to ovulation in women using ultrasonic, laparoscopic and biochemical measurements, *Br. J. Obstet. Gynecol.,* 88, 81, 1981.
22. **Picker, R. H., Smith, D. H., Tucker, M. H., and Saunders, D. M.,** Ultrasonic signs of imminent ovulation, *J. Clin. Ultrasound,* 11, 1, 1983.

23. **De Crespigny, L., O'Herlihy, C., and Robinson, H. P.,** Ultrasonic observation of the mechanism of human ovulation, *Am. J. Obstet. Gynecol.,* 139, 177, 1981.

24. **Hackeloer, B. J.,** The role of ultrasound in female infertility management, *Ultrasound Med. Biol.,* 10, 35, 1984.

25. **Sakamoto, C. and Nakano, H.,** The echogenic endometrium and alterations during the menstrual cycle, *Int. J. Gynecol. Obstet.,* 20, 255, 1982.

26. **Sakamoto, C.,** Sonographic criteria of phasic changes in human endometrial tissue, *Int. J. Gynecol. Obstet.,* 23, 7, 1985.

27. **Fleischer, A. C., Kalameris, C. C., and Entman, S. S.,** Sonographic depiction of the endometrium during normal cycles, in *Proc. 4th Meet. World Fed. for Ultrasound in Medicine and Biology,* Gill, R. W. and Dadd, M. J., Eds., Pergamon Press, Sydney, 1985, 281.

28. **Christie, A. D., Ed.,** *Ultrasound and Infertility,* Chartwel-Bratt, Bromley, 1981, 24.

29. **Polan, M. L., Totora, M., Caldwell, B. V., deCherney, A. H., Haseltine, F. P., and Kase, N.,** Abnormal ovarian cycles as diagnosed by ultrasound and serum estradiol levels, *Fertil. Steril.,* 37, 342, 1982.

30. **Coutts, J. R. T., Adam, A. H., and Fleming, R.,** Ovarian ultrasound and endocrine profiles in women with unexplained infertility, in *Ultrasound and Infertility,* Christie, A. D., Ed., Chartwel-Bratt, Bromley, 1981, 89.

31. **Jewelewicz, R.,** Management of infertility resulting from anovulation, *Am. J. Obstet. Gynecol.,* 122, 309, 1975.

32. **Liukkonen, S., Koskimies, A. I., Tenhunen, A., and Ylostalo, P.,** Luteinized unruptured follicle (LUF) syndrome, *J. Fr. Echogr.,* 3, 285, 1986.

33. **Bomsel-Helmreich, O. and Huyen, L. V. N.,** Delayed ovulation without inhibition of LH surge in the rabbit: a model of atresia of the preovulatory follicle, in *Follicular Maturation and Ovulation,* Rolland, R., van Hall, E. V., Hillier, S. G., McNatty, K. P., and Schoemaker, J., Eds., Excerpta Medica, Amsterdam, 1982, 295.

34. **Schenken, R. S., Werlin, L. B., Williams, R. F., Prihoda, T. J., and Hodgen, G. D.,** Histologic and hormonal documentation of the luteinized unruptured follicle syndrome, *Am. J. Obstet. Gynecol.,* 154, 839, 1986.

35. **Kerin, J. F., Kriby, C., Morris, D., McEvoy, M., Ward, B., and Cox, L. W.,** Incidence of luteinized unruptured follicle phenomenon in cycling women, *Fertil. Steril.,* 40, 620, 1983.

36. **Varnell, J. A., Balsch, J., Fuster, J. S., and Fuster, R.,** Ovulation in fertile women, *Fertil. Steril.,* 37, 712, 1982.

37. **Thomas, E. J., Lenton, E. A., and Cooke, I. D.,** Follicle growth patterns and endocrinological abnormalities in infertile women with minor degrees of endometroisis, *Br. J. Obstet. Gynecol.,* 93, 852, 1986.

38. **Brosens, I. A., Koninckx, P. R., and Corvelyn, P. A.,** A study of plasma progesterone, estradiol, prolactin and LH levels and luteal appearance of the ovaries in patients with endometriosis and infertility, *Br. J. Obstet. Gynecol.,* 85, 246, 1978.

39. **Koninckx, P. R., Heyens, W. J., Corvelyn, P. A., and Brosens, I. A.,** Delayed onset of luteinization as a cause of infertility, *Fertil. Steril.,* 29, 266, 1978.

40. **Hamilton, C. J. C. M., Evers, J. L. H., and Hoogland, H. J.,** Ovulatory disorders and inflammatory adnexal damage: a neglected cause of the failure of fertility microsurgery, *Br. J. Obstet. Gynecol.,* 93, 282, 1986.

41. **Coulam, C. B., Hill, L. M., and Breckle, R.,** Ultrasonic evidence for luteinization of unruptured preovulatory follicle, *Fertil. Steril.,* 37, 524, 1982.

42. **O'Herlihy, C., Pepperell, R. J., and Robinson, H. P.,** Ultrasound timing of human chorionic gonadotropin administration in clomiphene stimulated cycles, *Obstet. Gynecol.,* 59, 40, 1982.

43. **Marrs, R. P., Vargyas, J. M., and March, C. M.,** Ultrasonic and endocrinologic measurements in hMG therapy, *Am. J. Obstet. Gynecol.,* 145, 417, 1983.

44. **Muse, K. and Wilson, E. A.,** Monitoring ovulation induction: use of biochemical and biophysical parameters, *Semin. Reprod. Endocrinol.,* 4, 301, 1986.

45. **Haning, R. V., Austin, C. W., Kuzma, D. L., Shapiro, S. S., and Zweibel, W. J.,** Ultrasound evaluation of estrogen monitoring for induction of ovulation with menotropins, *Fertil. Steril.,* 37, 627, 1982.

46. **Mantzavinos, T., Garcia, J. E., and Jones, H. W.,** Ultrasound measurement of ovarian follicles stimulated by human gonadotropins for oocyte recovery and in vitro fertilization, *Fertil. Steril.,* 40, 461, 1983.

47. **Coulam, C. B., Hill, L. M., and Breckle, R.,** Ultrasonic assessment of subsequent unexplained infertility after ovulation induction, *Br. J. Obstet. Gynecol.,* 90, 460, 1983.

48. **Stanger, J. D. and Yovich, J. L.,** Failure of human oocyte release at ovulation, *Fertil. Steril.,* 41, 827, 1984.

49. **Sundstroem, P., Persson, P. H., Liedholm, P., and Wramsby, H.,** The ability of ultrasound to determine the time for harvesting preovulatory oocytes, *Acta Obstet. Gynecol. Scand.,* 62, 219, 1983.

50. **Messinis, I. E. and Templeton, A.,** Urinary estrogen levels and follicle ultrasound measurements in clomiphene induced cycles with an endogeneous luteinizing hormone surge, *Br. J. Obstet. Gynecol.,* 93, 43, 1986.
51. **Williams, R. F. and Hodgen, G. D.,** Disparate effects of human chorionic gonadotropin during the late follicular phase in monkeys: normal ovulation, follicular atresia, ovarian acyclicity and hypersecretion of follicle-stimulating hormone, *Fertil. Steril.,* 33, 64, 1980.
52. **McArdle, C., Siebel, M., Hann, L., Weinstein, F., and Taymor, M.,** The diagnosis of ovarian hyperstimulation (OHS): the impact of ultrasound, *Fertil. Steril.,* 39, 464, 1983.
53. **Rankin, R. N. and Hutton, L. C.,** Ultrasound in the ovarian hyperstimulation syndrome, *J. Clin. Ultrasound,* 9, 473, 1981.
54. **Holm, H. H.,** Interventional ultrasound, in *Recent Advances in Ultrasound Diagnosis,* Vol. 5, Kurjak, A. and Kossoff, G., Eds., Excerpta Medica, Amsterdam, 1986, 1.
55. **Lenz, S., Lauritsen, J. G., and Kjellow, M.,** Collection of human oocytes for *in vitro* fertilization by ultrasonically guided follicular puncture, *Lancet,* 1, 1163, 1981.
56. **Feichtinger, W. and Kemeter, P.,** Ultrasound-guided aspiration of human ovarian follicles for *in vitro* fertilization, in *Ultrasound Annual,* Sanders, R. C. and Hill, M., Eds., Raven Press, New York, 1986, 25.
57. **Renou, P., Trounson, A. O., Wood, C., and Leeton, J. F.,** The collection of human oocytes for *in vitro* fertilization. I. An instrument for maximizing oocyte recovery rate, *Fertil. Steril.,* 35, 409, 1981.
58. **Lauritsen, J. G., Lindberg, S., and Lenz, S.,** Instruments for human *in vitro* fertilization and embryo transfer, *Dan. Med. Bull.,* 30, 176, 1983.
59. **Dellenbach, P., Nisand, I., Moreau, L., Feger, B., Plumere, C., and Gerlinger, P.,** Transvaginal sonographically controlled follicle puncture for oocyte retrieval, *Fertil. Steril.,* 44, 656, 1985.
60. **Wikland, M., Enk, L., Hammarberg, K., and Nilsson, L.,** Use of vaginal transducer for oocyte retrieval in an IVF/ET program, *J. Clin. Ultrasound,* 15, 245, 1987.
61. **Parson, J., Booker, M., Goswamy, R., Akkermans, J., Riddle, A., Sharma, V., Wilson, L., Whitehead, M., and Campbell, S.,** Oocyte retrieval for *in vitro* fertilization by ultrasonically guided needle aspiration via the urethra, *Lancet,* 1, 1076, 1985.
62. **Lenz, S.,** Ultrasonic-guided follicle puncture under local anesthesia, *J. In Vitro Fertil. Embryo Transfer,* 1, 239, 1984.
63. **Lewin, A., Margalioth, E. J., Rabinovitz, R., and Schenker, J.,** Comparative study of ultrasonically guided percutaneous aspiration with local anesthesia and laparoscopic aspiration of follicles in an in vitro fertilization program, *Am. J. Obstet. Gynecol.,* 151, 621, 1985.

Chapter 12

THE ROLE OF ULTRASONOGRAPHY IN *IN VITRO* FERTILIZATION

Aby Lewin, Efraim Zohav, and Joseph G. Schenker

INTRODUCTION

A decade after the first announcement of a successful human pregnancy and birth after *in vitro* fertilization (IVF) by Steptoe and Edwards,[1] a major change in the role of ultrasonography (U/S) in IVF treatments can be marked. The use of U/S for the evaluation of infertility and the imaging of uterus and ovaries was documented for the first time in 1972 by Kratochwil et al.[2] At first, U/S imaging was limited to the diagnosis of follicular development in regular menstruating women attending oocyte retrieval by laparoscopy. This early stage was followed by the introduction in the IVF programs of induction of superovulation with the use of clomiphene citrate (CC), menopausal gonadotropins (hMG), pure follicle-stimulating hormone (hFSH), and gonadotropin-releasing hormone (GnRH) agonists. At this stage, U/S imaging was used as a main tool in the induction of controlled ovarian hyperstimulation. This was achieved by careful monitoring of the ovarian response to exogenous stimulation, enabling the individualization of treatment with the aim of maximal development of morphologically and functionally adequate follicles, timed administration of human chorionic gonadotropin (hCG), and the recovery of multiple mature oocytes. The third stage in the role of U/S in IVF followed the development of the new generation of high-resolution real-time scanners, with abdominal and vaginal transducers, and the introduction of U/S-guided oocyte recovery. This, together with the use of U/S imaging to facilitate the replacement of embryos and for early diagnosis of pregnancy and the complications of IVF, such as hyperstimulation syndrome, ectopic pregnancies, and multiple pregnancies with the possibility of their reduction, established the primary importance of U/S in present IVF.

LOCALIZATION OF THE OVARIES

Pelvic U/S may be performed with the use of either sector or linear scanners, although sector scanners are believed by some to be superior to linear array scanners, especially for the imaging of specific details within laterally positioned organs like the ovaries.[3]

Hackeloer et al.[4,5] described the technique employed for identifying the ovaries and measuring the follicles. A full bladder is the most important prerequisite for good visualization of the uterus and the ovaries when using an abdominal scanner. The uterus is the first pelvic organ which has to be identified as a reference point for the localization of the ovaries and for the exclusion of any abnormality that may prevent the continuation of treatment. Scanning is then performed to the sides of the uterus until the ovaries are demonstrated. The ovaries are localized medially to the side walls of the pelvis, in front of iliac vessels (Figure 1). Nevertheless, as a result of the variability in uterine position and the relative freedom of ovaries in the normal pelvis, the ovaries may be found in various locations within the pelvis and low abdomen during the same menstrual cycle. In the presence of pelvic adhesions, the ovaries may be abnormally located within the pelvis or behind the uterus, making their identification more difficult. These may be identified by their peculiar feature of cystic forms within a solid body. Other reasons for difficult imaging are the presence of abdominal scars and obesity. The recent introduction of the transvaginal (TV) transducer is especially indicated for the examination of these patients.[6] This approach avoids the need for a full

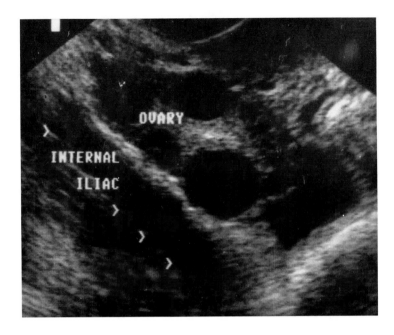

FIGURE 1.   The ovary located medially to the side wall of the pelvis, in front of the iliac vessels.

bladder, as the ovaries may be imaged directly through the vaginal vault, the distance between the transducer and the ovaries being very small. The high-frequency transducers used in vaginal U/S allow the identification of intraovarian structures as small as 2 to 3 mm. More details of this approach will be described when the technique of TV U/S-guided oocyte recovery will be described.

SPONTANEOUS CYCLES

The U/S visualization of the developing Graafian follicle throughout the normal cycle had been reported by several authors.[7-9] In the normal cycle, a cohort of hundreds of primordial follicles awakes under a hormonal stimulus and starts the way for ovulation throughout the process of recruitment, selection, and dominance.[10-12] Usually only one follicle overcomes the natural barrier of selection and becomes the dominant follicle, destined to ovulate (Figure 2). In only 5 to 10% of the cycles do two or more leading follicles develop. In over 80% of the cycles with a single leading follicle, a second subordinated group of follicles with limited development can be observed.[3,13] Smith et al.[8] observed the appearance and disappearance of small follicles over a period of a few days during the menstrual cycle, especially during anovulatory cycles (spontaneous as well as induced).

The intraovarian morphological changes during follicular development in the normal ovulatory cycles were described by Hackeloer et al.[14,15] and Renaud et al.[16] The daily rate of growth of the leading follicle diameter is linear and at the mean rate of 1 to 4 mm/d[7,17,18] during the last 5 d before luteinizing hormone (LH) surge. Nevertheless, the U/S measurement of the follicular diameter is of limited value as a predictor of the time of ovulation,[18-20] as the mean follicular diameter before ovulation ranges from 15 to 28 mm.[14-16]

The significance of the intrafollicular echos was also investigated. These echos represent the dissociation of the cumulus shortly before ovulation (Figure 3) and appear in more than 20% of the leading follicles >18 mm in diameter.[13] The demonstration of the echogenic

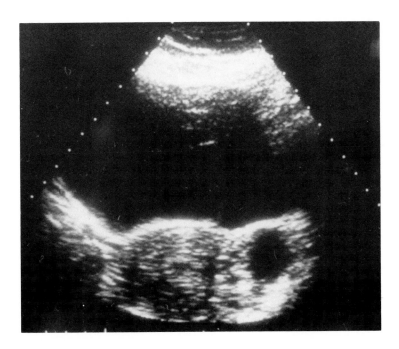

FIGURE 2. A dominant ovarian follicle, day 13 of a spontaneous cycle.

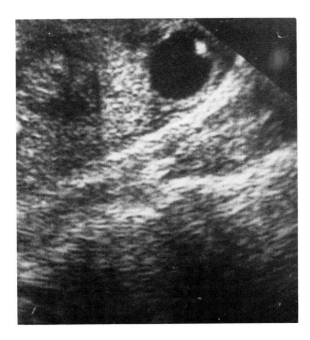

FIGURE 3. Intrafollicular echo, day 15 of a spontaneous cycle.

sign of the cumulus oophorus within a cystic formation in the ovary confirms the follicular nature of this cystic formation and may predict ovulation within 36 h.[21] Bomsel-Helmreich et al.[22] also demonstrated a correlation between the histological pattern of the cumulus and the U/S visualization of its echos within the leading follicle before ovulation. A linear correlation was also found between the growth rate of the dominant follicle and the rising serum levels of 17-β estradiol (E2).[5,8,23]

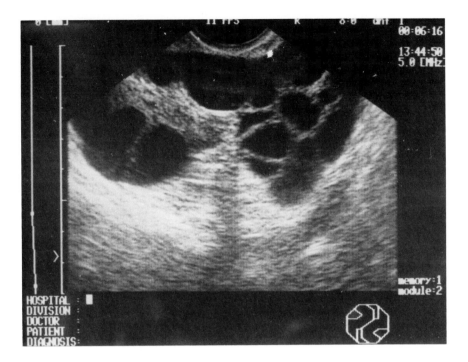

FIGURE 4.   Multiple follicular growth in hMG-induced cycle for IVF.

Although the first IVF pregnancies were achieved in spontaneous ovulatory cycles,[1,24] there are many disadvantages in unstimulated cycles. Frequent blood or urine sampling for the detection of LH surge, the need to perform oocyte pick-ups (OPU) out of regular working hours, and the low oocyte recovery rate and pregnancy rates[25,26] have made the IVF in spontaneous cycles an inefficient procedure and, therefore, was abandoned in favor of the use of induced cycles. Nevertheless, spontaneous cycles still have a role in the replacement of frozen/thawed embryos.[27]

INDUCED CYCLES

The successful use of stimulated cycles for IVF was first reported by Lopata et al.,[28] and thereafter, the use of controlled ovarian stimulation became the routine practice in IVF treatment. Various ovulation-inducing agents are used either alone or in combination, including CC, hMG, hFSH, and GnRH agonists.[29-32] The exogenous menopausal gonadotropins therapy is started as early as the 2nd or 3rd d of the menstrual cycle[33,34] in order to overcome the natural inhibition barrier of selection and dominance and to recruit a maximal number of follicles (Figure 4), allowing the recovery of more preovulatory oocytes, the replacement of a higher number of embryos, and the achievement of a higher pregnancy rate.[35-37] The positive correlation between the number of embryos replaced and the subsequent pregnancy rate has been reported by several authors.[35-39] Another aim of this therapy is to achieve synchronization of follicular maturity and, as a result, oocyte maturity.[39] The more synchronized the follicles are, the greater the ability to determine the accurate timing for hCG administration and, as a result, the achievement of a higher number of mature oocytes.

Assessment of the ovarian response during induction of ovulation for IVF includes a baseline U/S examination to exclude ovarian and pelvic pathology which may prevent or change the ovarian stimulation protocol, followed by serial U/S examinations and E2 assays. The goal of this monitoring is to achieve the stimulation of multiple follicles and adequately high E2 levels before hCG is administered, as serum E2 levels were shown to correlate with the pregnancy rate.[38,39] The ovarian response was also classified by the pattern of a rise in serum E2 levels around the time of hCG administration.[39] These authors showed that a rising pattern of E2 levels was associated with a higher pregnancy rate, while a decreasing pattern was associated with a low pregnancy rate. Yet, elevated serum levels of E2 may be found not only in the presence of large follicles, but also in the presence of many small follicles. This is especially true in stimulated cycles where there is no correlation between the size of the largest follicles and E2 levels, as there are usually multiple small follicles that are contributing to the peripheral E2 levels.[40] Therefore, titration of the induction drugs and the decision on the accurate timing of hCG administration cannot be based on the pattern or E2 levels only, nor can it be based on the follicular size only, but a combination of both parameters should be taken into account.

Although the pattern of individual follicular growth in each infertility subgroup, i.e., mechanical, unexplained, etc., is similar to that in the spontaneous cycle,[3,23] induction of ovulation usually results in multiple follicular growth. The number of follicles developing in any cycle reflect the dosage used, although fewer follicles usually develop with CC as compared to hMG therapy. In 80% of the cycles stimulated with hMG, there is multiple follicular growth, while only 35 to 60% of the CC cycles present multifollicular growth. Furthermore, not only the frequency of multifollicular cycles is higher with hMG therapy, but also the number of follicles.[3] The largest follicular diameter prior to ovulation ranges in CC cycles from 19 to 25 mm[8,41] and in hMG cycles from 16 to 30 mm.[42-44]

The anovulatory patients treated with IVF can be subclassified into patients with hypothalamic-pituitary failure, group I of the WHO classification, and patients with feedback disorders, group II of the WHO classification. The ovarian response to hMG stimulation is completely different in these two groups. In group I, the ovaries respond to exogenous hMG with the recruitment of a large cohort of synchronized follicles. The growth pattern of these follicles correlates in a linear fashion with the serum E2 pattern.[40] In group II patients, the exogenous hMG stimulation meets the ovarian follicles exposed to continuous stimulation of endogenous gonadotropins at various developmental stages, the stimulation thus resulting in the development of an asynchronous cohort of follicles with various levels of steroidogenic secretion. As a result, there is a dissociation between the number and size of the leading follicles and serum E2 levels,[40] and at OPU, the aspiration of follicles with a diameter ranging from 4 to 30 mm results in the recovery of an unpredictable number premature oocytes.[39] Furthermore, the largest follicles may not necessarily be those which contain the mature oocytes.[45] Rather, the follicles that contain higher concentrations of E2 tend to give rise to mature oocytes.[39]

The introduction of GnRH agonists for the induction of pituitary desensitization, as pretreatment before hMG or hFSH stimulation, was intended to achieve a "medical hypophysectomy", and thus induce artificially similar pituitary and ovarian conditions as in group I of the WHO classification. In this way, the exogeneous gonadotropins are expected to induce the development of a synchronous cohort of follicles with mature oocytes (Figure 5), while pituitary suppression prevents premature rise of LH and premature luteinization and ovulation before OPU takes place.[10,46-48] This points out a major improvement in IVF treatment, as up to 40% of the induced cycles may result in cancellation of the cycle due to either insufficient ovarian response or premature luteinization.[49,50]

In cycles where OPU was performed after premature luteinization, a reduced fertilization rate of the oocytes was reported.[39,51]

The premature progesterone (P) secretion may also affect the endometrium, resulting in asynchrony with the timing of embryo transfer.[52] The use of GnRH agonists combined with hMG or hFSH, either sequentially (after ovarian suppression) or concomitantly (the flare-up modality), resulted in an increase in the number of follicles, oocytes, and embryos, and in an increase in pregnancy rates.[53-58]

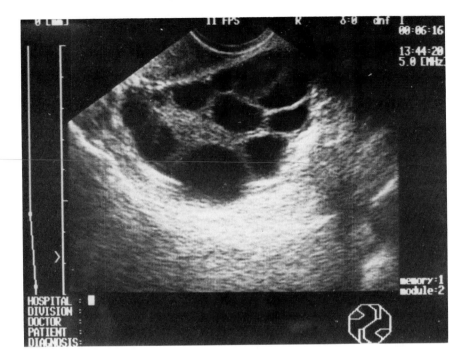

FIGURE 5.   Synchronous cohort of follicles in GnRH agonist/hFSH-induced cycle for IVF.

FOLLICULAR RECRUITMENT PROTOCOL FOR IVF

In our program, a depot preparation of GnRH agonist (Decapeptyl) is used concomitantly with hFSH or hMG in a flare-up modality (Figure 6). The agonist is administered intramuscularly on the 2nd d of the cycle, and hFSH or hMG are administered at a dose of three ampules per day from the 4th d of the cycle for 5 d and continued at an individual dosage according to the ovarian response. The use of GnRH agonists in this modality is aimed to augment the ovarian stimulation at the early follicular phase and prevent premature endogenous LH surge at the late follicular phase. As a result, the frequency of cancellations because of premature luteinization decreased from 29 to 0%.[57]

The first U/S scanning is usually performed at the beginning of menstruation to rule out the presence of ovarian cysts before ovarian stimulation is started. On the 9th d of the cycle, after 5 d of gonadotropins treatment, daily U/S measurements of follicular number and size are resumed, together with daily serum E2 assays. When follicular development is advanced, daily serum P assays are started for the detection of premature luteinization. A continuous growth pattern of the follicles, together with a continuous rise in E2 levels, without a rise in P levels is considered to be the ideal set-up for ovarian response.

OVULATION

The evaluation of the U/S features of spontaneous ovulation is of major importance in IVF. When signs of ovulation are demonstrated before OPU takes place, the procedure is usually cancelled, as the chances of collecting oocytes from the fluid in the cul-de-sac are low. Therefore, careful daily monitoring of follicular growth and E2 and P levels is usually performed, and the timing of ovulation is controlled by hCG administration. In our program, the decision on hCG administration is based on the number and size of follicles and the level of E2. When the leading follicle reaches 17 mm in diameter or at least two follicles

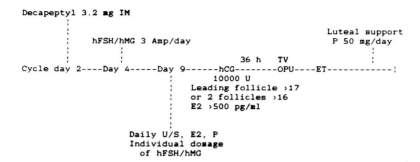

```
Decapeptyl 3.2 mg IM
                :
                :                                              Luteal support
                :          hFSH/hMG 3 Amp/day                  P 50 mg/day
                :                                              :
                :                             36 h    TV       :
Cycle day 2----Day 4-----Day 9------hCG--------OPU----ET-----------:
                :                    10000 U
                :                    Leading follicle >17
                :                    or 2 follicles >16
                :                    E2 >500 pg/ml
                :
        Daily U/S, E2, P
        Individual dosage
        of hFSH/hMG
```

FIGURE 6. Protocol for induction of superovulation for IVF with depot GnRH agonist (Decapeptyl) and hFSH/hMG. The flare-up modality.

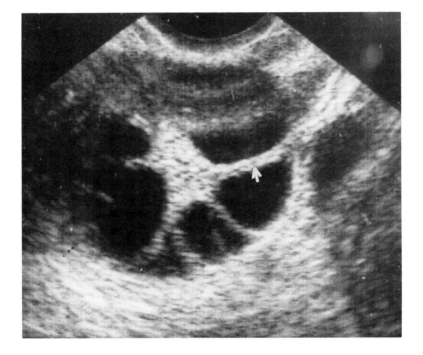

FIGURE 7. The double contour sign. Note the decreased reflectivity around the follicle (arrow), sign of imminent ovulation.

of 16 mm in diameter are present, and the serum E2 level exceeds 500 pg/ml, hCG is administered, and 36 h later, OPU is performed.[34,59]

SIGNS OF IMMINENT OVULATION

There are several U/S signs of ovulation.[3,17,22,60] These include (1) the appearance of echos on the internal surface of the follicular wall representing the dissociation of the cumulus oophorus shortly before ovulation; this may be imaged in more than 20% of follicles >18 mm in diameter;[13] and (2) edema and dissociation of the granulosa layer at the site of the expected expulsion of the ovum and hypervascularity and edema of the thecal layer, imaged sonographically as a line of decreased reflectivity around the follicle,[60] named "the double contour sign" (Figure 7).

SIGNS OF OVULATION

The following features may represent the occurrence of ovulation: (1) disappearance of the dominant follicle, (2) appearance of intrafollicular echos representing the formation of the corpus luteum and (3) appearance of fluid in Douglas's pouch. Another U/S sign which supports the diagnosis of ovulation is the imaging of a cystic corpus luteum in the luteal phase.[17]

ENDOMETRIAL VISUALIZATION DURING IVF CYCLES

Endometrial receptivity to implantation of the replaced embryos is one of the most important factors interfering with the success of IVF treatment. Nevertheless, relevant data on its development in induced cycles for IVF is scarce. Garcia et al.[61] performed early luteal phase endometrial biopsies in patients who underwent induction of ovulation with hMG for IVF and failed to undergo embryo transfer. In most patients, an advanced endometrium by 1 to 3 d was demonstrated. In another study[52] on 19 patients who were treated with a combination of CC and hMG and failed to conceive, an atrophic endometrium was found in almost half of the patients, in whom a poor correlation between the luteal phase serum E2 and P levels and endometrial development was observed, thus demonstrating the limited value of serum steroid hormones in predicting the endometrial response. In view of the potential risk in performing endometrial biopsies in conceptual cycles following ET, the role of the noninvasive ultrasonic measurement of endometrium has been investigated in our study[62] on a group of 47 patients undergoing IVF treatment. Measurements were performed in transverse scans at the level of the corpus uteri. Once the optimal level for the measurement was found, the picture was frozen. The endometrial halo appeared as an eliptical shadow with marked borderlines thought to represent the basalis-myometrial junction. A longitudinal central line appeared in part of the cases, representing the interface of the anterior and posterior superficial endometrial layers. The distance between the outer border of the two basalis layers was measured by the use of electronic calipers.

Three distinct endometrial growth phases were observed: (1) a rapid growth rate of about 0.5 mm/d from day −3 before hCG to day +2 after hCG (Figure 8); (2) a slow, almost linear growth pattern of 0.1 mm/d until day +11 (Figure 9); and (3) an accelerated rate of 0.4 mm/d in endometria harboring a conceptus (Figure 10). This period of accelerated growth coincided with the appearance of detectable serum β-hCG levels. In those patients who did not conceive, the slow growth rate was maintained until menstruation, at which time the visualization of the uterine cavity became blurred. The mean serum E2 levels in the patients who concieved was also consistently higher than the level in the patients who did not conceive. Our data, in nonconception cycles, corroborate previous similar U/S observations made by Sakamoto and Nakano,[63] Hackeloer,[17] Smith et al.,[64] and Fleisher et al.[65] in spontaneous cycles, in CC-induced cycles, in CC/hMG cycles, and hMG cycles. These studies demonstrated the same basic endometrial growth characteristics. Hackeloer[17] showed a good correlation between serum E2 and P levels and endometrial thickness in spontaneous cycles. We were not able to demonstrate any such correlation in hMG-induced cycles, either before or after OPU. This discrepancy between spontaneous and induced cycles may stem from two reasons. The first is the difference in response between ovarian steroids and endometrial growth. While the ovary responds to a wide range of serum hormone levels in induced cycles, the endometrium is restricted to a relatively small range of growth. Therefore, while at the time of hCG administration the E2 levels may vary among hMG-treated patients from 500 to 3500 pg/ml, the endometrial thickness may reach only 10 to 14 mm. The lack of correlation between serum hormones and endometrial growth may further be explained by asynchronous development of the endometrium in these cycles. It has been previously demonstrated that asynchrony exists between granulosa cell morphology and cumulus mor-

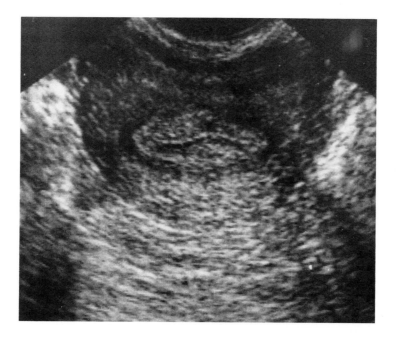

FIGURE 8.   Late proliferative endometrium.

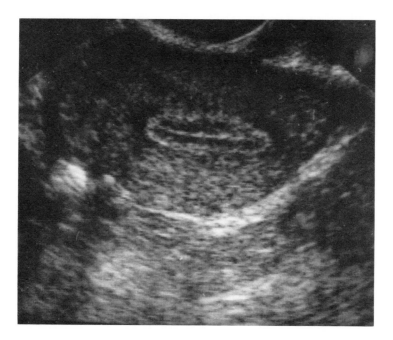

FIGURE 9.   Periovulatory endometrium.

phology as well as actual oocyte maturation.[66] It may therefore be that because of the hastened follicular development in hMG-induced cycles, there is a degree of asynchrony in endometrial development, leading, in turn, to discrepancies between serum hormone levels and endometrial thickness. Smith et al.[64] proposed the routine performance of endometrial measurements as an additional parameter for the monitoring of IVF cycles. In their study, it was

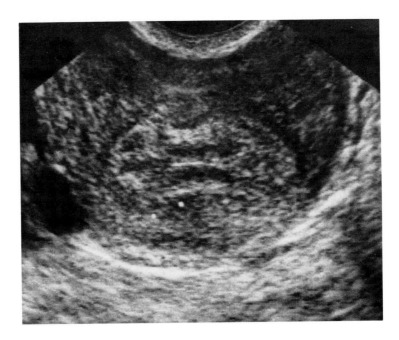

FIGURE 10.   Secretory endometrium.

claimed that preovulatory endometria of less than 10 mm in thickness were associated with retrieval of immature oocytes or failure in ovum retrieval. Yet, no correlation with fertilization or pregnancy rates could be demonstrated. We, however, did not find such a cut-off point in the preovulatory period, which has value in predicting the success of fertilization and conception following IVF. Yet, all conceptions following IVF occurred in women with an endometrial thickness of 13 mm or more on day +11. However, the same thickness was also found in 64% of women who did not conceive after the procedure. The failure to conceive in spite of an adequate ultrasonographic endometrial response is hypothesized to be due to defective embryonal quality.

We can conclude that endometrial thickness follows a distinct pattern of growth in hMG-induced cycles and does not correlate with serum hormones. This parameter does not seem to have any predictive value in the preovulatory phase, but a thickness exceeding 13 mm on day +11 seems to be conducive to conception after IVF.

TIMING OF OPU

In stimulated cycles, about 50% of the patients ovulate between 37 and 39 h after hCG administration. Only 3.4% of the patients have already ovulated when OPU is performed 36 h after the injection of HCG, and no ovulation usually occurs before 34 h after hCG.[67] Therefore, OPU is planned to take place shortly before the expected ovulation, about 36 h after hCG.[68,69] This way, a maximal number of mature oocytes is expected to be collected. Similarly, the collection of immature oocytes may be the result of an OPU performed too early, and the loss of some oocytes before OPU due to spontaneous ovulation may result from a procedure performed too late.

TECHNIQUES FOR ULTRASONICALLY GUIDED OOCYTE PICK-UP

The expansion of indications for IVF, to include mechanical, unexplained, male and immunological infertility, together with the relatively low pregnancy rates that make it neccessary for a couple undergoing IVF to be submitted several times to treatment before pregnancy is achieved. This has stressed upon the application of a low-risk, simple, and efficient ambulatory procedure for OPU. The introduction of ultrasonically guided oocyte collection by Lenz et al. in 1981,[70] and by other authors,[71-73,34] subsequently offered the potential advantage of a simple ambulatory procedure and the shortening of the distressing prolongation of waiting lists.

There are various techniques for U/S-guided OPU. These include the transabdominal-transvesical (TA) approach, the perurethral (PU) approach, and the transvaginal (TV) approach.

TRANSABDOMINAL-TRANSVESICAL OPU

The efficiency of the TA approach for OPU is by now well established. Several comparative studies have established the safety, efficiency, and low cost of this method (Table 1). In our two comparative studies,[46,59] we confirmed that in terms of pregnancy rate, the results of the U/S-guided OPU equal those of the laparoscopic method.

This procedure was introduced in our program in 1983 and shortly thereafter became the method of choice for OPU,[34] until the TV approach was introduced. Patients are admitted on the morning of the aspiration, and ultrasonic screening of ovaries is performed with a full bladder to verify that ovulation did not occur. After voiding, a no. 14 Foley catheter is inserted into the bladder. The bladder is rinsed with 200 to 300 ml of normal saline, emptied, and refilled under ultrasound monitoring with phosphate-buffered saline (PBS) with a pH of 7.4 and osmolarity of 280 mosmol/l. The bladder is refilled until a good visualization of the ovaries is obtained (usually 200 to 700 ml are needed). The transducer is covered by a sterile glove and sterile paraffin oil is applied to the abdominal skin. A cannula with a trocar is inserted at the abdominal midline, allowing access to both ovaries through a single percutaneous puncture (Figure 11). A 25-cm-long needle with an internal diameter of 1.6 mm is used for follicular aspiration. Both the cannula and the needle had their distal ends drilled to improve ultrasonic visualization (Figure 12). The follicular fluid is collected in a sterile disposable mucus aspirator with a 20-ml container connected to a suction aparatus at a negative pressure of 120 mmHg. The entire aspiration system is rinsed with heparinized culture medium. Sedation/analgesia is induced by Fentanyl (1 µg/kg) and Midazolam (2.5 mg) with inhalation of 50% nitrous oxide. Local anesthesia with 5 ml of 1% lignocaine is applied subcutaneously and a 3-mm skin incision is performed. The cannula with trocar are then inserted through the biopsy guide attached to the transducer into the bladder. The trocar is withdrawn and the needle inserted through the cannula into the bladder, pointed to the nearest follicle which is punctured through the posterior bladder wall. The aspirated follicular fluid is immediately examined microscopically for retreival of the oocytes. The needle is then advanced directly into the next follicle and the procedure repeated until all the follicles are aspirated. At times it is necessary to repuncture the bladder wall on the ipsilateral side in order to reposition the needle and give access to the maximal number of follicles. The needle is then withdrawn from the ovary into the bladder to puncture and aspirate the follicles within the contralateral ovary. Flushing of the follicles is performed using a 20-ml syringe filled with heparinized Ham's F-10. The flushing system is connected to the needle separately from the collecting system by a three-way tap (Figure 13). The whole procedure takes about 10 to 20 min.

ROLE OF NEEDLE DIAMETER IN OPU

In our previous study,[59] using a needle with an internal diameter (ID) of 1.4 mm, the mean number of oocytes recovered was only 4.0; but when we used a larger bore needle with an ID of 1.6 mm, the mean oocyte recovery rate was 6.5 oocytes per patient.[34] Consequently, there was an increase in the number of embryos transferred from a mean of

TABLE 1
Transabdominal OPU — Comparing Results with Laparoscopy

Author	Approach[a]	Needle diameter (internal diameter; mm)	Follicles/patient	Oocytes/follicle (%)	Oocytes/patient	Pregnancy rate (%)
Lenz and Lauritsen[71]	TA	0.6	1.9	42	0.8	
	TA	0.7	1.5	58	0.9	
Wikland and Hamberger[74]	TA	1.3	3.1	84	2.6	20
Robertson et al.[75]	TA	0.7	3.8	47	1.8	5
	LAP		3.6	86	3.1	13
Bellaisch-Allart et al.[93]	TA	1.2—1.5	2.9	41	1.2	32.6
	LAP	1.2	4.2	52	2.2	23.5
Sterzik et al.[76]	TA	0.8—1.2	3.4	72	2.5	42.8
Lewin et al.[46]	TA	1.4	2.8	75	2.1	10
	LAP	1.4	3.2	82.7	2.4	10
Lewin et al.[59]	TA	1.4	6.6	60.6	4.0	14.5
	LAP	1.6	7.1	74.6	5.3	12.5
Lewin et al.[34]	TA	1.6	8.7	74.7	6.5	19.2

[a] TA — transabdominal; LAP — laparoscopy.

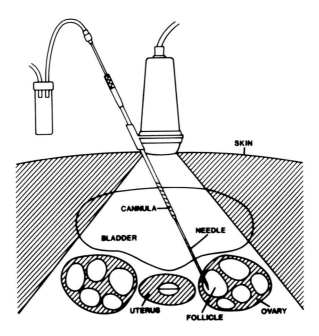

FIGURE 11. The U/S-guided transabdominal approach for oocyte collection. The use of the cannula enables the aspiration of follicles from both ovaries with a single percutaneous puncture.

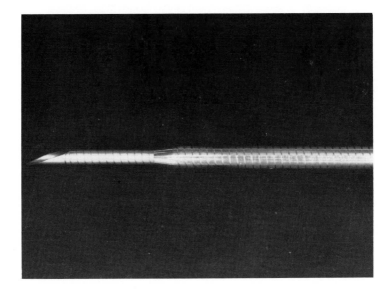

FIGURE 12. Drilling the distal end of the cannula and needle improves U/S visualization.

2.3 embryos per patient to 3.9 embryos per patient, and an increase in the pregnancy rate per transfer from 14.5 to 20%. Although experience may have contributed to a certain extent to the better results achieved in this group, it seems that this is not the only explanation. In comparing results from other studies (Table 2), it appears that as the needle diameter is increased, the number of oocytes recovered is also increased.

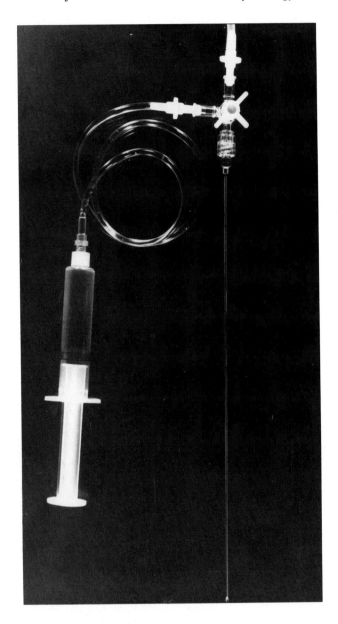

FIGURE 13.   Follicular aspiration system. The use of a three-way tap avoids interrupting the system when follicular flushing is performed.

TABLE 2
Effect of the Aspirating Needle Internal Diameter on the Oocyte Recovery Rate

Author	Internal diameter of needle (mm)	No. of oocytes per procedure
Lenz and Lauritsen[71]	0.6	0.8
Lenz and Lauritsen[71]	0.7	0.9
Feichtinger and Kemeter[77]	1.3	2.6
Wikland and Hamberger[74]	1.4	4.0
Lewin et al.[34]	1.6	6.5

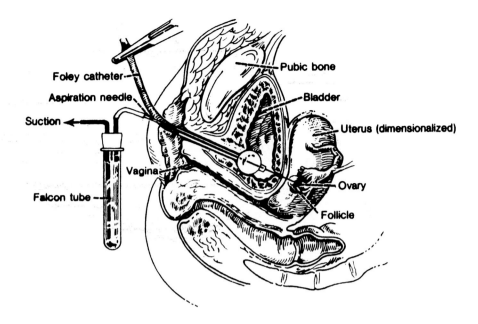

FIGURE 14. Diagram of the perurethral follicular aspiration system. (From Padilla, S. L., Butler, W. J., Boldt, J. P., Reindollar, R. H., Tho, S. P. T., Holzman, G. B., and McDonough, P. G., *Am. J. Obstet. Gynecol.*, 157, 622, 1987. With permission.)

BLADDER FILLING SOLUTION

There is an advantage in using PBS with a pH of 7.4 rather than normal saline with a pH of 5.7. The solution prevents the lowering of the pH in the follicular fluid aspirated by accidental leaks from the bladder filling solution into the aspiration system. In a preliminary study,[78] we observed a significantly better cleavage rate of the oocytes when PBS was used as compared to saline.

PERURETHRAL OPU

The U/S-guided PU OPU was reported by Parsons et al.,[79] Padilla et al.,[80] and Fateh et al.[81] as an alternative approach to the TA and TV methods.

The patient was placed in the lithotomy position with a full bladder filled with warm Ringer's lactate.[80] Pethidine (50 to 200 mg) or diazepam (5 to 20 mg) was administered intravenously for analgesia according to individual requirements.[79] A metal catheter[79] or a 20 French Foley catheter[80] was used to protect the urethra and to rinse the bladder and fill it with the Ringer's solution. Simultaneous ultrasound guidance was performed transabdominally by a sector scanner. Once the stimulated ovary was identified, the tip of the aspirating needle was guided to the posterior bladder wall adjacent to the follicle to be aspirated. The position of the needle tip was verified by transverse and longitudinal scanning, and the needle was then advanced into the follicle[80] (Figure 14). The needle used by Parsons et al.[79] and Fateh et al.[81] was a 16-gauge, 24-cm-long needle, and the needle used by Padilla et al.[80] was a 14-gauge, 22-cm-long needle. Continuous aspiration by wall suction at a pressure of 100 to 110 mmHg was used. The results of this method are presented in Table 3. These results indicate that the PU approach compares with the laparoscopic and transabdominal methods.

ADVANTAGES OF THE PU APPROACH

With the PU approach, there is no need to wrap the ultrasound equipment with sterile covers, the time for setting up the procedure is reduced, and there is no need for special

TABLE 3
Perurethral OPU — Comparing Results with Transabdominal and Laparoscopic OPU

Author	Approach	Needle	Follicles/patient	Oocytes/follicle (%)	Oocytes/patient	Pregnancy rate (%)
Parsons et al.[79]	Perurethral	16 gauge	7.9	70	5.5	
	Transabdominal			67		
Padilla et al.[80]	Perurethral	14 gauge	6	75	4	18
	Laparoscopy		8	85	7	25
Fateh et al.[81]	Perurethral		4.5	64	2.9	10.7
	Laparoscopy		5.1	68	3.5	13.3

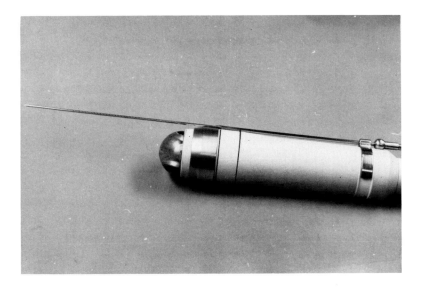

FIGURE 15. Vaginal transducer (Pie Medical, model 1120) with biopsy guide.

instruments. Skin wounds can be avoided, and the PU approach has a very low morbidity rate and avoids exposure of the oocyte to CO_2.

SIDE EFFECTS AND LIMITATIONS

Some side effects and limitations associated with the PU approach are transient hematuria and dysuria that usually settles in 24 h, minimal extravasation of urine into the paravesical tissues, and low efficiency when the ovaries are free and high or behind the uterus.

TRANSVAGINAL OPU

The TV approach for oocyte retrieval had been introduced initially as a modification of the transabdominal approach.[82-84] Originally, the aspiration procedure had been separated from the abdominal transducer and performed ''free hand'' through the vaginal fornix while guided by abdominal scanning. Then followed the production of vaginal probes equipped with a biopsy guide (Figure 15) that made the TV approach a simple and easy procedure, such that it became the present method of choice in most IVF centers (Table 4).

The excellent U/S imaging achieved with the high-frequency (5 to 7.5 MHz) vaginal transducers and scanning performed in close proximity to the ovaries enables precise identification of intraovarian and uterine structures and vessels, allowing better estimation of follicular and endometrial maturation. The recent introduction by Steer et al.[95] of transvaginal flow Doppler may allow a better understanding of the uterine and ovarian perfusion response and may identify the reason for some of the poor ovarian and endometrial responses in IVF in particular and in infertility in general.

Due to the fact that vaginal U/S does not require a full bladder and allows superior imaging, it became the preferred mode of monitoring follicular growth by physicians and patients. In our program, a substantial portion of the follicular monitoring is performed using this approach with a 7.5-MHz transducer.

For OPU, the TV probe is wrapped with a sterile nylon cover, and the vagina is cleaned with chlorhexidine solution and irrigated with 1000 ml of normal saline. After both ovaries are scanned to exclude premature ovulation, the sedation/analgesia including intravenous administration of fentanyl (1 μ/kg) and midazolam (2.5 mg) and nitrous oxide by mask is administered.

TABLE 4
TV OPU — Comparing Results with Laparoscopic and Transabdominal OPU

Author	Approach[a]	Needle	Oocytes/patient	Oocytes/follicle (%)	Fertility rate (%)	Pregnancy rate (%)
Russell et al.[85]	TV	22 gauge	6.8	87	70	
Lenz et al.[86]	TV		5.1	58		
Feichtinger and Kemeter[87]	LAP		4.7	77		
Torode et al.[88]	TV		4.5	86	63	
	TV		3.9	74	78	
	LAP		4.7	84	68	
Evers et al.[89]	TV	30 gauge	4.2	65		
Deutinger et al.[90]	TV	20 gauge	4.8	91	66	16.7
Daya et al.[91]	LAP		3.7	85	52	21.4
	TV		6.6		82	22
Schulman et al.[92]	TV		2.4		80	20
Seifer et al.[94]	TV	16 gauge	5.9	76	60	
	TA	18 gauge	4.9	92	73	
	LAP	14 gauge	6.2	97	45	
Lewin et al.[57]	TV	16 gauge	9.5	99	77	43

[a] TV — transvaginal; LAP — laparoscopy.

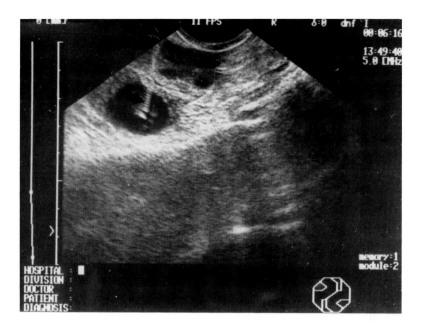

FIGURE 16.   Transvaginal OPU. Note the clear imaging of the aspirating needle within the follicle (arrow).

The needle, 30 cm long, 16 gauge, connected to a suction system, as described earlier, is introduced through the biopsy guide into the vaginal fornix at the nearest point to the ovary (Figure 16). All the follicles, of any size, are aspirated. This way, in our experience, one can reduce significantly the risk of ovarian hyperstimulation syndrome (OHSS).

ADVANTAGES OF THE TV APPROACH

This procedure can be performed even when the ovaries are covered by severe adhesions. The procedure is less painful than the TA procedure, especially because there is no need to penetrate the bladder wall, which is particularly painful,[98] and, therefore, only light anesthesia[86,90,57] or local anesthesia[85,96] is required.

The prevention of general anesthesia is one of the main advantages of the TV approach. Boyers et al.[97] reported a higher fertilization and cleavage rate of those oocytes retrieved first during general anesthesia as opposed to the oocytes retrieved last. A theorethical explanation for this may be the prolonged exposure of the last oocytes retrieved to the systemic anesthetic agents. TV allows easy monitoring in obese patients and patients with abdominal scars, where abdominal U/S offers poor imaging. The needle has a greater freedom of maneuverability as compared to the TA approach, since there is only one point of attachment (lateral fornix) instead of two points (the abdominal wall and the posterior bladder wall).

DISADVANTAGES OF TRANSVAGINAL OPU

Some authors reported initially lower results for TV oocyte aspiration as compared to laparoscopy,[68] but recent studies reported better oocyte retrieval rates related to improvement in the technique and equipment (Table 4). Another problem is the possible pelvic contamination from the bacterial flora of the vagina that may cause infection or abscess formation.[85] Inaccessibility to ovaries located high in the pelvis is yet another disadvantage of TV OPU.

COMPLICATIONS AND PROBLEMS RELATED TO U/S-GUIDED OPU

The U/S-guided techniques for oocyte aspirations have gained popularity because of their simplicity, efficacy, and reduced cost and time consumption. Yet, these techniques are not devoid of complications. Ashkenazi et al.[98] reported the frequency of complications and side effects of TA OPU in 102 punctures, in comparison to 38 cases of laparoscopy. Abdominal pain was found to be the most frequent side effect (11.6%) in the U/S method, as compared to 7.8% after laparoscopy. Urinary tract infection (UTI) and transient hematuria occurred in 5.8% of the U/S group, and none in the laparoscopy group. The frequent UTI after TA OPU was attributed to direct contamination by the Foley catheter used for bladder filling. Other complications are rare. Puncture of ovarian vessels or flushing of the follicles with culture medium containing heparin, which may result in damage to the fine vascular network of the theca interna, are the causes of mild hemoperitoneum reported in 2.9% of the cases, although one should bear in mind that severe bleeding that may lead to shock and death may also occur. Pelvic inflammatory disease (PID) is reported to occur in a relatively low incidence and may result from a recurrence of chronic PID.

In the TV approach for OPU, the complications are minor. Evers et al.[89] recorded no major complications in 181 TV OPU procedures. Bleeding from the puncture site occurred only in 24% of cases. Usually, bleeding stopped by the end of the procedure. In less than 2% of the cases, additional measures had to be taken in order to stop the bleeding (pressure with a dry swab). Side effects such as respiratory depression, dizziness, nausea, vomiting, local skin reactions, and collapse due to vagal reflex were encountered in less than 2% of the cases. Cohen et al.[96] reported the puncture of an iliac vein without sequelae in two patients. Accidental perforation of the intestine or rectum could result in infection of the culture medium or, more seriously, of the pelvis.[96] Feichtinger and Kemeter[87] found evidence of infection in 5.9% of the cultures following TV OPU, but the origin of the infection may have been caused by infected semen. Yet, the possibility of contamination from the bacterial flora in the vagina was also reported,[85,86] and the prophylactic administration of antibiotics significantly reduced the incidence of contaminations.[85-87,96]

OHSS is a frequent complication in IVF cycles, due to the multifollicular development with elevated serum E2 levels. Lindner et al.[99] reported an incidence of 10 to 40% of moderate OHSS in IVF cycles induced with hMG and GnRH agonist/hMG. In our program, we encountered an overall incidence of 12.2% of OHSS, including mild cases.[100] It is our impression that the complete aspiration of follicles during OPU may prevent OHSS in the majority of patients, including those with multiple follicles and high E2 levels.

U/S-GUIDED EMBRYO TRANSFER

The transfer of embryos (ET) to the uterine cavity is usually performed by loading the embryos, suspended in 90% serum-enriched culture medium, into a Teflon® catheter.[34] The embryos are aspirated in a 15- to 20-μl droplet placed between two air bubbles. Before ET, we ask the patients to fill their bladder as for abdominal U/S. The distended bladder straightens the uterus when anteroflexed, facilitating the transcervical introduction of the catheter, and enables U/S assistance when difficulty is encountered in introducing the catheter (Figure 17). The catheter is advanced to reach the uterine fundus, withdrawn a few millimeters, and the fluid containing the embryos is injected into the uterine cavity.

In an attempt to improve the relatively low pregnancy rates achieved in IVF, being in the range of 20 to 40%, in spite of the major advances in induction of ovulation, oocyte retrieval, and culture methods, various ET techniques were applied. The transcervical route is the most common, with the use of many different types of catheters, among which the

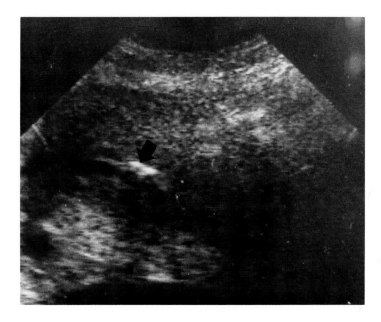

FIGURE 17.   Ultrasound-guided embryo transfer. The catheter tip is imaged about
1 cm from the uterine fundus (arrow).

most popular are the Tomcat and the Bourn hall catheters. Various positions of the patients
are also used, depending on whether the uterus is anteroverted or retroverted.

Various factors may interfere with embryo implantation in the uterine cavity. Among
these are, of course, the quality of embryos and the adequacy of the endometrium, but also
the introduction of microorganisms from the cervical mucus into the endometrial cavity[101]
and the release of prostaglandins that may cause uterine contractions and expel the embryos
to the vagina or into the Fallopian tubes, resulting in ectopic pregnancy. Yovich et al.[102]
studied the relationship between ectopic pregnancy and ET technique. The transfer of embryos with more than 50 μl of culture medium and injection of the embryos in proximity
of the uterine fundus correlated with a high frequency of ectopic pregnancies.

Another approach described was the surgical transfer through the uterine wall under U/S
guidance. Animal studies have shown a higher implantation rate using this approach.[103,104]
This approach may prevent the introduction of bacteria from the cervical canal. Parsons et
al.[101] reported a successful pregnancy following surgical ET carried out using the U/S-guided
PU approach (Figure 18A). With the patient in the lithotomy position, sedation/analgesia
with intravenous Pethidine (50 mg) and diazepam (5 mg), a 16-gauge, 25-cm-long needle
rinsed with culture medium was introduced into the bladder in the tip of a 14-gauge self-
retaining catheter. The bladder was filled with Hartman's solution. After identification of
the endometrial cavity using a mechanical sector scanner, the needle was passed with a
single rapid movement through the posterior bladder wall into the anterior myometrial wall.
It was advanced slowly until loss of resistance to the injection of culture medium was noted.
The embryos were then loaded into the end of an ET catheter passed through the needle
and injected in a 20-μl droplet of culture medium. The same author[101] also described a
successful implantation after surgical TV ET (Figure 18B). In this case, the vagina was
cleaned with a solution containing 0.15% cetrimide and 0.015% chlorehexidine. A 16-gauge
needle, primed with culture medium, was passed through the biopsy guide and the vaginal
fornix and the uterine wall into the uterine cavity. The embryos were transferred in 10 μl
of culture medium using a transfer catheter. U/S imaging of the small air bubbles injected
with embryos confirmed the site of transfer. Lenz et al.[105] described the transabdominal

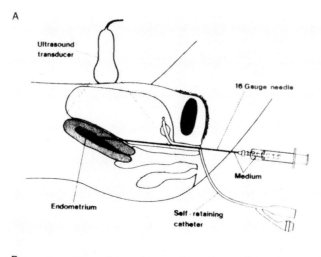

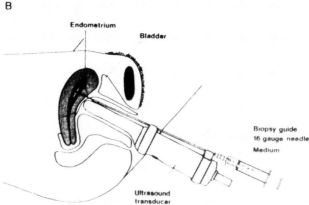

FIGURE 18.   Diagram illustrating ultrasound-guided surgical embryo transfer. (A) Perurethral; (B) transvaginal. (From Parsons, J. H., Bolton, V. N., Wilson, L., and Campbell, S., *Fertil. Steril.,* 48, 691, 1987. With permission.)

surgical transfer of embryos in ten patients. With the patients having a full bladder, a 16-gauge needle was introduced under U/S guidance through the abdominal wall, the posterior bladder wall, and the anterior uterine wall into the uterine cavity. Embryos were transferred in a transfer catheter introduced through the needle. No pregnancy was achieved. It is difficult to draw conclusions from these studies on only small numbers of patients concerning the future role of the surgical TA or TV approach for ET, and further evaluation is needed. For the time being, these procedures may be considered in cases where transcervical passage is difficult or traumatic.

ULTRASONICALLY GUIDED REDUCTION OF MULTIPLE PREGNANCIES

Multiple pregnancies are considered one of the major complications of IVF treatment, their incidence being of about 20%.[106] The successful implantation of multiple embryos increases the risk of maternal health and to the survival and outcome of these pregnancies. Late abortions, prematurity, high perinatal morbidity, and mortality are frequently associated with multiple pregnancies. The incidence of multiple pregnancy can be controlled to a certain

TABLE 5
Selective Reduction of Multiple Pregnancies

Authors	Approach[a]	Needle	Procedure[b]	Gestational age (weeks)	No. embryos reduced
Hansmman et al.[108]	TA	22 gauge	AF Aspiration, fetal injection	9 (5% NaCl)	5 to 2
Farquharson et al.[109]	TA		Fetal injection	(5% NaCl)	
Brandes et al.[110]	TA	21 gauge	1 ml Dolosal + Xylocain 1%	10	5 to 3
Lopez et al.[111]	TV	16 gauge	Fetal aspiration	8—11	
Dumez and Oury[112]	TV	16 gauge	Fetal aspiration	8—11	
Kanhai et al.[113]	TA		Fetal trauma	11	
Itskovitz et al.[114]	TV	16 gauge	AF aspiration	7	5 to 3
Lewin and Zohav[115]	TV	17 gauge	Fetal trauma	10	4 to 2
Breckwoldt et al.[116]	TA		Fetal trauma	8—10	9 to 3

[a]   TA — transabdominal; TV — transvaginal.
[b]   AF — amniotic fluid.

extent by (1) frequent monitoring of the ovarian response to stimulation and strict titration of drugs used for the induction of superovulation, although multiple pregnancies may occur despite intensive monitoring,[107] and (2) by restricting the number of embryos transferred. It is well accepted that the transfer of more than four to five embryos does not improve the pregnancy rate, but increases the risk of multiple implantation.[37] Therefore, most centers limit the number of embryos transferred to three to five at most. The spare embryos are frozen and can be thawed and transferred in later cycles.

In those cases were multiple embryos implant, selective reduction of embryos can be offered. There are several methods of U/S-guided selective embryocide (Table 5; Figure 19). The decision of which embryo or gestational sac to reduce is only a technical one. The anatomic position and the proximity to the puncture site are the factors to be considered.

U/S-GUIDED FALLOPIAN TUBE CANNULATION FOR GAMETE TRANSFER

This technique was described by Anderson and Jansen[117] after evaluation on a group of 20 patients. A 25-cm 3-French-gauge Teflon® cannula drawn out to 2 French gauge was successfully inserted, with the aid of a guiding cannula and metal obturator and under scanning with a 7-MHz vaginal transducer, through the cervix and the uterine cavity into the Fallopian tubes. No sedation was required. This procedure seems to have the potential of being a reasonable alternative to the laparoscopic gamete intra-Fallopian transfer (GIFT) procedure.

THE SAFETY OF DIAGNOSTIC AND OPERATIVE U/S IN IVF

Ultrasound has become a major diagnostic and operative tool, with advanced technology enabling high-quality imaging. Yet, the massive involvement of ultrasound in monitoring follicular growth, OPU, and ET has raised concerns about the safety of its use regarding oocytes and early embryos.

The diagnostic systems currently used are the continuous wave mode and the pulsed wave mode. In the real-time imaging devices, such as linear-array and sector scanners, used in IVF programs, the pulsed ultrasound mode is used. Their intensity output is 0.1 to 60

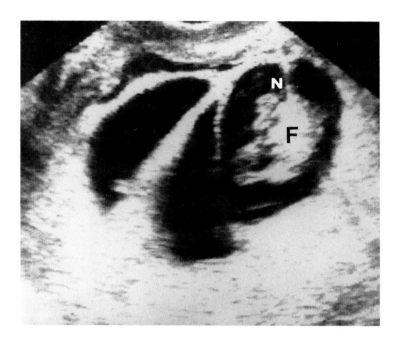

FIGURE 19.   Ultrasound-guided transvaginal reduction of a 10-week quadruplet pregnancy. Needle (N); fetus (F).

mW/cm^2 (spatial peak, temporal average intensity).[118] The ovaries and oocytes are exposed to sound waves during the stimulation phase and during the OPU procedure. The sensitivity threshold of the ovaries varies during the follicular phase according to the tissue density, blood supply, the amount of air and liquid around and within the ovary, and the multiplication rate of the cells. The amount of absorbtion of the ultrasound waves depends mainly on the frequency of the wave, the output intensity of the sound waves, and the duration of exposure. The physical effects of ultrasound are the outcome of interaction between ultrasound waves and the tissue.

Two distinct phenomena are noted: cavitation and temperature elevation. Cavitation is the result of the propagation of ultrasound waves through the tissue that causes expansion and shrinkage of air bubbles within the tissue, resulting in mechanical damage to the surrounding structures. There is evidence that cavitation does not appear in the mammalian organized tissues, but at a peak intensity of over 1500 W/cm^2 with continuous wave mode.[119] This includes tissues immersed in liquid, like oocytes in follicular fluid or fetus in amniotic fluid. As for the pulsed ultrasound mode, the threshold for mechanical damage in terms of output intensity is even higher, and the safety margin from cavitation is at least doubled.

Temperature elevation is caused by absorbtion of the acoustic energy of ultrasound waves by the tissue. The potential risk of heat caused by diagnostic ultrasound devices is very low. It was shown that temperature elevation to 42° for 8 h by continuous waves did no harm to mammalian tissues such as muscle, liver, kidney, and testes,[119,120] and an insonation by pulsed wave ultrasound at a frquency of 3.2 MHz for up to 1 h caused no histological damage.[119] It is evident that there is no real risk of ultrasonic hyperthermic teratology associated with current clinical practice unless the patient is febrile and the insonation prolonged for over 60 min.[121] Daya et al.[91] studied the U/S effects on the reproductive function of oocytes using a transvaginal probe of 7 MHz. No effect on fertilization and cleavage of oocytes exposed to the sound waves was demonstrated. A possible adverse effect is the premature rupture of follicle, reported when U/S monitoring was performed after the endogenous LH surge or after the administration of hCG.[121] This phenomenon was not demonstrated by other authors.[91,34] The safety of diagnostic ultrasound has been supported by *in vivo* human studies in which no genetic abnormalities were observed in fetuses and children that were exposed *in utero* to U/S waves.[122] The minimal intensity of U/S waves found to produce morphological abnormalities is 600 mW/cm^2 with pulsed ultrasound.[123] This intensity is much higher than the intensities used in human diagnostic ultrasound, being less then 100 mW/cm^2.

The Bioeffects Committee of the American Institute of Ultrasound in Medicine (AIUM) has stated that in the low-frequency-range insonations, there have been no independently confirmed significant biological effects in mammalian tissues exposed to intensities below 100 mW/cm^2.[124] The intensity used over an average exposure time of 20 to 30 min produces an energy exposure that is, at most, only 10% of that allowed by the AIUM statement.[91] Mahadevan et al.[125] reported that in 39 patients who underwent a combined laparoscopic and U/S OPU, there was no difference in the fertilization rate and embryonic development following IVF and ET, comparing the oocytes that were exposed to U/S to those aspirated by laparoscopy in the same cycle. Lenz et al.[126] evaluated the effect of ultrasound and flushing during OPU, after the report by Cartensen and Flymn[127] that the injection of media into the follicles introduces micro-air bubbles which might oscillate and explode under sonication, with the possible result of a cavitation-like effect. No difference was found in the cleavage rate between oocytes collected in the first aspirate and oocytes obtained after flushing.

To conclude, it seems that all the studies reporting sonication damage to experimental animal cells *in vivo* and *in vitro* and to human cells *in vitro* have employed energy levels and duration of sonication greater than would be expected to exist in clinical use.[128] There is evidence that the application of diagnostic ultrasound does not cause any bioeffects or chromosomal abnormalities to exposed cells.[129,130] From the human IVF literature we reviewed, it appears that there is no valid proof to doubt the safety of the currently used U/S techniques in IVF, and there is no evidence, despite the widespread use of diagnostic and operative U/S in IVF-ET, of any adverse effect that could be related to the use of U/S imaging.

CONCLUSION

After the first successful fertilization of human oocytes recovered laparoscopically was achieved in 1977 by Steptoe and Edwards, this method became the standard procedure worldwide during the first years of IVF treatment. Yet, in spite of the successful results, it soon became clear that the laparoscopy procedure had many disadvantages when used for an elective minor procedure such as OPU: (1) the need for general anesthesia with endotracheal intubation and abdominal inflation with CO_2 and the morbidity associated with it; (2) the risk of damage to bowel, bladder, and other abdominal organs; (3) the use of CO_2 may alter the follicular fluid pH and damage the oocytes; and (4) severe pelvic adhesions may prevent access to the ovaries.

The advent of the simple, low-cost, and low-risk U/S-guided OPU, with its various approaches, offered an efficient alternative and is established by now as the first-choice technique for OPU.

Nevertheless, laparoscopic OPU still remains a practical alternative, especially when combined with diagnostic laparoscopy for infertility investigation.

REFERENCES

1. **Steptoe, P. C. and Edwards, R. G.,** Birth after reimplantation of a human embryo, *Lancet,* 2, 366, 1978.
2. **Kratochwil, A., Urban, G., and Friedreich, F.,** Ultrasonic tomography of the ovaries, *Ann. Chir. Gynaecol. Fenn.,* 61, 211, 1972.
3. **Ritchie, W. M.,** Ultrasound in the evaluation of normal and induced ovulation, *Fertil. Steril.,* 43, 167, 1985.
4. **Hackeloer, B. J., Nitsche-Dabelstein,** Ovarian imaging by ultrasound. An attempt to define a reference plane, *J. Clin. Ultrasound,* 9, 275, 1980.
5. **Hackeloer, B. J. and Robinson, H. P.,** Ultrasound examination of the growing follicle and corpus luteum, *Geburtshilfe Frauenheilkd.,* 38, 163, 1978.
6. **Yee, B., Barnes, R. B., Vargyas, J. M., and Marrs, R. P.,** Correlation of transabdominal and transvaginal ultrasound measurements of follicle size and number with laparoscopic findings for *in vitro* fertilization, *Fertil. Steril.,* 47, 828, 1987.
7. **Ylostalo, P.,** Measurement of the ovarian follicle by ultrasound in ovulation induction, *Fertil. Steril.,* 31, 651, 1979.
8. **Smith, D. H., Picker, R. H., Sinosich, M., and Saunders, D. M.,** Assessment of ovulation by ultrasound and E2 levels during spontaneous and induced cycles, *Fertil. Steril.,* 33, 387, 1980.
9. **de Crespigny, L. J., O'Herlihy, C., Hoult, I. J., and Robinson, H. P.,** Ultrasound in an *in vitro* fertilization program, *Fertil. Steril.,* 35, 25, 1981.
10. **Hodgen, G. D., Kenigsberg, D., Collins, R. L., and Schenken, R. S.,** Selection of the dominant ovarian follicle and hormonal enhancement of natural cycle, *Ann. N.Y. Acad. Sci.,* 442, 23, 1985.
11. **di Zerega, G. S. and Hodgen, G. D.,** Folliculogenesis in the primate ovarian cycle, *Endocrinol. Rev.,* 2, 27, 1981.
12. **Di Zerega, G. S., Niyon, W. E., and Hodgen, G. D.,** Intercycle serum follicle stimulating hormone elevations: significance in follicle and assessment of corpus luteum normalcy, *J. Clin. Endocrinol. Metab.,* 50, 1046, 1980.
13. **Kerin, J. F., Edmonds, D. K., Warmes, G. M., Cot, L. W., Seamark, R. F., Mattheus, C. D., Young, G. B., and Baird, D. T.,** Morphological and functional relationships of graafian follicle growth to ovulation in women using ultrasonic, laparoscopic and biomedical measurements, *Br. J. Obstet. Gynecol.,* 88, 81, 1981.
14. **Hackeloer, B. J., Nitsche, S., Daumme, E., Sturm, G., and Buchholz, B.,** Ultraschalldorstellung von ovaeranderungen, *Geburtshilfe Frauenheilkd.,* 37, 185, 1977.
15. **Hackeloer, B. J., Fleming, R., Robinson, H. P., Adam, A. H., and Coutts, R. T.,** Correlation of ultrasonic and endocrinologic assessment of human follicular development, *Am. J. Obstet. Gynecol.,* 135, 122, 1979.
16. **Renaud, R., Macler, J., Dervain, I., Ehret, M., Aron, C., Plas-Roser, S., Spria, A., and Pollack, H.,** Echographic study of follicular maturation and ovulation during the normal menstrual cycle, *Fertil. Steril.,* 33, 272, 1980.
17. **Hackeloer, B. J.,** Ultrasound scanning of the ovarian cycle, *J. In Vitro Fertil. Embryo Transfer,* 1, 217, 1984.
18. **Bryce, R. L., Shuter, B., Sinosich, M. J., Stiel, J. N., Picker, R. H., and Saunders, D. M.,** The value of ultrasound, gonadotropins and estradiol measurements for precise ovulation prediction, *Fertil. Steril.,* 37, 42, 1982.
19. **O'Herlihy, C., De Crespigny, L. H., and Robinson, H. P.,** Monitoring ovarian follicular development with real-time ultrasound, *Br. J. Obstet. Gynecol.,* 87, 613, 1980.
20. **Queenan, J. T., O'Brien, G. D., Bains, L. M., Simpson, J., Collins, W. P., and Campbell, S.,** Ultrasound scanning of ovaries to detect ovulation in women, *Fertil. Steril.,* 34, 99, 1980.
21. **Hackeloer, B. J.,** The roll of ultrasound in female infertility management, *Ultrasound Med. Biol.,* 10, 35, 1984.
22. **Bomsel-Helmreich, O., Bessis, R., Huyon, L. U. N.,** Cumulus oophorus of the preovulatory follicle assessed by ultrasound, in *Infertility,* Christie, A. D., Ed., Chartwel-Bratt, Bromley, 1981, 105.
23. **Templeton, A., Messinis, I. E., and Baird, D. T.,** Characteristics of ovarian follicle in spontaneous and stimulated cycles in which there was an endogenous luteinizing hormone surge, *Fertil. Steril.,* 46, 1113, 1986.
24. **Lopata, A., Johnston, I. W. H., Hoult, I. J., and Speirs, A. I.,** Pregnancy following intrauterine implantation of an embryo obtained by in vitro fertilization of a prevovulatory egg, *Fertil. Steril.,* 33, 117, 1980.
25. **Trounson, A. O., Leeton, J. F., Wood, C., Webb, J., and Wood, J.,** Pregnancies in human by fertilization in vitro and embryo transfer in the controlled ovulatory cycle, *Science,* 212, 681, 1981.

26. **Testart, J., Frydman, R., DeMounzon, J., Lassale, B., and Belaisch, J. C.,** A study of factors affecting the success of human fertilization *in vitro.* I. Influence of ovarian stimulation upon the number and condition of oocytes collected, *Biol. Reprod.,* 28, 415, 1983.

27. **Cohen, J., DeVane, G. W., Elsner, C. W., Fehilly, B. C., Kort, H. I., Massey, J. B., and Turner, T. G.,** Cryopreservation of zygotes and early cleaved human embryos, *Fertil. Steril.,* 49, 283, 1988.

28. **Lopata, A., Broun, J. B., Leeton, J. F., Talbot, J., and Wood, C.,** *In vitro* fertilization of preovulatory oocytes and embryo transfer in infertile patients treated with clomiphene and human chorionic gonadotropin, *Fertil. Steril.,* 30, 27, 1978.

29. **Jones, H. W., Jr., Jones, G. S., Andrews, M. C., Acosta, A. A., Bundren, C., Garcia, J., Sandow, B., Veeck, L., Wilkes, C., Witmyer, J., Wortham, J. E., and Wright, G.,** The program for in vitro fertilization at Norfolk, *Fertil. Steril.,* 38, 14, 1982.

30. **Lopata, A.,** Concepts in human *in vitro* fertilization and embryo transfer, *Fertil. Steril.,* 40, 289, 1983.

31. **Jones, G. S. Acosta, A. A., Garcia, J. E., and Rosenwaks, Z.,** The effect of follicle stimulating hormone without additional luteinizing hormone on follicular stimulation and oocyte development in normal ovulatory women, *Fertil. Steril.,* 43, 696, 1985.

32. **Shaw, R. W. Ndukwe, G., Imoedemhe, D., Burford, G. C., and Han, R.,** Stimulation of multiple follicular growth for *in vitro* fertilization by administration of pulsatile luteinizing hormone releasing hormone during midfollicular phase, *Fertil. Steril.,* 46, 135, 1986.

33. **Laufer, N., Decherney, A. H., and Haseltine, F. P.,** Human in vitro fertilization employing individualized ovulation induction by human menopausal gonadotropins, *J. In Vitro Fertil. Embryo Transfer,* 1, 56, 1984.

34. **Lewin, A., Laufer, N., Rabinowitz, R., and Schenker, J. G.,** Ultrasonically guided oocyte recovery for *in vitro* fertilization: an improved method, *J. In Vitro Fertil. Embryo Transfer,* 3, 370, 1986.

35. **Trounson, A. O., Leeton, J. F., Wood, C., Webb, J., and Wood, J.,** Successful human pregnancies by IVF and ET in the controlled ovulatory cycles, *Science,* 212, 681, 1981.

36. **Speirs, A. C., Lopata, A., Gronow, M. G., Kellow, G. N., and Johnston, W. I. H.,** Analysis of the benefits and risks of multiple embryo transfer, *Fertil. Steril.,* 34, 468, 1983.

37. **Laufer, N., Less, A., Lewin, A., Rabinowitz, R., Margalioth, E. J., Elmalech, U., and Schenker, J. G.,** A multivariant analysis for the prediction of conceptions following IVF-ET, abstr. presented at the 5th World Congr. on In Vitro Fertilization and Embryo Transfer, Norfolk, VA, April 5 to 10, 1987, Abstr. PP-141.

38. **Laufer, N., DeCherney, A. H., and Tarlatzis, B. C.,** The association between preovulatory serum 17 b-estradiol pattern and conception in HMG/HCG induced cycles for human in vitro fertilization, *Fertil. Steril.,* 46, 73, 1985.

39. **DeCherney, A. H., Tarlatzis, B. C., and Laufer, N.,** Follicular development: lessons learned from human in vitro fertilization, *Am. J. Obstet. Gynecol.,* 153, 911, 1985.

40. **Tarlatzis, B. C., Laufer, N., DeCherney, A. H.,** The use of ovarian ultrasonography in monitoring ovulation induction, *J. In Vitro Fertil. Embryo Transfer,* 1, 226, 1984.

41. **Joyce, M., Vargyas, M. D., and Mishell, D. R.,** Correlation of ultrasonic measurement of ovarian follicle size and serum E2 Levels in ovulatory patients following clomiphene citrate for IVF, *Am. J. Obstet. Gynecol.,* 1, 569, 1982.

42. **Marrs, R. P., Vargyas, J. M., and March, C. M.,** Correlation of ultrasound and endocrinology measurements in human menopausal gonadotropin therapy, *Am. J. Obstet. Gynecol.,* 145, 417, 1983.

43. **Mantzavinos, T., Garcia, J. E., and Jones, H. W., Jr.,** Ultrasound measurement of ovarian follicles stimulated by human gonadotropins for oocyte recovery and in vitro fertilization, *Fertil. Steril.,* 40, 461, 1983.

44. **Cabau, A. and Bessis, R.,** Monitoring of ovulation induction with human menopausal gonadotropin and human chorionic gonadotropin by ultrasound, *Fertil. Steril.,* 36, 178, 1981.

45. **Trounson, A. O.,** Current perspectives of in vitro fertilization and embryo transfer, *Clin. Reprod. Fertil.,* 1, 55, 1982.

46. **Lewin, A., Margalioth, E. J., Rabinowitz, R., and Schenker, J. G.,** Comparative study of ultrasonically guided percutaneous aspiration with local anesthesia and laparoscopic aspiration of follicles in an in vitro fertilization program, *Am. J. Obstet. Gynecol.,* 151, 621, 1985.

47. **De Ziegler, D., Cedars, M. I., Randle, D., Lu, J. K., Judd, H. L., and Meldrum, D. R.,** Suppression of the ovary using a gonadotropin releasing-hormone agonist prior to stimulation for oocyte retrieval, *Fertil. Steril.,* 48, 807, 1987.

48. **Albert, P. J., Schlafke, J., Kaesemann, H., and Gille, J.,** Pregnancy following induction of ovulation with pure FSH after suppression of endogenous gonadotropins with subcutaneous buserelin, *Arch. Gynecol. Obstet.,* 241, 53, 1987.

49. **Kerin, J. F. and Warnes, G. M.,** Monitoring of ovarian response to stimulation in in vitro fertilization cycles, *Clin. Obstet. Gynecol.,* 29, 158, 1986.

50. **Vargyas, J. M., Morente, C., Shangold, G., and Marrs, R. P.,** The effect of different methods of ovarian stimulation for human in vitro fertilization and embryo replacement, *Fertil. Steril.,* 42, 745, 1984.

51. **Trounson, A. O.,** Factors controlling normal embryo development and implantation of human oocytes fertilized in vitro, in *Fertilization of the Human Egg In Vitro,* Beier, H. M. and Lindner, H. R., Eds., Springer-Verlag Berlin, 1983, 235.

52. **Cohen, J., Debache, C., Pigeau, F., Mandelbaum, J., Plachot, M., and De Brux, J.,** Sequential use of clomiphen citrate, human menopausal gonadotropin and human chorionic gonadotropin in vitro fertilization. Study of luteal adequacy following Aspiration of the preovulatory follicles, *Fertil. Steril.,* 42, 360, 1984.

53. **Barriere, P., Lopes, P., Boiffard, J. P., Pousset, C., Quentin, M., Sagot, P., L'hermite, A., Lerat, M. F., and Charbonnel, B.,** Use of GnRH analogues in ovulation induction for in vitro fertilization: benefit of a short administration regimen (letter), *J. In Vitro Fertil. Embryo Transfer,* 4, 64, 1987.

54. **Neveu, S., Hedon, B., Bringer, J., Chinchole, J. M., Arnal, F., Humeau, C., Cristol, P., and Viala, J. L.,** Ovarian stimulation by a combination of a gonadotropin-releasing hormone agonist and gonadotropins for in vitro fertilization, *Fertil. Steril.,* 47, 639, 1987.

55. **Porter, R. N., Smith, W., Craft, I. L., Abdulwahid, N. A., and Jacobs, H. S.,** Induction of ovulation for in-vitro fertilisation using Buserelin and gonadotropins (letter), *Lancet,* 2, 1284, 1984.

56. **Palermo, R., Amadeo, G., Navot, D., Rosenwaks, Z., and Cittadini, E.,** Concomitant gonadotropin-releasing hormone agonist and menotropin treatment for the synchronized induction of multiple follicles, *Fertil. Steril.,* 49, 290, 1988.

57. **Lewin, A., Zohav, E., Yanay, N., Berger, M., Simon, A., Laufer, N., and Schenker, J. G.,** What should be the preferred method for using combined long-acting GnRH analogue (decapeptyl) and hFSH (metrodin) for induction of ovulation in IVF? Comparison between concomitant and sequential protocols, presented at the 4th Meet. of the European Soc. of Human Reproduction and Embryology, Barcelona, July 3 to 6, 1988, Abstr. 183.

58. **Lewin, A., Zohav, E., Yanay, N., Berger, M., Simon, A., Laufer, N., and Schenker, J. G.,** Combined early follicular phase GnRH analogue and hFSH for induction of ovulation in IVF — comparison between a daily subcutaneous regimen and a single injection of a long-acting preparation, presented at the 4th Meet. of the European Soc. of Human Reproduction and Embryology, Barcelona, July 3 to 6, 1988, Abstr. 185.

59. **Lewin, A., Laufer, N., Rabinowitz, R., Margalioth, E. J., Bar, I., and Schenker, J. G.,** Ultrasonically guided oocyte collection under local anesthesia: the first choice method for in vitro fertilization — a comparative study with laparoscopy, *Fertil. Steril.,* 46, 257, 1986.

60. **Picker, R. H., Smith, D. H., Tuker, M. H., and Saunders, D. M.,** Ultrasonic signs of imminent ovulation, *J. Clin. Ultrasound,* 11, 1, 1983.

61. **Garcia, J. E., Acosta, A. A., and Jones, H. W., Jr.,** Advanced endometrial maturation after ovulation induction with human menopausal gonadotropins human chorionic gonadotropin for in vitro fertilization, *Fertil. Steril.,* 41, 31, 1984.

62. **Rabinowitz, R., Laufer, N., Lewin, A., Navot, D., Bar, I., Margalioth, E. J., and Schenker, J. G.,** The value of ultrasonographic endometrial measurement in the prediction of pregnancy following in vitro fertilization, *Fertil. Steril.,* 45, 824, 1986.

63. **Sakamoto, C. and Nakano, H.,** The echogenic endometrium and alterations during menstrual cycles, *Int. J. Gynecol. Obstet.,* 20, 255, 1982.

64. **Smith, B., Porter, R., Ahuja, K., and Craft, I.,** Ultrasonic assessment of endometrial changes in stimulated cycles in an in vitro fertilization and embryo transfer program, *J. In Vitro Fertil. Embryo Transfer,* 1, 233, 1984.

65. **Fleischer, A. C., Herbert, C. M., Sacks, G. A., Wentz, A. C., Entman, S. S. and James, A. E., Jr.,** Sonography of the endometrium during conception and nonconception cycles of in vitro fertilization and embryo transfer, *Fertil. Steril.,* 46, 442, 1986.

66. **Laufer, N., Tarlatzis, B. C., DeCherney, A. H., Masters, J. T., Haseltine, F. P., MacLusky, N., and Naftolin, F.,** Asynchrony between human cumulus corona cell complex and oocyte maturation after human menopausal gonadotropin treatment for in vitro fertilization, *Fertil. Steril.,* 42, 366, 1984.

67. **DeCherney, A. H. and Lavy, G.,** Oocyte recovery methods in in-vitro fertilization, *Clin. Obstet. Gynecol.,* 29, 171, 1986.

68. **Garcia, G. E., Jones, G. S., and Wright, G. L.,** Predicting the time of ovulation, *Fertil. Steril.,* 36, 308, 1981.

69. **Lopata, A., Gronon, M. J., Johnston, W. I. H., McBain, J. C., Speirs, A. L., and Leung, P. S.,** In vitro fertilization embryo implantation, in *Infertility,* Insler, V. and Lunenfeld, B., Eds., Churchill Livingstone, Edinburgh, 1986, 507.

70. **Lenz, S., Lauritsen, J. G., and Kjellow, M.,** Collection of human oocytes for in vitro fertilization by ultrasonically guided follicular puncture (letter), *Lancet,* 1, 1163, 1981.

71. **Lenz, S. and Lauritsen, J. G.,** Ultrasonically guided percutaneous aspiration of human follicles under local anesthesia: a new method of collecting oocytes for *in vitro* fertilization, *Fertil. Steril.,* 38, 673, 1982.

72. **Wikland, M., Nilsson, L., Hansson, R., Hamberger, L., and Janson, P. O.,** Collection of human oocytes by the use of sonography, *Fertil. Steril.,* 39, 603, 1983.

73. **Feichtinger, W. and Kemeter, P.,** Laparoscopic or ultrasonically guided follicle aspiration for in vitro fertilization? *J. In Vitro Fertil. Embryo Transfer,* 1, 244, 1984.

74. **Wikland, M. and Hamberger, L.,** Ultrasound as a diagnostic and operative tool for in vitro fertilization and embryo replacement (IVF/ER) programs, *J. In Vitro Fertil. Embryo Transfer,* 1, 213, 1984.

75. **Robertson, R. D., Picker, R. H., O'Neill, C., Ferrier, A. J., and Saunders, D. M.,** An experience of laparoscopic and transvesical oocyte retrieval in an in vitro fertilization program, *Fertil. Steril.,* 45, 88, 1986.

76. **Sterzik, K., Jonatha, W., Keckstein, G., Rossmanith, W., Traub, E., and Wolf, A.,** Ultrasonically guided follicle aspiration for oocyte retrieval in an in vitro fertilization program: further simplification, *Int. J. Gynecol. Obstet.,* 25, 309, 1987.

77. **Feichtinger, W. and Kemeter, P., Eds.,** In vitro fertilization and embryo transfer an outpatient office procedure, in *Recent Progress in Human In Vitro Fertilization,* Cofese, 1984, 285.

78. **Lewin, A., Laufer, N., Rabinowitz, R., Margalioth, E. J., Bar, I., and Schenker, J. G.,** The effect of different isotonic solutions for bladder filling on the results of ultrasonically guided oocyte aspiration for IVF, presented at the 4th World Conf. on In Vitro Fertilizaiton, Melbourne, November 18 to 22, 1985, Abstr. 54.

79. **Parsons, J., Riddle, A., Booker, M., Sharma, V., Goswamy, R., Wilson, L., Akkermans, J., White-head, M., and Campbell, S.,** Oocyte retrieval for in vitro fertilisation by ultrasonically guided needle aspiration via the urethra, *Lancet,* 1, 1076, 1985.

80. **Padilla, S. L., Butler, W. J., Boldt, J. P., Reindollar, R. H., Tho, S. P., Holzman, G. B., and McDonough, P. G.,** Transurethral ultrasound-guided oocyte retrieval for in vitro fertilization, *Am. J. Obstet. Gynecol.,* 157, 622, 1987.

81. **Fateh, M., Ben Rafael, Z., Blasco, L., Tureck, R. W., Meloni, F., and Mastroianni, L., Jr.,** Comparison of ultrasonographic transurethral and laparoscopic guided oocytes retrieval, *Fertil. Steril.,* 46, 653, 1986.

82. **Dellenbach, P., Nisand, I., Moreau, L., Feger, B., Plumere, C., Gerlinger, P., Brun, B., and Rumpler, Y.,** Transvaginal sonographically controlled ovarian follicle puncture for egg retrieval (letter), *Lancet,* 1, 1467, 1984.

83. **Gleicher, N., Friberg, J., Fullan, N., Giglia, R. V., Mayden, K., Kesky, T., and Siegel, I.,** Egg retrieval for in vitro fertilisation by sonographically controlled vaginal culdocentesis (letter), *Lancet,* 2, 508, 1983.

84. **Wikland, M., Enk, L., and Hamberger, L.,** Transvesical and transvaginal approaches for the aspiration of follicles by use of ultrasound, *Ann. N.Y. Acad. Sci.,* 442, 182, 1985.

85. **Russell, J. B., DeCherney, A. H., and Hobbins, J. C.,** A new transvaginal probe and biopsy guide for oocyte retrieval, *Fertil. Steril.,* 47, 350, 1987.

86. **Lenz, S., Leeton, J., and Renou, P.,** Transvaginal recovery of oocytes for in vitro fertilization using vaginal ultrasound, *J. In Vitro Fertil. Embryo Transfer,* 4, 51, 1987.

87. **Feichtinger, W. and Kemeter, P.,** Transvaginal sector scan sonography for needle guided transvaginal follicle aspiration and other applications in gynecologic routine and research, *Fertil. Steril.,* 45, 722, 1986.

88. **Torode, H. W., Picker, R. H., Porter, R. N., Robertson, R. D., Smith, D. H., O'Neil, C., and Saunders, D. M.,** Oocyte pick-up by laparoscopy replaced by transvaginal aspiration in an in vitro fertilization program, *J. In Vitro Fertil. Embryo Transfer,* 4, 148, 1987.

89. **Evers, J. L., Larsen, J. F., Gnany, G. G., and Sieck, U. V.,** Complications and problems in transvaginal sector scan guided follicle aspiration, *Fertil. Steril.,* 49, 278, 1988.

90. **Deutinger, J., Reinthaller, A., Csaicsich, P., Riss, P., Fischl, F., Bernaschek, G., Muller, and Tyl, E.,** Follicular aspiration for in vitro fertilization: sonographically guided transvaginal versus laparoscopic approach, *Eur. J. Obstet. Gynecol. Reprod. Biol.,* 26, 127, 1987.

91. **Daya, S., Wikland, M., Nilsson, L., and Enk, L.,** Fertilization and embryo developement of oocytes obtained transvaginally under ultrasound guidance, *J. In Vitro Fertil. Embryo Transfer,* 4, 338, 1987.

92. **Schulman, J. D., Dorfmann, A. D., Jones, S. L., Pitt, C. C., Joyce, B., and Patton, L.,** Outpatient in vitro fertilization using transvaginal ultrasound guided oocyte retrieval, *Obstet. Gynecol.,* 69, 665, 1987.

93. **Belaisch-Allart, J. C., Hazout, A., Guillet, Rosso, F., Glissant, M., Testart, J., and Frydman, R.,** Various techniques for oocyte recovery in an in vitro fertilization and embro transfer program, *J. In Vitro Fertil. Embryo Transfer,* 2, 99, 1985.

94. **Seifer, D. B., Collins, R. L., Paushter, D. M., George, C. R., and Quigley, M. M.,** Follicular aspiration: a comparison of an ultrasonic endovaginal transducer with fixed neelde guide and other retrieval methods, *Fertil. Steril.,* 49, 462, 1988.

95. **Steer, C., Campbell, S., Mason, B. A., and Pampiglione, J.,** Transvaginal colour flow doppler studies of the uterine arteries, presented at the 4th Meet. of the European Soc. of Human Reproduction and Embryology, Barcelona, July 3 to 6, 1988, Abstr. 137.

96. **Cohen, J., Debache, C., Pez, J. P., Junca, A. M., and Cohen-Bacrie, P.,** Transvaginal sonographically controlled ovarian puncture for oocyte retrieval for in vitro fertilization, *J. In Vitro Fertil. Embryo Transfer,* 3, 309, 1986.

97. **Boyers, S. P., Stronk, J. N., Fino, L., Russell, J. B., Lavy, G., and DeCherney, A. H.,** The time interval between laparoscopic aspiration of mature oocytes affects fertilization rate, presented at the 42nd Annu. Meet. of the American Fertility Soc., Toronto, September 27 to October 2, 1986, 83.

98. **Ashkenazi, J., Mordechai, B. D., Feldberg, D., Shelef, M., Dicker, D., and Goldman, J. A.,** Abdominal complications following ultrasonically guided percutaneous transvesical collection of oocytes for in vitro fertilization, *J. In Vitro Fertil. Embryo Transfer,* 4, 316, 1987.

99. **Lindner, C. H., Braendle, W., Lichtenberg, V., and Bettendorf, G.,** Analysis of 500 GnRH-agonist/HMG cycles for in vivo fertilization, IVF and GIFT, presented at the 4th Meet. of the European Soc. of Human Reproduction and Embryology, Barcelona, July 3 to 6, 1988, Abstr. 8.

100. **Rabinowitz, R., Laufer, N., Lewin, A., Amran, H., Margalioth, E. G., Simon, A., and Schenker, J. G.,** Ovarian hyperstimulation syndrome (OHSS) in in vitro fertilization attempts following human menopausal gonadotropin (hMG) and human chorionic gonadotropin (hCG) administration and follicular aspiration, presented at the 5th World Congr. on In Vitro Fertilization and Embryo Transfer, Norfolk, VA, April 5 to 10, 1987, Abstr. AP-500.

101. **Parsons, J. H., Bolton, V. N., Wilson, L., and Campbell, S.,** Pregnancies following in vitro fertilization and ultrasound directed surgical embryo transfer perurethral and transvaginal techniques, *Fertil. Steril.,* 48, 691, 1987.

102. **Yovich, J. L., Turner, S. R., and Murphy, A. J.,** Embryo transfer technique as a cause of ectopic pregnancies in in vitro fertilization, *Fertil. Steril.,* 44, 318, 1985.

103. **Iuliamo, M. F., Squires, E. L., and Cook, V. M.,** Effect of age of equine embryos and method of transfer on pregnancy rate, *J. Anim. Sci.,* 60, 258, 1985.

104. **Seidel, G. E. and Seidel, S. M.,** The embryo transfer industry, in *New Technologies in Animal Breeding,* Bracket, B. G., Seidel, G. E., Jr., and Seidel, S. M., Eds., Academic Press, New York, 1981, 41.

105. **Lenz, S., Leeton, J., Rogers, P., and Trounson, A.,** Transfundal transfer of embryo using ultrasound, *J. In Vitro Fertil. Embryo Transfer,* 4, 13, 1987.

106. **Kerin, J. F., Quin, P. J., Kirby, C., Seamark, R. F., Warmes, G. M., Jeffrey, R., Matthews, C. D., and Cox, L. W.,** Incidence of multiple pregnancy after in vitro fertilization and embryo transfer, *Lancet,* 2, 537, 1983.

107. **Fedorkow, D. M., Corenblum, B., Pattinson, H. A., and Tylor, P. J.,** Septuplet gestation following the use of human menopausal gonadotropin despite intensive monitoring, *Fertil. Steril.,* 49, 364, 1988.

108. **Hansmman, M., Hackeloer, B. J., and Staudach, A.,** *Ultrasound Diagnosis in Obstetrics and Gynecology,* Springer-Verlag, Berlin, 1985, 73.

109. **Farquharson, D. F., Wihmann, B. K., Hansmman, M., Yuen, B. H., Balduin, V. J., and Lindhal, S.,** Management of quintuplet pregnancy by selective embryocide, *Am. J. Obstet. Gynecol.,* 158, 413, 1987.

110. **Brandes, J. M., Itskovitz, J., Timor-Tritsch, I. E., Drugon, A., and Frydman, R.,** Reduction of the number of embryos in a multiple pregnancy: quintuplet to triplet, *Fertil. Steril.,* 48, 326, 1987.

111. **Lopez, P., Talmaart, C., Thiery, M.,** Partial termination of a quintuplet pregnancy, *Z. Geburtshilfe Perinatol.,* 189, 239, 1985.

112. **Dumez, Y. and Oury, J. F.,** Method for first trimester selective abortion in multiple pregnancy, *Contrib. Gynecol. Obstet.,* 15, 50, 1986.

113. **Kanhai, H. H., Van Russel, E. J. C., and Meerman, R. J.,** Selective termination in quintuplet pregnancy during first trimester, *Lancet,* 2, 1447, 1986.

114. **Itskovitz, J., Buldes, R., Taler, J., Lytman, A., Erlich, J., and Brandes, J.,** Reduction of quituplet pregnancy to triplet by vaginal approach, presented at the 9th Congr. of the Israel Assoc. of Obstetrics and Gynecology, Tel-Aviv, December 2 to 4, 1987, Abstr. 4.

115. **Lewin, A. and Zohav, E.,** Transvaginal Reduction of Quadruplet Pregnancy after IVF, unpublished data.

116. **Breckwoldt, M., Geisthovel, F., Neulen, J., and Schillinger, H.,** Management of multiple conceptions after gonadotropin-realising hormone analog/human menopausal gonadotropin/human chorionic gonadotropin therapy, *Fertil. Steril.,* 49, 713, 1988.

117. **Anderson, J. C. and Jansen, R. P. S.,** Fallopian tube cannulation without anesthesia utilizing phased-array transvaginal echography, presented at the 5th World Congr. on In Vitro Fertilization and Embryo Transfer, Norfolk, VA, April 5 to 10, 1987, Abstr. OC-404.

118. **National Institutes of Health,** National Institutes of Health Consensus Development Conf: Consensus Statement, Diagnostic Ultrasound in Pregnancy, U.S. Government Printing Office, Washington, DC, 1984.

119. **Lele, P., De Hazzard, G., and Litz, M. L., Eds.,** Thresholds and Mechanisms of Ultrasonic Damage to Organized Animal Tissues. Symposium on Biological Effects and Characterization of Utlrasound Sources, HEW Publ. U.S. Department of Health, Education and Welfare, Washington, DC, 1977, 224.

120. **Frizzell, L. A., Linke, C. A., Carstensen, E. L., and Fridd, C. W.,** Tresholds for focal ultrasonic lesions in rabbit kidney, liver and testicle, *IEEE Trans. Biomed. Eng.,* BME-24, 393, 1977.

121. **Lele, P. P.,** Safety and potential hazards in the current applications of ultrasound in obstetrics and gynecology, *Ultrasound Med. Biol.,* 5, 307, 1979.

122. **Emoulin, A., Bologne, R., Hustin, J., and Lambotte, R.,** Is ultrasound monitoring of follicular growth harmless?, *Ann. N.Y. Acad. Sci.,* 442, 146, 1985.

123. **Sakamoto, S., Mukuboh, M., Okai, T., and Hara, K.,** Safety of pulsed ultrasound — experimental and epidemiological studies, *Jpn. J. Ultrasound Med.,* 283, 1981.

124. **American Institute of Utlrasound in Medicine,** Safety Considerations for Diagostic Ultrasound, AIUM Publ. No. 316, Bioeffects Committee, Bethesda, MD, 1984.

125. **Mahadevan, M., Chalder, K., Wiseman, D., Leader, A., and Taylor, P. J.,** Evidence for an absence of deleterious effects of ultrasound on human oocytes, *J. In Vitro Fertil. Embryo Transfer,* 4, 277, 1987.

126. **Lenz, S., Lindenberg, S., Fehilly, C., and Petersen, K.,** Are ultrasonic-guided follicular aspiration and flushing safe for the oocyte?, *J. In Vitro Fertil. Embryo Transfer,* 4, 159, 1987.

127. **Cartensen, E. L. and Flynn, H. G.,** The potential for transient cavitation with microsecond pulses of ultrasound, *Ultrasound Med. Biol.,* 8, 720, 1982.

128. **Lewin, A. and Schenker, J. G.,** On the safety of diagnostic ultrasonography in obstetrics and gynecology, *Rev. Environ. Health,* 5, 129, 1985.

129. **Baker, M. L. and Dalrymple, G. U.,** Biologic effects of diagnostic ultrasound: a review, *Radiology,* 126, 479, 1978.

130. **Bioeffects Committee of the American Institute of Ultrasound in Medicine,** Safety Considerations for Diagnostic Ultrasound, AIUM Publ. 316, AIUM, Washington, DC, 1984, 12.

Chapter 13

TRANSVAGINAL COLOR DOPPLER

Asim Kurjak and Ivica Zalud

INTRODUCTION

The past 15 years have given the medical world a number of extraordinary imaging techniques, such as dynamic ultrasound scanning, CT scanning, and NMR scanning which provide high resolution sectional images and accurate morphological information on a completely different physical basis. More than any other available method, diagnostic ultrasound has a unique potential for the noninvasive study of fetal and maternal circulation. Furthermore, endosonography has evolved into an important imaging modality which has significantly changed the profile of diagnostic ultrasound. Esophageal, rectal, and vaginal probes provide for superb visualization of the organ of interest and are now widely used in clinical practice, significantly increasing the sensitivity and specificity of ultrasound diagnosis. Transvaginal probes have been used extensively in the assessment of gynecological and obstetrical patients. The first comparisons of vaginal sonography with abdominal ultrasound have shown a significant improvement in the detection and characterization of pelvic masses (tumors, extrauterine pregnancy, etc.).[1] Transvaginal sonography was widely introduced into clinical practice simultaneously with the clinician's growing awareness of the diagnostic value of blood flow studies by Doppler ultrasound. Therefore, the introduction of vaginal Doppler studies has almost coincided with the first reports on vaginal sonography. The vaginal approach now provides for a clear definition of pelvic structures, and their characterization has become the primary goal of many clinical investigations.

However, the most exciting recent development in the field of diagnostic ultrasound in obstetrics and gynecology is transvaginal color Doppler. The most important advantage of color Doppler is the display of blood flow across the whole scanning plane, as compared with only one line of sight available with conventional pulsed Doppler. Pulsed Doppler combined with real-time ultrasonic imaging, the so-called duplex method, permits the accurate localization of deep vessels and the positioning of the Doppler sample volume within them. The duplex technique is now widely used to detect blood flow in the human fetus but it can also be used in the study of normal pelvic blood flow. However, the combination of high quality B-mode images, pulsed Doppler, and color Doppler in the same vaginal probe produces a superb simultaneous visualization of structural and flow information about the female pelvis. The first promising results obtained with this new diagnostic facility have already been reported.[2-9]

INFERTILITY

Transvaginal color Doppler provides a promising new tool for the study of reproductive physiology and pathophysiology. The functional activity of the ovaries and uterus is of particular importance in infertility and the clinical assessment of its therapy. For this purpose, the study of blood flow in pelvic vessels seems to be very important. The color Doppler signal from both uterine arteries can be easily seen in all patients laterally to the cervix at the level of the cervicocorporeal junction of the uterus. The artery and the vein are distinguished according to the pulsation and brightness of color flow. Ovarian vessels are the most difficult to obtain but an experienced operator using modern color Doppler equipment can detect them in most patients. Conversely, the internal iliac vessels can be visualized easily in the entire population. They can be observed in the side wall of the pelvis, often lying deep close to the ovary. During the proliferative phase of the normal menstrual cycle the appearance of uterine vessels appeared similar to that of other arteries in the body, and there is a prominent notch and little or no end-diastolic velocity in the Doppler velocity waveform.[10] Close to the end of the secretory phase, changes in vessel compliance begin and an end-diastolic component is usually present. The resistance index falls with a rise in estrogen level during the early follicular phase and then increases in the preovulatory phase along with the periovulatory drop in estrogen levels. There is subsequently a fall in the resistance index with rising levels of progesterone indicating a positive uterine response to rising estrogen and progesterone levels during the ovarian cycle.[7] Uterine perfusion increases and color flow are much more prominent in response to rising levels of estrogen in the follicular phase, and of estrogen and progesterone in the luteal phase. It should be stressed that the uterine response to endogenous endocrine changes can be clearly assessed using transvaginal color and pulsed Doppler. Increased diastolic color and pulsed Doppler flow would indicate increased uterine perfusion.

Animal studies have suggested that older animals are less fertile because of decreased uterine perfusion.[12] It may be hypothesized that the fertility of older animals could be enhanced by improving uterine perfusion, and that similarly, women may be infertile because of decreased uterine perfusion due to aging and pelvic surgery, which could make poor uterine perfusion a cause of embryo implantation failure.[13,14]

Taylor et al. have demonstrated characteristic waveforms of ovarian, uterine, and iliac vessels as well as changes in these waveforms associated with hormonal changes.[15] Transvaginal ultrasound produces images of a better resolution than transabdominal ultrasound, primarily through better preservation of the beam pattern and utilization of higher frequencies. The use of transvaginal color Doppler permits accurate placement of sample volume. By using Doppler waveforms it is possible to distinguish the ovary containing an active corpus leteum from the inactive ovary.[16] Since an increasing resistance index reflects some reduction in the blood flow distal to the point at which the Doppler recording was made, namely in the corpus leteum, one might postulate that this reflects a reduction in corpus leteum function which is incompatible with pregnancy. IVF treatment failure can be predicted by transvaginal color Doppler ultrasound at an earlier stage than has previously been reported and this could reflect an inadequacy of the corpus leteum.[17]

ADNEXAL MASSES

Ultrasonography has been an indispensable diagnostic tool in the field of gynecology, and there are numerous reports of its use in the diagnosis of benign and malignant pelvic disease.[18,19] Transvaginal color Doppler is a recent advantage in the field of oncology, and the first clinical investigations were concentrated particularly on the study of ovarian malignancy and blood flow supply of the tumor.[2]

The differentiation of benign and malignant tumors *in vivo* still involves many clinical problems. However, there are known features that characterize this difference. Many of them, such as the mitotic index and pleomorphism, are of histologic nature and are not amenable to current imaging methods. One feature of malignancy is the bizarre vascular morphology which characterizes many malignant tumors. Tumor vessels have a relative paucity of smooth muscle in their walls in comparison with their caliber.[20] Due to this lack of normal muscle components, the amount of vasoconstriction by sympathetic stimulation cannot be increased. This could be the basis for differentiation between benign and malignant tumor vascularity. The importance of tumor vascularity was first recognized by Judah Folkman in 1972, when he proposed the hypothesis that increased cell population must be preceded by the production of new vessels.[21] These vessels must be formed very early on in the development of the tumor and are therefore early markers of tumor presence. Several substances have been identified as angiogenic factors.[22] Such factors are secreted by the tumor and induce the formation of new vessels by the host tissue. As noted in morphologic studies, these vessels have an abnormal vascular morphology, including the frequent presence of arteriovenous anastomoses and vascular walls deficient in muscular elements. The lack of muscular elements is reflected in the low impedance to flow leading to high diastolic flow and, in some tumors, in the absence of systolic/diastolic variation.

Neovascularization is the process by which new blood vessels are induced and it occurs in the corpus leteum, in embryogenesis, in tumors, and in wound healing. It is, therefore, a process of some interest in relation to the application of color Doppler to maternal and fetal medicine. The changes in impedance seen in association with the development of the corpus luteum are due to neovascularization.[23] Since functioning ovarian tissue has a characteristic luteal waveform associated with low impedance and high flow requirements, a similar finding would be expected in functioning tumors of the ovary. A small functioning tumor is capable of modifying blood flow supply to a degree that can be easily detected by color and pulsed Doppler techniques. Neovascular signals have been described in many different types of tumors, notably of the breast.[24] Neovascularization is an essential prerequisite for tumor growth and must therefore occur very early in the life of a tumor. Taylor et al. detected neovascular Doppler signals in tumors weighing as little as 50 mg in experimental animals.[23]

Numerous studies of experimentally induced tumors and angiographic findings in human tumors have shown that tumor vessels display characteristics permitting a presumptive diagnosis of malignancy.[25,26] Some of these characteristics may vary with the tumor type. In experimental tumors the morphologic features of neovascularization are certainly so characteristic of different tumor types that the histologic type can be predicted from the tumor pattern alone by experienced observers.[23] Pathologic vessels show an irregular course without progressive caliber diminution. Other features include the presence of arteriovenous shunting and bizarre thin-walled vessels lined by tumor cells which end in amorphous spaces constituting "tumor lakes" that retain contrast material.[25]

Doppler time-velocity waveforms also provide a semiquantitative estimate of distal impedance. Tumors often contain abnormal vascular channels lacking muscle in the wall. Because smooth muscle in the arterioles is the site of peripheral resistance in normal vessels, it might be expected that abnormal, thin-walled vessels would exhibit low-impedance signals with little systolic-diastolic variation, thus providing another opportunity for characterizing tumor blood flow.

Doppler studies and transvaginal color Doppler sonography seem to produce a better characterization of pelvic tumor vascularity. The results obtained at the Ultrasonic Institute of the University of Zagreb have shown that it is easy to demonstrate color flow in small vascular branches within tissues in pathological conditions.[2,5] These vessels are detectable by transvaginal color Doppler due to higher blood velocity and consequently increased flow volumes (Plates 6 and 7).* Being very thin and randomly dispersed within the tissue, such vessels are difficult to find unless color Doppler is used. Our own study has shown that tumor vascularity can be successfully used for the characteriztion of pelvic tumors (Table 1). Sensitivity, specificity, and accuracy are acceptably high, and it seems that we should be concerned about false-negative rather than about false-positive findings (Table 2). Waveform analysis of signals obtained from the "hot" color coded area within masses produced excellent results. All malignant tumors had a resistance index lower than 0.50 and all benign tumors, which showed color flow, a resistance index higher than 0.50. The resistance index of 0.50 is used therefore, as a cut-off point to differentiate malignant vs. benign lesion.

---

* Plates 6 and 7 follow page 38.

TABLE 1
Blood Flow in Adnexal Tumor (N = 390)

PHD	N	Color Flow Yes	Color Flow No	RI
Cystadenocarcinoma	14	14	0	0.34 ± 0.09
Metastatic follicular Ca of the thyroid gland	1	1	0	0.25
Metastatic rectal Ca	1	1	0	0.30
Granulosa cell tumor	2	2	0	0.35 ± 0.10
Dermoid cyst	6	0	6	
Simple ovarian cyst	27	5	22	0.68 ± 0.12
Hydrosalpinx	9	1	8	0.71
Cystadenoma	10	2	8	0.65 ± 0.13
Endometriosis	7	0	7	
Abscess	1	0	1	
Sactosalpinx	3	0	3	
Pseudocyst	1	1	0	0.41
Other adnexal mass	308	59	249	0.69 ± 0.11

TABLE 2
Evaluation of Diagnostic Criteria of Adnexal Tumor

Color Flow and R.I.	Final diagnosis Malignant	Final diagnosis Benign
Malignant	18	1
Benign	0	63

Note: Sensitivity = 94.7%; specificity = 100%; accuracy = 98.8%.

The goal of transvaginal color Doppler sonography should be to identify ovarian tumors which are not significantly enlarged. This new technique may be used as a screening method in the early detection of ovarian malignancy. So far no diagnostic imaging technique has been adequate enough in this respect. Color Doppler ultrasound is a pertinent diagnostic tool which can also be used to observe changes in the vascularity of gynecologic malignant tumors before and after treatment.

UTERINE MASSES

The presence of uterine tumor vascularity is often associated with an increased number of vessels within a tumor, or hypervascularity. Neovascularity may be further characterized as fine or coarse.[27] Histopathologically, these vessels are primitive avascular channels, lacking smooth muscle and often consisting of an endothelial layer and connective tissue alone. Low resistance to flow must be expected in such vessels, since they lack normal arteriolar smooth muscle, the recognized site of peripheral resistance. Another vascular alteration in malignancy is the presence of arteriovenous shunting. The small vessels around the periphery of a tumor have blood flow velocities many time greater than those in the normal aorta.[25]

Transvaginal color Doppler is helpful in diagnosing uterine malignancy. Patients with suspected uterine tumors have been examined using 5 MHz transvaginal color Doppler. Color flow inside the endometrium and myometrium has been detected in all of five cases with endometrial carcinoma. The peripheral impedance was very low (RI $= 0.34 \pm 0.06$).[7] In four cases of carcinoma *in situ* of the uterine cervix no abnormality has been found. It can be speculated that newly formed vessels are too small and velocity and volume flow below the resolution power of the equipment. In several uterine fibroids color flow was detected in the border of the tumor (Plate 8).* However, when peripheral impedance was compared in cases of myoma uteri and carcinoma endometrii, a significantly lower resistance index was obtained in the latter. Transvaginal color Doppler offers an acceptable sensitivity, specificity, and accuracy in the diagnosis of uterine malignancy. Transvaginal color Doppler appears to be an accurate noninvasive diagnostic tool for the early detection of endometrial carcinoma.[3,13]

EARLY PREGNANCY

Ultrasound is already an essential component of obstetric evaluation, but it is winning even more attention as Doppler techniques open new paths in the diagnosis of blood flow disturbances in the embryo and fetus. Transvaginal ultrasonography has increased the amount of morphologic information, and color Doppler the amount of functional information obtained during the first trimester of pregnancy.

It has been found that Doppler waveform patterns in the first trimester differ markedly from those found later in pregnancy. Thus, the umbilical artery waveform has absolutely no diastolic component early in the first trimester. This is in contrast to the third trimester where the absence of diastolic flow is associated with a poor fetal outcome. Diastolic flow begins to increase around the 12th to 17th week, indicating the decrease in placental resistance. It seems that color Doppler could increase the reproducibility of measurement expecially in feto-maternal circulation. With this modality it is possible to clearly visualize even small vessels thus permitting accurate placing of pulsed Doppler sample volumes. Transvaginal sonography provides superb visualization of early pregnancy morphology. Color Doppler studies could contribute to visualizing blood flow in the trophoblast, umbilical cord, and vessels of the embryo (Figure 1).[6,28] In the future such information could play an important role in diagnosing normal early pregnancies or pregnancy failures.

ECTOPIC PREGNANCY

The incidence of ectopic pregnancy has increased due to the higher incidence of pelvic inflammatory disease and the activities of infertility clinics. Transvaginal sonography has been proven to be very useful in the diagnosis of ectopic pregnancy. The normality of embryonic development can be assessed approximately 1 week earlier than by the transabdominal route. However, many ectopic gestations do not develop a fetus so that these specific findings are not seen, and the presence of an adnexal cystic mass may be ambiguous. Thus, other means to identify the nature of an adnexal mass become useful.

The trophoblast actively invades the maternal tissues eroding blood vessels which bleed into the intervillous space and thereby start a primitive placental circulation. The hemodynamics involved in the process provides the basis for the characteristic flow observed. The fact that the intervillous space lacks any muscle wall will also result in low impedance flow. These characteristics are found in ectopic pregnancies and can be analyzed by pulsed Doppler.[28]

Transvaginal color Doppler is a new important innovation in the diagnosis of ectopic pregnancy. However, color and pulsed Doppler can help to characterize the nature of the adnexal mass thus permitting preoperative diagnosis when the ectopic fetus and its characteristic heartbeat cannot be visualized. The corpus leteum can be identified by transvaginal sonography. Fetuses invade the maternal tissues, and it is possible to get a very high blood

* Plate 8 follows page 38.

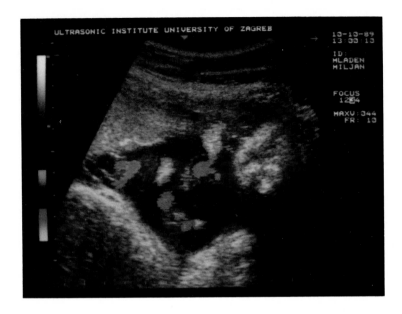

FIGURE 1.   Umbilical cord of the 14th week fetus detected by transvaginal color Doppler.

TABLE 3
Diagnostic Accuracy of
Transvaginal Color Doppler
and Pulsed Doppler in the
Detection of Ectopic Pregnancy

Color flow and	Ectopic pregnancy	
RI > 0.50	Yes	No
Yes	17	1
No	2	14

Note: Sensitivity = 94.4%; specificity = 87.5%; accuracy = 91.2%.

flow from the maternal arteries into spaces around them. Thus, it basically is worthwhile to use this vascular signature of trophoblastic flow as a way of tissue-characterization of the adnexal mass.

The results obtained by transvaginal color Doppler diagnosis of ectopic pregnancy have been good enough to justify its clinical application (Table 3).[2] We have examined 34 patients with suspected ectopic pregnancy. Two false-nagative findings were observed in cases of tubal abortion. Color flow could not be visualized due to an inactive trophoblast. In these patients beta HCG has been measured and found to be decreased. The highest value was 200 mUI/ml and the lowest one 80 mUI/ml. One false-positive finding was obtained in the case of a corpus luteum cyst. The current policy would be to wait with management if there is no trophoblast flow outside the empty uterus in amenorrhoic patients. On the contrary, if there is color flow in the adnexal region with a resistance index <0.50 the patient is scheduled for laparoscopy regardless of clinical signs. The hypothesis is that the absence of color flow from the trophoblast and corpus luteum may indicate that the ectopic pregnancy is no longer viable. There is no doubt that some extopic embryos die and are resorbed.

Color Doppler signals might then prove helpful in predicting which ectopic embryos could be treated expectantly. Nevertheless, in the absence of free fluid in the cul-de-sac, this policy suggests that the population without color flow involves ectopic pregnancies which are nonviable, and, therefore, best suited for medical therapy, i.e., methotrexate.[29]

With ultrasound it is not always possible to see the embryo, but it is possible to see an adnexal mass. However, color flow around and inside of the mass gives a positive identification that it is an ectopic gestation.

CONCLUSION

The most exciting recent developments in the field of diagnostic ultrasound in obstetrics and gynecology are color Doppler and transvaginal sonography. The combination of high quality B-mode imaging, pulsed wave Doppler and color Doppler in the same vaginal probe provides for superb simultaneous visualization of structural and flow information and offers new insights in dynamic studies of blood flow within the female pelvis. In all malignant tumors the presence of neovasularization has been documented preoperatively by color Doppler. The characteristic findings include prominent color flow and a very low resistance index. Analyses of tumor vascularity have shown considerable accuracy in the preoperative assessment of tumor nature. The obvious differences in vascularity between benign and malignant lesions demonstrated in the study can be explained by the abnormal vascular morphology of the newly formed vessels in malignant tumors. The vessels are characterized by the frequent presence of arteriovenous anastomoses and a deficiency in the development of muscular elements of the vascular wall. This results in low resistance and high blood flow velocities in abnormal vessels and permits their detection by ultrasound Doppler. We believe that color Doppler assessment of tumor vascularity can be used for a better noninvasive characterization of pelvic masses and, furthermore, that it may be potentially useful as a screening test for ovarian malignancy in populations at risk of this disease. The results obtained in early pregnancy have shown that blood flow in major embryonic vessels can be analyzed as early as the 6th week of gestation. Embryonic vessels can be easily visualized by color Doppler, and the pulsed Doppler beam can thus be easily guided to the vessel of interest. Color Doppler has been found to be particularly useful in demonstrating trophoblastic flow. If only pulsed Doppler is used, the localization of blood flow in the trophoblast is a time-consuming and relatively difficult procedure. The guidance of a pulsed Doppler beam by color flow mapping helps to locate areas of the most abundant flow and makes examination much faster and easier. In terms of the foregoing it seems that transvaginal color Doppler sonography can hardly be called a luxury. For the time being, it is a useful convenience which can very easily become a necessity in the near future.

REFERENCES

1. **Fleischer, A. C., Gordon, A. N., and Entman, S.,** Transabdominal and transvaginal sonography of pelvic masses, *Ultrasound. Med. Biol.,* 15, 529, 1989.
2. **Kurjak, A., Zalud, I., Alfirevic, Z., and Jurkovic, D.,** The assessment of abnormal pelvic blood flow by transvaginal color Doppler, *Ultrasound. Med. Biol.,* in press.
3. **Kurjak, A., Jurkovic, D., Alfirevic, Z., and Zalud, I.,** Transvaginal color Doppler, *J. Clin. Ultrasound,* in press.
4. **Kurjak, A., Miljan, M., Jurkovic, D., Alfirevic, Z., and Zalud, I.,** Color Doppler in the assessment of fetomaternal circulation, *Rech. Gynecol.,* 1, 269, 1989.
5. **Kurjak, A., Zalud, I., Jurkovic, D., Alfirevic, Z., and Miljan, M.,** Transvaginal color Doppler in the assessment of pelvic circulation, *Acta. Obstet. Gynecol. Scand.,* 68, 131, 1989.

6. **Alfirevic, Z. and Kurjak, A.**, Transvaginal color and pulsed wave Doppler in the assessment of blood flow in the first trimester of pregnancy, *J. Perinat. Med.*, in press.

7. **Kurjak, A., Zalud, I., and Crvenkovic, G.**, Transvaginal color Doppler in the assessment of maternal and fetal circulation, in Proceeding of the International Symposium: Transvaginal Sonography, Rotterdam, 1989, 93.

8. **Kurjak, A.**, Transvaginal color Doppler in the assessment of pelvic circulation, *Jpn. J. Med. Ultrasound*, 16 (Suppl. II), 1, 1989.

9. **Kurjak, A. and Zalud, I.**, Early diagnosis of ovarian tumors: transvaginal color Doppler ultrasound, in *ECO Italia*, Napoli, 1989, 189.

10. **Deutinger, J., Rudelstorfer, R., and Bernarschek, G.**, Vaginosonographic velocimetry of both main uterine arteris by visual vessel recognition and pulsed Doppler method during pregnancy, *Am. J. Obstet. Gynecol.*, 159, 1072, 1988.

11. **Goswamy, R. K. and Steptoe, P. C.**, Doppler ultrasound studies of the uterine artery in spontaneous ovarian cycles, *Hum. Reprod.*, 3, 721, 1988.

12. **Finich, C. E. and gosden, R. G.**, Animal models for the human menopause, in *Ageing Reproduction and the Climacteric*, Mastroiani, L. J. and Pulsen, C. A., Eds., Plenum Press, New York, 1986, 3.

13. **Siddle, N., Sarrel, P., and Whitehead, M. I.**, The effect of hysterectomy on the age of ovarian failure: identification of a subgroup of women with premature loss of ovarian function and literature review, *Fertil. Steril.*, 47, 94, 1987.

14. **Goswamy, R. K., Williams, G., and Steptoe, P. C.**, Decreased uterine perfusion — a cause of infertility, *Hum. Reprod.*, 3, 955, 1988.

15. **Taylor, K. J. W., Burns, P. N., Wells, P. N. I., and Conway, D. I.**, Ultrasound Doppler flow studies of the ovarian and uterine arteries, *Br. J. Obstet. Gynaecol.*, 92, 240, 1985.

16. **Baber, R. J., McSweeney, M. B., Gill, R. W., Porter, R. N., Picker, R. H., Warren, P. S., Kossoff, G., and Saunders, D. M.**, Transvaginal ultrasound assessment of blood flow to the corpus luteum in IVF patients following embryo transfer, *Br. J. Obstet. Gynaecol.*, 95, 1226, 1988.

17. **Kurjak, A. and Jurkovic, D.**, Transvaginal color Doppler in the assessment of pelvic massess, in 6th World Congress of In Vitro Fertilization and Alterate Assisted Reproduction, Jerusalem, 1989. 26.

18. **Hata, T., Hata, K., Senoh, D., Makihara, K., Aoki, S., Takamiya, O., and Kitao, M.**, Doppler ultrasound assessment of tumor vascularity in gynecologic disorders, *J. Ultrasound Med.*, 8, 309, 1989.

19. **Fleisher, A. C.**, Transvaginal sonography helps find ovarian cancer, *Diagn. Imag.*, 10, 124, 1988.

20. **Gammil, S. L., Shipkey, R. B., Himmelfarb, E. H., et al.**, Roentgenology-pathology correlative study of neovascularity, *Am. J. Roentgenol.*, 126, 376, 1976.

21. **Folkman, J.**, Anti-angiogenesis: new concept for therapy of solid tumors, *Ann. Surg.*, 175, 409, 1972.

22. **Folkman, J., Nerler, E., Abernathy, C., and Williams, G.**, Isolation of tumor factor responsible for angiogenesis, *J. Exp. Med.*, 33, 275, 1971.

23. **Taylor, K. J. W., Grannum, P. A. T., and DeCherney, A. H.**, Research lessons for maternal-fetal research from reproductive system studies, in *Doppler Ultrasound Measurement of Maternal-Fetal Hemodynamics*, Maulik, D. and McNellis, D., Eds., Perinatology Press, New York, 1986, 185.

24. **Lambert, S. J., Russell, J. B., Taylor, K. J. W., and DeCherney, A. H.**, Androgen producing hilus cell tumor of the ovary in a post-menopausal women detected by duplex Doppler scanning, *JAMA*, 123, 1225, 1986.

25. **Taylor, K. J. W., Ramos, I., Carter, D., Morse, S. S., Snower, D., and Fortune, K.**, Correlation of Doppler US tumor signals with neovascular morphologic features, *Radiology*, 166, 57, 1988.

26. **Ney, F. G., Feist, J. N., Altemus, L. R., and Ordinario, V. R.**, Characteristic angiographic criteria of malignancy, *Radiology*, 104, 567, 1972.

27. **Levin, D. C., Watson, R. C., and Baltaxe, H. A.**, Arteriography in the diagnosis and management of acquired peripheral soft-tissue masses, *Radiology*, 103, 53, 1972.

28. **Schaaps, J. P. and Soyeur, D.**, Pulsed Doppler on a vaginal probe: necessity, convenience, or luxury?, *J. Ultrasound Med.*, 8, 315, 1989.

29. **Taylor, K. J. W.**, New techniques for the diagnosis of ectopic pregnancy — transvaginal sonography and Doppler, in *ECO Italia*, Napoli, 1989, 135.

INDEX